Melanie Mehta

November 2005

CU00919999

The Voice Clinic Handbook

The Voice Clinic Handbook

by
Tom Harris, Sara Harris, John S Rubin,
and David M Howard

with
Jacob Lieberman, Dinah Harris
and Phiroze Neemuchwala

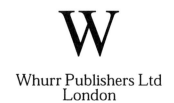

Whurr Publishers Ltd
London

© 1998 Whurr Publishers Ltd
First published 1998 by
Whurr Publishers Ltd
19b Compton Terrace, London N1 2UN, England

Reprinted 2000 and 2002

All rights reserved. No part of this publication may be
reproduced, stored in a retrieval system, or transmitted
in any form or by any means, electronic, mechanical,
photocopying, recording or otherwise, without the
prior permission of Whurr Publishers Limited.

This publication is sold subject to the conditions that it
shall not, by way of trade or otherwise, be lent, resold,
hired out, or otherwise circulated without the
publisher's prior consent in any form of binding or
cover other than that in which it is published and
without a similar condition including this condition
being imposed upon any subsequent purchaser.

British Library Cataloguing in Publication Data
A catalogue record for this book is available from the
British Library.

ISBN 1-86156 034 6

Printed and bound in the UK by Athenaeum Press Ltd,
Gateshead, Tyne & Wear

Contents

Introduction

Part 1
Outline of the structure and function of the vocal tract

Part 2
Treatment modalities

Part 3
Equipment for measuring voice: uses and limitations

Contributors

Tom Harris MA FRCS is a consultant laryngologist. Together with his wife, Sara, he set up the multidisciplinary voice clinic at the Radcliffe Infirmary in Oxford in 1982 and subsequently those at Queen Mary's Hospital, Sidcup and University Hospital Lewisham where he now works. Other current appointments include overseas affiliate of the Center for Voice Disorders, New York Eye and Ear Infirmary. In April 1985 he was one of the co-founders and first chairman of the Voice Research Society, later to become the British Voice Association.

Sara Harris MRCSLT is a speech and language therapist who has specialised in voice disorders since 1978. Together with Tom Harris, she set up a multidisciplinary voice clinic first at the Radcliffe Infirmary in Oxford and later at Queen Mary's Hospital in Sidcup. She was also one of the founder members of the Voice Research Society, now the British Voice Association. She has a particular interest in singers and performers and is an associate member of the Collegium Medicorum Theatri as well as a member of the Voice Committee of the British Association of Performing Arts Medicine.

John S Rubin MD FACS FRCS is a consultant laryngologist. He is the lead clinician of the Voice and Laryngology Department at the Royal National Throat Nose and Ear Hospital, London, a consultant ENT surgeon at The Royal Free Hospital, St. Bartholomew's Hospital and University Hospital Lewisham. He is also Honorary Senior Lecturer at the Institute of Laryngology and Otology, University College London, and a visiting associate professor at the Albert Einstein College of Medicine, New York. Mr Rubin is a member of the Speech, Voice and Swallowing committee of the American Academy of Otolaryngology-Head and Neck Surgery and a member of the Scientific Advisory board of the Voice Foundation. He is the editor of the major textbook *The Diagnosis and Treatment of Voice Disorders*.

David M Howard BSc (Eng), PHD (London), CEng is Professor of Electronics and Head of the Department of Electronics at the University of York. Previously he was a lecturer in Experimental Phonetics at University College London for 11 years. His main research interests are the acoustics and psychoacoustics of speech, singing and music. He is a founding member of the International Association of Forensic Phoneticians, a Fellow of the Institute of Acoustics, a Member of the Audio Engineering Society, and the 1997/98 President of the British Voice Association.

Jacob Lieberman DO MA is qualified both as an osteopath and psychodynamic psychotherapist. He is the member of the Queen Mary's voice clinic team responsible for the manual therapy services for dysphonic patients. He is also a member of the research faculty at the British School of Osteopathy, and has a specialist osteopathic practice for the treatment of hyperfunctional voice disorders in South-East London.

Dinah Harris ARCM is a singing teacher and voice coach. She has been a member of the Queen Mary's voice clinic team since 1990. Between 1971 and 1990, she was a professional opera and concert singer both in Europe and the United Kingdom, her work including records for Erato and EMI, BBC broadcasts, concerts with the BBC Symphony Orchestra, The Philharmonia, the CBSO, and performances with the English National Opera.

Phiroze Neemuchwala MA Adv.Dip.PC Adv.Cert.PG BAC is a psychotherapist and counsellor. His practice in psychosomatic psychotherapy is based in Southeast London. His training and qualifications include cognitive-behavioural, analytical psychotherapy and Gestalt models. Since 1992 he has organised and run weekend workshops to introduce groups to the psychotherapeutic approach to dealing with symptoms. He has been associated with the Queen Mary's Hospital voice clinic since 1992.

Acknowledgements

To Ingrid and Gunnar Rugheimer for persuading us to write it all down. To the Primary Health Care South East Thames RHA Fund for Research and Development Projects, which funded our initial trial between 1990 and 1992 into the association between head, neck and shoulder-girdle tension and dysphonia, and enabled us to provide objective evidence that manual therapy is an extremely valuable addition to the therapeutic armamentarium. To our long-suffering partners without whose tolerance and (sometimes) constructive criticism the book would have taken even longer. To Mrs Jo Mills for transcribing endless rewrites without complaint and reminding us about the necessity for support staff. To Janet Preston whose cartoons put things into proper perspective. To friends and colleagues, Jo Estill, Jayne Comins, Kirsten Thyme-Frøkjær, Alison Bagnall, Gillyanne Kayes, Gordon Stewart, Linda Hutchison, Mark Meylan and Kristine Rubin and who have all read rough drafts to excise inaccuracy and grammatical malfeasance.

Foreword

We certainly have come along way. I first grappled with the intricacies of voice disorders back in the early 1960s – not so long ago that events are nostalgically shrouded in the softening mists of time, but far enough away that an overall perspective is possible. And my recollection is that "voice" was clearly on the sidelines of the rehabilitation game. It wasn't that it was unimportant, exactly. There was meaningful, sometimes important work for the vocal therapist to do. Laryngectomees were plentiful in those days, and there was always the hoarse schoolteacher, clergyman, or salesman. But – at least on this side of the Atlantic – vocal rehabilitation was certainly not in the spotlight, which, as I recollect, was pretty much fixed on stammering and aphasia. West, Ansberry, and Carr's *Rehabilitation of Speech*, a then-prominent American text for beginning students, devoted all of 11 of its 688 pages to "remedial procedures for dysphonia" and another six and a half pages to rehabilitation of the laryngectomee. Therapy for aphasia got twice as much play.

There were three major groups involved with vocal dysfunction back then. The medical people dealt with, from their perspective, the "real" problems. The lesions, paralyses, infections. The psychologists laid claim to all those situations that were not the province of the medicosurgical arts, apparently believing, in those Freud-dominated years, that all – vocal nodes, aberrant vocal mutation, spasmodic dysphonia, you name it– all was psychoneurosis. And finally there were the speech therapists who, in North America, were just starting to metamorphose into more-impressive "speech pathologists." Their education in voice disorders was often limited to part of a one-semester course called "Voice and Articulation", but to them fell the role of patching up the postsurgical patient and of remediating the persistent vocal problems of the psychologized-but-still-dysphonic. Members of the three professional groups talked to each other, of course, and they sometimes referred patients back and forth, but, at least in my experience, their professional actions were perhaps better described as parallel, rather than cooperative, play. Each Profession had its own set of background assumptions, its own rules of engagement, its own remedial-world view, and, of paramount import, its own turf to defend.

There were a few relatively good ways of getting an accurate assessment of vocal tract function and of obtaining better physiological insight into the patient's problem, but they were for the professional elite. The venerable Sonograph, progenitor of almost all of today's spectral insight, was, for those times, horifically expensive. (It could also spew clouds of noxious black grit and electrocute the fingers of the unwary). Stroboscopy was only nascent, and, in the pre-VCR era, provided no permanent record for careful analysis. Even getting and accurate reading of the fundamental frequency was difficult and the perturbation measurement was out of the question. Research labs had ways of sorting out the physiological bases of a given dysphonia, but little that could be economically and conveniently applied in the average clinical setting. So, for most of us, assessment of vocal function meant not very much more than listening to vocal production.

Voice is much more "in" today. We have, as I said, come along way. To be sure, laryngology still doesn't have the cachet of, let us say, brain surgery, and speech pathology still has a whole lot more psycholinguistics groupies than voice specialists. But, unobtrusively, the treatment of voice disorders has moved decidedly forward on the rehabilitative stage, if not into the centre spotlight then at least into the brighter illumination of the footlights. Doing something about vocal problems has become more important: witness the number of specialised voice clinics that are sprouting up. Social scientists will no doubt postulate various reasons for this: the greater importance of spoken communication in an increasingly white-collar workplace; a more affluent society indulging in more vocally-deleterious entertainments and amusements; changes in medical economics, and so on. But there are other (I like to think more important) propelling forces, and they are manifest in the construction, content, and tone of this book.

For one thing, we know a great deal more about vocal mechanisms. We've learnt from models, from sophisticated probes of physiological function, in vitro and in vivo, from epidemiological and genetic analysis, from highly sophisticated acoustic analysis, from the vast array of advanced techniques made possible by explosive advances of technology. And, most important, we've been blessed with a generation of very gifted theorists.

We can also offer our patients much more. Phonosurgery comes to mind, as does an enriched palette of behavioural approaches to vocal restoration and rehabilitation. That we can do so is due to the better integration of the insights of careful research, highly-structured clinical observation, and everyday exingencies of the clinical world.

And then, of course, we can understand the patient's particular problem better than we ever hoped to 35 years ago. Thanks largely to a revolution in technology interacting with advancing physiological and acoustic theory, we can obtain a much more complete picture of how and why the vocal system is malfunctioning. The clearer the picture, the more targeted the intervention can be.

Which brings me, finally, to this book, a well-endowed child that much-more-mature science of voice, Its very tone – self-confident enough to undertake an authoritative survey of the field without being laborious or pedantic, shows how far we have indeed come. More substantially, this book is impressive in the unique way in which it weaves together insights and understandings from so many of the basic and applied sciences that inform the practice of vocal rehabilitation, and in the way in which it brings that integration to bear on such a broad spectrum of clinical problems. With clarity, conciseness, and a leavening of wit, this tome deals with whatever the question that the vocal professional might pose. (If an answer is not here, the question must, I think, be very odd indeed.) Achieving this is an accomplishment of very significant magnitude. An accomplishment that merits real congratulation.

Uniquely, however, along with a thorough survey of the canonical interventions – medicosurgical, behavioural, and psychological – this text includes approaches and therapies not heretofore emphasised in the context serious literature on vocal dysfunction. And it does so with a careful rationality and persuasiveness that have not generally been characteristic of therapeutic writing in our field. And for that, this book warrants enthusiastic applause.

But there is, at base, something very different about this text. And that is that its several authors have not simply come together (or, as is more common, remained apart!) for the purpose of writing a book. What we have here is an explanation of practice by a functioning *team*, a group of professionals who do not simply share a common understanding for their endeavour but who *do* it together. There results in their book a unification of approach, a consistency of understanding, an obvious mutual respect, and a professional interdependence that are, in my experience, unparalleled in any similar publication in our profession. And for that achievement: Bravissimo!

R.J. Baken, PhD.
Department of Otolaryngology
The New York Eye and Ear Infirmary
New York, NY
1997

Preface

A scientific approach does NOT mean a patient must be treated as a mere biochemical machine. It does NOT mean the exclusion of spiritual, psychological and social dimensions of human beings.
But it DOES mean treating these in a rational manner.

DR Laurence, Clinical Pharmacology 1: 9.

This book is divided into an Introduction and three main parts. The Introduction outlines the structure and function of a voice clinic. Part 1 reviews the structure and function of the vocal tract and outlines the commoner forms of voice disorder likely to be encountered in a clinic. Part 2 provides brief descriptions of the various forms of therapy available for the treatment of non-cancerous voice disorders, attempts to provide a rationale for their use and, where appropriate, outlines suitable approaches for specific problems. Part 3 contains an overview of the instrumentation available for the investigation and documentation of voicing.

In Parts 1 and 2 we have included anatomical, physiological and acoustic detail only where it is felt that the reader might benefit from a fresh look at what they may already know. We, the authors, do not intend this primer for clinical voice practice to compete with the excellent books that already cover these basic sciences and how they relate to voice. We particularly admire *The Anatomical and Physiological Bases of Speech* by Dickson and Maue-Dickson (1982, Little, Brown and Co.), *Principles of Voice Production* by Ingo Titze (1993, Prentice Hall) and *The Science of the Singing Voice* by Johan Sundberg (1987, N. Illinois University Press). Our aim has been to outline the ways in which we believe 'normal' voicing becomes abnormal and to provide a basis on which the disorder can be corrected or resolved. To this end we have attempted to provide a summary of the collective experience of all the members of a single voice clinic and we therefore include much material that is so far based only in experience.

Experimental verification of all aspects of our treatment modalities will take a lifetime to demonstrate in appropriately blinded trials, and although we have made a start on the objective evaluation of what we do, we wish to share some of what we feel are significant advances with other practitioners and allow them to evaluate the techniques as they will. Where patterns of muscular activity are hypothesized from observations of clinical patterns of misuse, this is made clear. If future experimental evidence proves us wrong, we will be among the most enthusiastic to examine how patterns of misuse may be better interpreted.

Part 3 is based entirely in science, and is intended to help practitioners who have hitherto been limited to perceptual observations of voicing to familiarize themselves with the hardware of instrumental evaluation of voice. The aim is to enable them to understand better the particular merits and limitations of different apparatus, to encourage the objective assessment of clinical findings and to help the reader achieve reliable, meaningful results by choosing appropriate investigations when assessing a subject's voice using instrumentation. We sympathize with computerphobes whose efforts are governed by Osborne's Law ('Variables won't. Constants aren't') and we have tried to make the outline of instrumental evaluation as approachable as possible.

Who is this book aimed at?

The book is aimed at laryngologists with an interest in voice but little or no experience in running a voice clinic; speech and language therapists, especially those who have not previously worked together with professionals from other therapeutic modalities in an integrated team; teachers of singing and voice coaches who might wish to work in such an environment where a pedagogic pursuit of excellence can be reinforced by a sound basic approach to what may be happening when a voice seems to be failing; and practitioners of manipulative therapies who want to base their therapy on better understanding of the mechanics of an efficiently working vocal tract.

We hope that this book may also be useful to those responsible for the planning of future training curricula in any of the specialities mentioned, and that they may find things worthy of consideration. Indeed, we hope that any voice user interested in the possibility of using his or her instrument more effectively or safely, or wishing to translate things they have been told about voicing into more 'user friendly' language will find this book helpful.

Because we wish to attempt to find some common ground for a variety of specialities related to voice care and pedagogy, we have quite deliberately tried to keep language simple and to keep to an absolute minimum the professional jargon, which in our view has for so long been the bugbear of those wishing to communicate what they know about voice to other professions. We have used metaphor freely where we feel that it provides a useful illustration or will help readers to understand a concept.

We do not intend to present this book in a coherent 'house style' that should be read from cover to cover; it is intended to be helpful to a wide variety of voice care professionals who may only wish to use specific sections. Indeed, it is anticipated that almost all the readers of this book will find that those sections relating to their own speciality appear rather reductionist or simplistic: we beg their indulgence; the work is intended to assist them in the understanding of diagnostic and management problems of voice disorder from the point of view of specialisms other than their own. For this reason, there are apparent repetitions within the text. For instance, elements relating to history-taking appear several times within the text. This is not an editorial oversight, it merely reflects the different requirements and interpretations of each therapeutic specialism.

Why should anyone wish to treat voice disorders anyway?

I think that if a person can't communicate, then the very least they can do is shut up.

Tom Lehrer

The species *Homo sapiens* has the ability to communicate complex messages containing an individual's knowledge and invention as well as emotional content, such that another individual listening to those messages could be made aware of the sum total of human experience given time.

This, above all other factors, has made man the dominant species on earth. This ability to voice our experience to others has given us great power to do as we will, but, as a result, breakdown of this communication system is treated very harshly by all other members of society. We all make snap judgements in a fraction of a second about a person's gender, age, emotional state, physical health and intentions towards ourselves from their voice quality alone. Views on the speaker's nationality, race, background, upbringing, sexual orientation and more will all have been formed after the speaker has uttered a very few phrases. In order to be permitted to take an appropriate place in society, all humans need to have a voice and speech appropriate to that place. Any discrepancy between the expected and the actual voice will very rarely be judged charitably. Although good manners, if not common decency, forbid us to make comments to a disabled person about any missing or deformed parts of their anatomy, blindness or other personal disabilities, no such taboos seem to exist to prevent our commenting to a total stranger that they have a hoarse voice or that they may be infectious. Even for a person who may not be described as a professional voice user, it is difficult both to get a job and keep it, let alone make friends, if the voice does not fit. For anyone whose voice is integral to their livelihood, deterioration in voice quality for any reason, no matter how trivial, is always seen as a potential end to a career. We feel that a good voice clinic should be able to deal with any vocal catastrophe no matter how small.

What is different about dysphonia?

Most diseases have multiple symptoms; dysphonia, a symptom, may have multiple causes. Moreover, not all patients with a given dysphonic symptom will be suffering from the same predisposing factors.

A patient may have a husky or otherwise innappropriate voice that is related to their work, overuse, gastro-oesophageal reflux, a vocal cyst or poor technique, which may be habitual or learned. Around 60% of all the hoarseness you will see is due to inefficient vocal function. This is often described as 'functional dysphonia' in general ENT practice, and usually carries with it the stigma that the patient is probably 'psychological'. In fact, the aforementioned 60% of clinic attenders are not all mad (we find that the number of true hysterical dysphonias coming to the clinic is nearer 0.4%); it is just that in normal practice around 60% of patients may not receive an accurate functional diagnosis.

For this reason, we have tended to concentrate on the management of dysfunction rather than dwell on the finer details of the pathogenesis, classification and operative treatment of lesions; these will be covered in outline only, as other books already provide the detail in a manner that we could not hope to emulate. We particularly value *Diagnosis and Treatment of Voice Disorders* edited by Rubin, Sataloff, Korovin and Gould (1995, Igaku-Shoin, New York), *Phonosurgery* by Isshiki (1989, Springer-Verlag, Tokyo) and the integrated teaching video-book *Phonosurgery* by Cornut and Bouchayer (1993, The Three Ears Co Gibralter). We would strongly recommend that any surgeon wishing to start a new career in phonosurgery should read/view these.

Because of the very fine control required to produce normal voice, vocal disorder is an extremely sensitive indicator of the early stages of many diseases. The voice clinic is the ideal place to pick up on these minimal signs and start appropriate management at the earliest possible moment.

Enough of the rationale and even the excuses for writing this book. When all is said and done the principal driving force has been our common fascination with the whole panoply of problems that present to us, the simply staggering possibilities that the human voice offers and our enthusiasm to share what little we know and what we have guessed.

The Clinic

What/who constitutes a voice clinic?

A voice clinic can be defined as a place to which a person complaining of a voice disorder can go to receive expert help in the diagnosis of their problem, and treatment appropriate to their particular needs.

This definition should be taken to imply that the clinic will offer the skills of more than one practitioner, and that the complainant will be seen for their initial appointment by a team. It should also be understood that, at the very minimum, there will always be a competent, medically qualified person present who, using appropriate techniques, can either exclude a pathological process or arrange any necessary medical treatment. There will also be a member of staff present who is able to offer at least symptomatic treatment for those dysphonias that are not due to medical disorder.

The staff

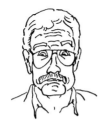 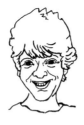 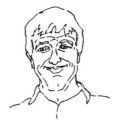 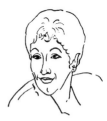

The rather stolid definition of a voice clinic offered above seeks to include all the help that is available. Of necessity, we all use what (or who) we've got. Voice clinic personnel vary internationally depending on the country's traditional management of voice disorder. In most of Europe, there is a strong tradition of medical specialization in disorders of communication, which is referred to as phoniatrics or

phoniatry. A phoniatrician is a doctor who has been trained in ENT surgery, audiological medicine and all aspects of speech and language therapy (logopedics).
Although this speciality is considered essential in most of Europe and Scandinavia,
for the most part the English speaking nations do not acknowledge the need for
this speciality and divide the responsibility for management of voice problems
between ENT surgeons and speech therapists, with the predictable wide variation
in expertise available to the patient.

This situation allows ignorance to persist about the role and contribution of
each team member and, not infrequently, there is confusion as to what is the most
appropriate management of communication disorders and, most especially,
phonation problems. There are many speech and language therapists in Britain for
whom a normal letter of referral gives only the information 'I can see nothing
wrong with this patient's larynx, please see and treat.' (In general, ENT surgeons
are trained to detect the structural changes associated with disease, but have only
the most rudimentary training as to the origins of laryngeal dysfunction.)

The situation might be acceptable if the therapist to whom the patient is
referred has spent considerable time as a compulsory part of his or her formal
training learning about diagnosis and treatment. The reality, however, is that many
highly competent voice specialized therapists in the UK and elsewhere have, like
the ENT surgeon, learned their phoniatric skills much later in a hit-and-miss
manner while actually at work. The working of most voice clinics in Britain when
they first open for business could reasonably be described as 'the blind leading the
blind'. This was certainly the case where we were concerned, and what is more, it
is liable to remain the case in the near future unless postgraduate training courses
are developed and are accorded proper professional recognition.

If the clinic is staffed by a phoniatrician or ENT surgeon and a speech therapist
who are competent in what they do, then the system of referral will inevitably bring
them patients who are harder to treat effectively and efficiently. There will for
instance be the professional voice users with unusual and very demanding voicing
requirements, not to mention all the patients in whom there is a significant psychological or social component in the production and maintenence of their symptoms.
Although the clinic is set up to deal with acute voicing problems, one of its aims is
bound to be the correction of dysphonia in such a way that it does not recur. To
this end, clinics all develop their own 'short list' of voice professionals, e.g. singing
teachers, voice coaches, psychotherapists et al., whom they know to be expert in
their own fields, and to whom they are happy to refer the patient for further
management.

The next logical step is to ask these willing professionals to join the clinic team
on a regular basis, so that they may learn more about the medical/scientific background to their clients' disorders and so that the other members of the team may
learn something of their skills.

There are of course certain obvious problems with this stage: What skills are
available locally? How do you interest these other professionals enough in this
particular enterprise to give up time on a regular basis? How do you persuade

hospital management that these people have skills that are marketable in a medical context, profitable to the hospital and who therefore should be added to the payroll? The important thing to grasp is that although it is not easy to jump these hurdles, it *is* possible. We found that a good way to demonstrate the usefulness of these new colleagues was to 'slide them in sideways' as it were, by finding research money from unrelated sources to get things started, and by producing research results that proved that these 'additional' personnel had an important role to play in improving the efficiency of treatment. If you can persuade a director of finance that a potential member of staff's activities can be self-financing, then you are halfway there.

Our case-load and available expertise has led us to a position where we now have a 'core team' of ENT surgeon, speech therapist, voice coach/singing teacher and specialist osteopath/psychotherapist. Other voice clinics will of course meet their patients' requirements rather differently. The clinic at the Vancouver General Hospital consists of an ENT surgeon, speech therapist, psychiatrist and singing teacher. Configurations vary; what is important is that members of staff are prepared to see patients in joint consultation; it is not intended that patients are seen in isolation by a series of specialists who refer patients on to each other for further management. This was the system that prevailed in the past. It is slow and inefficient, it does not put patients through the system and discharge them fully recovered nearly fast enough, and it does not allow staff to learn from one another.

In today's atmosphere of contractual commitments it is no longer possible simply to announce to a stunned world that you are going to open a new clinical service. Help has to be organized and paid for. Do not forget that as well as the additional case-load for the Appointments Desk and the Medical Records Department, and the general unhappiness about taking on an 'extra' clinic, there will of course be a requirement for additional support staff.

Patients, when they arrive, need a warm and reassuring welcome that they are in the right place and 'in good hands'. A relaxed and efficient atmosphere goes a long way towards helping to reduce anxiety and fear, especially for new patients. There must be a clinic coordinator/administrator to ensure the smooth running of the clinic for patients and staff alike – someone to make sure everything and everybody is in the right place at the right time. Important little things like tea and biscuits to soothe the nerves and reduce the tension are a valuable adjunct to any voice clinic.

Never underestimate the 'hidden' tasks required to run the clinic administratively. There has to be someone who can liaise with the patients, the voice clinic team and the other departments, as well as get together the case notes, questionnaires, letters and the forms – please don't forget the forms! It cannot rest with a professional member of the team, for instance the speech therapist or voice coach, to fulfil this role; it is too time consuming, and of course the administration goes on long after the clinic has finished for the day.

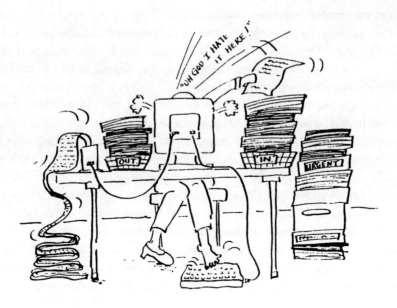

Best use of personnel

If all the professionals involved in the clinic see the patient at his or her initial interview, then, very rapidly, the team will develop its own consensus view of exactly
what the patient is complaining about, what his or her needs are and how they
might be most efficiently met. Clearly, after the initial interview, each involved
professional may wish to assess the patient in more detail. We would not wish to
pretend that objective measures relating to voice quality – tape recordings, electroglottography, spectrograms, phonetograms, airflow measurements or whatever
– can all be gathered at a diagnostic and planning interview. Experience tells that
examination by videostrobolaryngoscopy with or without fibre endoscopy is all
there is time for on this first occasion. Quite separate time has to be found for
further analysis on another occasion. This time constraint is no different from any
other form of medical consultation; the patient is usually seen without a blanket
battery of tests, and further management is decided upon on the basis of the
history and examination.

   In other traditions, voice clinics are much more hierarchical; the diagnosis and
formulation of a treatment plan are decided by one person, usually a phoniatrician,
and the game plan is rigidly adhered to until the patient has been seen for further
review by the same individual. We feel that this takes no account of the special skills
brought to the clinic by disciplines other than ENT and speech therapy. In our
view, all the personnel involved in the clinic should be actively involved in formulating a treatment plan. To say that the ultimate responsibility for the patient's care
rests with the doctor and therefore he or she should dictate what is to happen
simply negates the possibility of any further interdisciplinary learning.

Survival as a team

We must indeed all hang together, or, most assuredly, we shall all hang separately.

Benjamin Franklin

In the clinic

If and when the voice clinic has become a successful fact of life, and the weeks have started becoming years, then inevitably there will be episodes of friction between staff members. For the clinic to work, its multidisciplinary nature requires that it is a clinic of equals, and the opinions of all must be heard and included in any 'game plan'. This internal rule applies regardless of any traditional hierarchical rules of healthcare provision as to 'Who is the boss'.

Problems can, and do, arise when there are sincere differences of opinion about the best course of action concerning a patient's treatment plan. No one person ever has all the right answers, therefore it is imperative that a consensus is reached in each and every case. Every clinic develops its own *modus vivendi* to deal with this. It is obviously not acceptable to argue at length over an already confused patient. This demands a certain degree of self-discipline. Everyone should be allowed to make their own comments about the findings from the history and examination and to explain it aloud to the patient. This being done, it is almost inevitable that the team members will have a clear idea as to whether any part of the treatment is within their personal remit or not. (Working together regularly develops the ability to second-guess the other members of the team quite accurately.) If a team member thinks he has noticed a factor that may have escaped the others, he must of course voice the observation. If the other members agree, then it will automatically be taken into account by all, and the patient is usually much reassured by the general agreement. If, on the other hand, there is one of the rare occasions when the other team members do not agree, then the dissenting member must (a) refrain from further argument until the patient has left, and (b) equally importantly, discuss it with all the other members afterwards until all the reasons for and against have been given by all concerned and a genuine consensus has been reached. If members take gripes and disagreements home unresolved, then resentment builds rapidly and the person feeling wronged will start looking for opportunities elsewhere and the team will die as a true multidisciplinary entity.

Once the primary course of action is agreed, the appropriate spokesperson explains the management plan to the patient. This will normally be the therapist or surgeon who is going to organize or undertake the treatment; it is not automatically the titular 'head' of the clinic.

Beyond the clinic

If this discipline holds good within the clinic, the patients are normally impressed. They spread the word, and the clinic members will, over time, achieve a certain notoriety for their skills. All team members, of course, have their own individual careers and lives to get on with, and there will be competing commitments elsewhere, which may strain even the most loyal members of the clinic. We would strongly suggest that members air their future plans and ambitions together frequently and openly. This is not simply a matter of a chat over coffee should the opportunity arise; it is vitally important if the clinic is to continue to work as a unit. If there is no convenient time for this, make it. We would further suggest that if members are asked to talk about individual aspects of voice treatment or research that are not pertinent to their own particular domain within the clinic, they should suggest that, whenever possible, the appropriate member or members should do it instead. A truly multidisciplinary clinic cannot survive in the long term if members of the staff feel that they are being 'used' by any of the others.

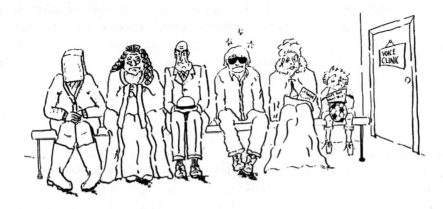

The patients

Who comes to a voice clinic? Patterns of referral: Service-related considerations in the UK

Once the decision has been taken to organize a specialist voice clinic, the question 'Exactly *who* shall we see in the clinic?' arises. After the Oxford Voice Clinic was established in 1982, we found that while approximately 8% of patients passing through a general ENT outpatient department were presenting with dysphonia that required further assessment, only the more severely dysphonic patients without any apparent neoplastic pathology were being referred internally by members of the department for further management. It was not until we had gained the confidence of our colleagues that we felt able to comb out all the dysphonias referred by GPs to the department (Harris et al., 1987). When a voice clinic has been established for some time, however, it inevitably becomes well known and begins to establish its own clientele. Patients come via tertiary referrals from colleagues outside the area as well as from distant GPs whose patients may have bullied them into a referral for a 'second opinion' or for specialist management. The clinic runs the risk of being swamped with work, unless:

(a)   all the members of the clinic are able to come together for more than a single clinic per week and are also able to find additional time to deal with the treatment of the extra patients that the increased clinic capacity will engender; or

(b) the clinic accepts that there will have to be some primary screening by colleagues in the general ENT service.

For all these reasons the eventual pattern of referrals within the UK seems to suggest that clinic patients will be drawn from a mix of:

(i) internal referrals from ENT colleagues within the local department;
(ii) internal referrals from speech therapists who have problem patients who have been seen in an ENT department already. The patient may have self-referred for therapy, in which case the therapist needs to have the patient checked for organic pathology. (Be courteous, be careful to check that the patient's own doctor is amenable first);
(iii) external referrals from GPs within the clinic's catchment area, who know of the voice clinic's existence and who have made a direct referral;
(iv) external referrals from distant GPs who have been 'persuaded' to make an extracontractual referral (ECR). The hospital should have a system in place for collecting the ECR monies attracted by the clinic before the clinic can see these patients. Management is not keen on the idea of 'loss leaders' any more;
(v) external referrals from ENT surgeons outside the catchment area for which there is a contract. This is not the problem that it used to be: as long as the colleague has filled in an appropriate *PU1* form, the referring unit is bound to honour the contractual implications of the contract.

There are of course other categories that do not readily fit into the above description, for instance the medico-legal referrals sent for independent assessment and others. These latter will not, however, make up the bulk of the case-load.

Finance
It will be noted when reading the list above, that, sadly, it is no longer adequate metaphorically to hang out a sign saying 'We treat dysphonia'. In the current climate dominated by financial considerations the clinic must be seen to be financially advantageous to the unit in which it is housed. Business plans indicating the type of patients to be seen and the origin of their referral will have to be submitted to management, otherwise there will be no financial backing for the acquisition of apparatus or for hiring staff not normally found in departments of ENT surgery. Judicious suggestion that the expected case-mix of patients who will be attracted to the clinic will prove 'a nice little earner' of extra revenue for the hospital does help a proposal for such a clinic to be regarded in a more favourable light. If it can be demonstrated that the throughput of such patients is more efficient than it would be if patients continue to be shuffled between a general ENT clinic and a speech therapy department, then the commissioners buying healthcare for the local population can also be satisfied at the same time. It may be suggested that a price of around £150 for a half hour clinical appointment for an ECR is realistic (the video-laryngostroboscopy routinely performed in-clinic is regarded as an integral minor outpatient procedure by healthcare comissioners and private insurance companies

alike). This also offers some small incentive to those who hold the financial reins to equip the proposed clinic with appropriate apparatus.

Appointments

How much time does an interview take? (How long is a piece of string?)

Do not forget that a voice clinic is one in which a minor surgical procedure – endoscopic assessment – is undertaken on every patient. Instrumental assessment always takes longer than the team would like. The patient needs to be prepared and the procedure explained. In addition to performing the endoscopy, sterilization of instruments is required afterwards and the findings must be explained to the patient, all of which takes *time*. Do not imagine that the clinic can perform to the best of its collective ability if much less than half an hour is allocated for every patient, new and old alike.

Running late

Eventually, even in a 'closed' clinic there will be extra patients – the emergencies, the force-booked postoperative follow-ups, the 'walk-ins' and the truly desperate professionals with genuinely career-threatening work commitments that cannot be ducked. The clinic will tend to become overloaded even if the original number of patient slots is adhered to as strictly as possible. We feel that as a tertiary referral centre we should endeavour to give each patient as much time as it takes to understand fully the nature of the problem and arrange a suitable treatment plan. This means that it is not always possible to stick rigidly to appointment times. This matters less than it might do as long as new patients are forewarned that the clinic may run a little late, that they should certainly bring something to read and that they should *definitely* not arrange other appointments timed for less than an hour after they were due to be seen in clinic. If patients are thus forewarned they do not get restless if an overloaded clinic is running late.

Tools for finding out about the patient

History-taking: freestyle question and answer versus the structured questionnaire

History-taking is a much more detailed business in a voice clinic than it would be in a more general outpatient setting. It is certainly one of the factors that requires a longer appointment time than is allocated for a general ENT clinic. In addition to the referral letter and any other related correspondence, there are areas of history-taking that are absolutely germane to the management of the patient and that must be covered in every case. According to the style of the clinic, it may be felt that a questionnaire can be given to the patient for filling out prior to the consultation, and the answers to the questions can then be 'gone over' in the clinic in less time than free-form questioning requires.

Some of the advantages of a proforma based interview are that history-taking is quicker, the form guarantees that factors are not overlooked and that negative and 'normal' findings are always written into the notes (a very important consideration in these days when 'evidence-based medicine' is the 'politically correct' term for good clinical practice). If questions of scale are sought, then the patient is actually obliged to quantify his or her perceptions at a given moment in time, and this is of great value in the record as patients' memories of symptoms are notoriously unreliable. It is also true that the completed forms make any subsequent analysis for audit and research purposes very much easier.

The obvious disadvantage with the proforma is that the questions, by their very nature, always tend to limit the answer to an area within a preconceived range. The questions tend to beget yes/no type answers and it is extremely difficult to produce questions that open up a new line of thinking or that beget further searching questions. This can be more of a hindrance than is at first apparent, especially when there are specialists from several disciplines in the clinic who will pick up on even small nuances of language in the patient's answers and who may wish to probe a little further.

The Sidcup Voice Clinic is only one of many clinics that routinely use proformas. It is essential, however, always to bear in mind the convergent thinking that accompanies such questionnaires and hence in the consultation to try to expand on any areas that may be concealed by the form of the answers required by the document. Having 'ears to hear' what the patient is trying to express is exceedingly important, and for this reason there will be several further sections relating to the history in the chapters on therapy.

The purpose of paper

The purpose of a preliminary history questionnaire is merely to establish and document a number of agreed facts. This is also the aim of assessment protocols for recording the facts relating to an examination (see for example the speech therapy questionnaires and the Lieberman protocol for examination of posture and laryngopharyngeal set appended to the chapter on manual therapy, pp. 134–137). The purpose of this type of document is therefore not the same as that of specialist protocols designed to elicit information about and perhaps quantify such factors as stress and anger, of which the patient may be entirely unaware. The difference in approach for the psychological inventory is that the precise wording of each question has been demonstrated to elicit a reliable and appropriate response, and is therefore absolutely not to be changed if it is to be used for scoring purposes. We are particularly impressed by The Nottingham University Department of Psychology questionnaires for assessing levels of stress at work.

It is not necessarily a good idea to become wedded to the use of proformas, no matter how beguiling the thought that the patient does more of the work. From a clinical point of view, the data will always be recorded and accessible, and from a research point of view protocols allow the data to be shuffled into (maybe) statistically significant bins. However, this must be offset against the extra time that this added activity will require. The next inevitable step is to consider what to do with all this painstakingly acquired data.

The trouble with data

Data is a Latin word meaning 'Things given'. Of course data are not really given, they are sort of 'extracted' with varying degrees of difficulty and tedium both for the subject and enquirer alike. When establishing a voice clinic it is a very good idea to have some long-term plans about both clinical practice and future research. If the questions 'What data do we really want or need? For now? and (perhaps) for the future?' are posed, then it will be possible to identify the path you wish the clinic to take without wasting enormous amounts of time in the acquisition of useless data.

If data are required, where will they be stored? In the patient's notes? For clinical purposes we keep the history proforma and a downloaded photograph (Mavigraph®) from the videostrobolaryngoscopy tape in the patient's notes; all other documents are kept on file, on digital tape, on video or in the memory of the clinic computer. Experience has shown that material necessary for research should *never* be entrusted to hospital notes – copy it from the notes if necessary (we assume that permission will have been sought and given), and keep the copy securely in the clinic. The same applies to all material gathered specifically for research.

So much for the paper and basic investigations. Now what about the ever increasing torrent of electronic data that require storage in a manner that allows for retrieval when required? Even the first 10 years' videotape of sundry patients' larynges can prove burdensome to look through when seeking particular pieces of taped examples. Archiving is the new name of the game, and to do this you need to be able to examine a collection longitudinally as well as latitudinally. Tape is great for saving gigabytes of data, but it is mind-bogglingly tedious to search through. What you will be seeking when time and cash allow is a read–write optical disk, and accompanying frame grabber, computer and software. Market prices are falling all the time, and it is always expensive to be the first kid on the block, but at some point in the future, you will probably be driven to make enquiries. Then there will be the problem of transferring all your existing data to the new system, if you have the patience. For further comments please see the section on videostrobolaryngoscopy (p. 312).

Tailoring a treatment plan to individual patient requirements

To every complex problem there is a simple solution. – And it's wrong.

Dysphonia is a symptom, not a disease entity. Hence different patients with a similar voice disorder will not all be managed with equal efficiency by a standard treatment plan if the several factors that have played a part in producing the problem are of different orders of importance (see Morrison, Rammage et al., 1994).

The obese patient with severe gastro-oesophageal reflux and periodic nocturnal laryngospasm may well present with the same pattern of hyperfunctional voicing as an angry super-fit athlete. The treatment plan is clearly not going to be identical for both, because the priorities are different. The same is true for different voice requirements: an epidermoid cyst in a vocal fold is a catastrophe for an aspiring opera singer, but may be an absolute boon for a character actress of a certain age. Just because a lesion has been identified does not necessarily mean it must be fixed.

References

Harris T, Collins S, Clarke D (1987) The effectiveness of the voice clinic. In Transcripts of symposium, Recent Advances in Voice Conservation. Naerum, Denmark, Bruel & Kjaer. pp 40–51.

Morrison M, Rammage L (1994) The Management of Voice Disorders, San Diego, Singular Publishing Group. pp 1–2.

Part 1
Outline of the Structure and Function of the Vocal Tract

The Structural Anatomy of the Larynx and Supraglottic Vocal Tract: A Review

JOHN S RUBIN

This chapter is primarily intended as an 'aide-mémoire' for doctors and manipulative therapists; the descriptive language has therefore not been modified for more general readership.

The larynx

The larynx is an intrusion into the pharynx, rather like the rearwards-pointing ventilation funnel of an old-fashioned ship pushed into an inverted cone. It subsumes several functions.

1. Airway protection: this is the larynx's most important function. The larynx is a complex sphincter that acts to protect the upper airway from saliva and food particles. The supraglottic structures act both passively and actively to direct the food bolus in streams away from the glottic chink, towards the pyriform fossae and thence, through a relaxing cricopharyngeus muscle, into the oesophagus. Many of the intrinsic laryngeal muscles act predominantly in this capacity, thereby depressing and tilting the epiglottis posteriorly. This mechanism, together with adduction and medial compression of the true vocal folds, cannot be overly emphasized as it is the critical phylogenetic role of the larynx, and thus essential to survival. Maladaption of the involved structures is common, and represents one of the more frequent causes of visits to voice clinics.

2. Pressure-valving: this function is also of particular importance from a survival standpoint. Here, the larynx functions in the role of closing off the airway to prevent ingress or egress of air. This allows for sudden increases in intra-thoracic and intra-abdominal pressures and thus permits such activities as

childbirth, defaecation, weight-lifting, forceful micturition and vomiting. It is also integral in the protective act of coughing, whereby forced laryngeal closure permits build-up of subglottic pressure followed by sudden larygeal release with forceful expulsion of air. It has been observed that pressure-valving involves not only closure at the level of the true vocal fold, but also at the level of the false vocal fold (Dickson and Maue-Dickson, 1982). Again, hyperfunction of this mechanism represents a common cause of patient visits to the voice clinic.

3.   Phonation: although phonation is also important for survival (screaming to frighten off an attacking animal or to attract attention), in animals other than man this function has far less intrinsic importance than airway protection and pressure-valving, and is phylogenetically a more recent activity. The capacity to produce very complex phonatory activity is limited to human beings and has been related by Laitman et al. (1995) to the lowering of the laryngeal complex from the basicranium. This function is primarily subsumed by intrinsic laryngeal muscles related to the arytenoid cartilages, by the medial portion of the thyroarytenoid muscle (the vocalis) and by one 'extrinsic' muscle, the cricothyroid muscle. More will be written of these muscles and the biomechanical activities necessary for phonation later in this chapter and in subsequent chapters.

In general, it is useful to think of the larynx as a structure consisting of cartilaginous, bony and membranous components into which a series of muscles connect, and which is draped by mucous membrane; then to visualize this structure suspended from the skull base and mandible above by muscles, membranes and ligaments, and from the trachea directly and from the clavicles and sternum by muscles below.

In infancy, the larynx is located at C2–3. It proceeds thereafter to descend throughout life to C5–6 in adulthood and perhaps as low as C8 in senescence.

We prefer to structurally review the larynx from below up.

Cartilages and bones

Cricoid cartilage

The cricoid is the only completely circumferential structure in the larynx and thus is essential for the provision of adequate rigidity of the laryngeal framework. It can be thought of as the foundation upon which the larynx is built.

The cricoid is named from the Greek description implying 'signet ring-shaped'. It consists of hyaline cartilage and is narrow anteriorly and very broad posteriorly. The narrower anterior portion is known as the arch. The posterior body when seen from the rear is like a vertical trapezoid with the lower margins of the sides chamfered off. In the posterior midline, a vertical ridge separates the lamina into two halves; inferiorly, this ridge broadens. According to Maue (1970), and Maue and Dickson, (1971)), the average posterior height is 25 mm in the male and 19 mm in the female.

i) From above

posterior   Articular
                   facet for
                   arytenoid

Articular
facet for
thyroid

anterior

ii) From right side

anterior

posterior

iii) From the rear

Articular
facet for
arytenoid

Articular
facet for
thyroid

iv) From above with
arytenoid cartilages mounted
on their facets

v) From right side

vi) From rear with arytenoid and
thyroid cartilages in place

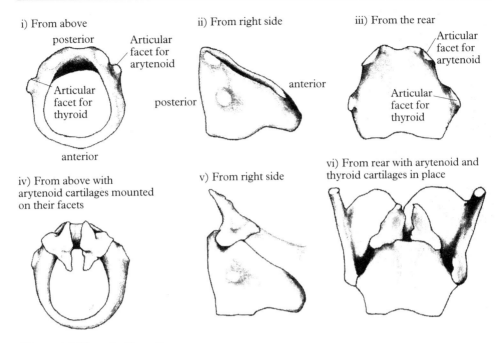

Figure 1.1 The cricoid cartilage

The inferior edge of the cricoid cartilage is firmly attached to the first tracheal ring. Anteriorly, the superior aspect of the cricoid arch is attached to the thyroid cartilage via a thin, avascular membrane, and its anterior condensation, the anterior (median) cricothyroid ligament. Laterally, at or near the junction between the arch and the body of the cricoid, are the **cricothyroid articular facets**. These articulate with corresponding facets on the inferior horns of the thyroid cartilage to form the cricothyroid joints. The joints are plane synovial in type; the facets on each side of the larynx are frequently grossly asymmetric, one to the other. They face dorsolaterally and slightly superiorly (Dickson and Maue Dickson 1982, p. 156). In addition to the joint capsule, there are two ligaments stabilizing the joint, the posterior cricothyroid and lateral cricothyroid ligaments. The former ligament prevents spreading of the inferior thyroid horns and the latter limits but does not abolish, posterior displacement of the thyroid over the cricoid. The functional potential of this joint is governed by the obliquity of the joint facets that somewhat limit the posterosuperior to anteroinferior motion. Rotation in a vertical plane is possible with opening or closure of the cricoid arch and lower margin of the thyroid angle being limited by the anterior cricothyroid ligament or by contact between the same structures. Through an investigation on fresh human cadaver larynges, Dickson has identified correlative vocal fold changes in length through vertical movement of this joint of approximately 25% (Dickson and Dickson 1971 and Maue Dickson 1982).

Thyroid cartilage

The thyroid cartilage is shield-shaped (thus its name in Greek). It consists of hyaline cartilage, which begins to ossify in the third decade of life. It is constituted by two pentagonal laminae that meet in the midline, the angle at the join being more acute (90 degrees) in the male than the female (120 degrees) and accounting for the 'Adam's apple'. Superior and inferior horns arise from the posterior edges of the laminae. The inferior horns have already been noted to articulate with the cricoid cartilage. The superior horns, as well as the entire superior edge of the cricoid cartilage, are connected by the **thyrohyoid membrane** to the hyoid bone. Laterally, this membrane condenses to form the paired lateral thyrohyoid ligaments. Medially, it gives rise to the medial thyrohyoid ligament. Laterally the thyrohyoid membrane is pierced by the superior laryngeal nerve (internal branch) and vessels. On the lateral aspects of the two pentagonal laminae of the thyroid are the two oblique lines. These serve as the origin of the deep layers of the strap muscles (the thyrohyoid and sternothyroid muscles).

The thyroid cartilage is covered externally by heavy perichondrium and internally by thinner perichondrium that is dehiscent over a small prominence where the anterior commissure of the true vocal folds attaches.

Hyoid bone

The thyrohyoid membrane connects the thyroid cartilage to the hyoid bone. Although not truly a laryngeal structure, and originating from a different embryologic anlage, the hyoid bone will be mentioned here because it is important to laryngeal fixation and, thus, function.

The hyoid bone is a more or less horseshoe-shaped bone consisting of a central body anteriorly with two lateral projections, the greater and lesser cornua, the greater being the arm of the horseshoe and the lesser being a small posterosuperior projection from the superior surface of the junction between body and greater cornu. The hyoid bone attaches the larynx to the tongue musculature, the mandible and to the skull base via a series of muscular attachments. These muscles are important in laryngeal elevation given their capacity to pull the tongue body posteriorly and larynx either anteriorly or posteriorly. They include such muscles as the myoglossus, hyoglossus and geniohyoid, not to mention the mylohyoid, digastric muscles, stylohyoid, etc. The hyoid bone is also attached to most of the strap muscles (sternohyoid, omohyoid, thyrohyoid), which, upon contraction, act as laryngeal depressors (sternohyoid, omohyoid) or elevators (thyrohyoid). Although these muscles have a significant but minor role in the microcontrol of laryngeal pitch (Vilkman et al., 1996), by controlling the absolute length and configuration of the supraglottic vocal tract, they are more important in the production of the formants (enhanced resonances) of the supraglottic vocal tract.

These muscles are frequently misused in singing, and persistent hyperfunction may lead to a pitch-locked, fatigued voice with loss of appropriate vocal timbre. (See Chapters 5, 6, 7 and 8 for detail.)

Epiglottis

The epiglottis is a large, leaf-shaped structure made up of fibroelastic cartilage. The vocal folds insert, as previously mentioned, onto the inner surface of the thyroid cartilage. Just above this insertion is the petiole or attachment of the epiglottis via the thyroepiglottic ligament. The epiglottis extends superoposteriorly to the level of the base of the tongue where it overhangs the larynx. Its perichondrium is more tightly bound on its laryngeal than its lingual surface. Mucous glands are present on both surfaces although more are located on the laryngeal surface.

Superiorly, above the level of the hyoid bone, the epiglottis forms the vallecula with the base of the tongue via a series of mucosal condensations. Inferiorly, it defines the laryngeal inlet together with the arytenoid cartilages, via a series of mucosal folds (the aryepiglottic folds). As will be noted later in this chapter, a series of intrinsic laryngeal muscles insert into the epiglottis and are concerned mainly with laryngeal protection during swallowing. These muscles frequently contribute to the persistent hyperfunctional state.

Arytenoid cartilages

The paired arytenoid cartilages perch atop the posterior signet ring portion of the cricoid cartilage. Each cartilage is a dynamic pyramidal-shaped structure, apex up, which is integral to vocal fold motion. According to Maue (1970), the average height in adult males is 18 mm and in adult females 13 mm. Antero-posterior dimensions are, respectively, 14 mm and 10 mm.

The arytenoid cartilage is somewhat conical in shape, although its medial surface is flat, its posterior and inferior surfaces are concave and its antero-lateral surface is irregularly rounded. It has three pronounced angles: a sharp anterior angle, the vocal process (which makes up 40% of vocal fold length in the adult); a blunt postero-lateral angle, the muscular process; and a recurved superior angle, the apex (Boileau Grant, 1972).

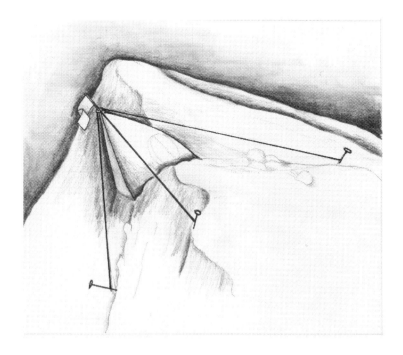

Figure 1.2 The arytenoid cartilage perches on the cricoid cartilage 'like a tent on the ridge of a mountainside'

The cricoarytenoid joint is a synovial load-bearing joint. An elliptical joint facet, 6 mm in length, sits on the posterior aspect of the rounded upper border of the cricoid. It slopes laterally, downwards and forwards. The deeply grooved base of the arytenoid cartilage has a corresponding facet that articulates with it, with the long diameter of the cartilage being set at right angles to that of the cricoid (Boileau Grant, 1972). This facet is on the inferior surface of the muscular process.

Two ligaments affect motion of the cricoarytenoid joint, the posterior cricoarytenoid ligament and the vocal ligament. The former is contiguous with the joint, attaches to the superior rim of the cricoid lamina between the two cricoarytenoid facets and extends anteriorly to the medial surface of the arytenoid cartilage. The latter attaches to the vocal process and extends anteriorly to insert onto the thyroid cartilage. There is also a tight fibrous articular capsule enclosing the cricoarytenoid joint (Dickson and Maue Dickson, 1982). We think that the primary function of the posterior cricoarytenoid ligament is prevention of lateral dislocation of the arytenoid on forced abduction of the vocal folds.

Motion permitted in the cricoarytenoid joint includes sliding along the long flat axis of the cricoid facet and rocking about the short convex axis of the cricoid facet. In fresh cadaver specimens, Dickson and Maue Dickson (1982) have demonstrated that only a few millimetres of sliding is possible due to the limiting joint capsule. Rocking (rotation), however, is quite free with the ligaments acting as guide wires.

Corniculate/cuneiform cartilages

The corniculate cartilages are very small pieces of elastic cartilage, roughly conical in shape, lying on, and frequently fused with, the apex of each arytenoid cartilage. The cuneiform cartilages (cartilages of Wrisberg) are very small bits of cartilage lying within the aryepiglottic fold, extending from the arytenoid to the epiglottis.

Membranes

Thyrohyoid membrane

The thyrohyoid membrane has already been described in its relation to the thyroid cartilage (see page 18).

Cricothyroid membrane

The cricothyroid membrane is a bilateral triangular-shaped structure; thus it has been referred to as the triangular membrane. To confuse the issue further, it has also been called the cricovocal ligament and the cricothyroid ligament. For the purposes of this discussion, the cricothyroid ligament will be considered to be the anterior (median) condensation of the cricothyroid membrane that extends between the cricoid arch and the deep inferior border of the thyroid cartilage back to the level of the cricoarytenoid facet. The borders of the cricothyroid membrane can be defined as follows: superior border, vocal ligament, anterior border, anterior cricothyroid ligament; inferior border, superior rim of the cricoid arch; poste-

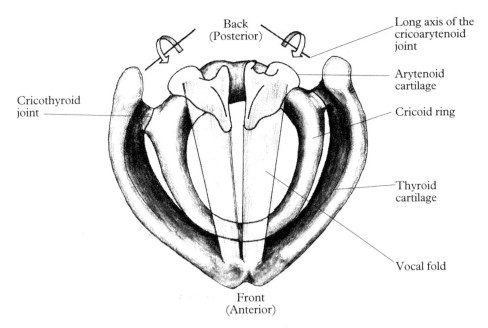

Figure 1.3 Principal cartilages of the larynx seen from above

rior border, posterior end of the vocal ligament, attaching to the vocal process and inferior fossa of the arytenoid cartilage (Dickson and Maue Dickson, 1982). The body of this membrane is known as the 'conus elasticus' and is the supporting structure for the deeper surfaces of the vocal folds below the vocal ligaments.

Vocal ligaments

The vocal ligament is the condensation of the superior edge of the cricothyroid membrane. It extends from the end of the vocal process of the arytenoid and passes horizontally forward. Its anterior attachment to the thyroid cartilage is known as Broyle's ligament. It maintains the positional integrity of the true vocal fold.

Quadrangular membrane

The quadrangular membrane is a fibroelastic sheath. It is more delicate than the cricothyroid membrane. It extends bilaterally from either side of the epiglottis and curves backwards to the lateral border of the arytenoid cartilage. Its free upper edge is slightly thickened to form the aryepiglottic ligament. Its free lower border condenses to form the vestibular ligament, the basis for the false vocal (vestibular) fold. Its anterior vertical height is greater than its posterior vertical height.

Mucous membranes

Folds of mucous membrane clothe the cartilaginous and membranous structures of the larynx. Reviewing this on a coronal basis, mucosa lines the thyrohyoid membrane and a portion of the thyroid cartilage; folding upward, it ascends over the lateral border of the quadrangular membrane and then descends, draping over the medial aspect of the quadrangular membrane, thus creating the aryepiglottic fold superiorly and the vestibular fold inferiorly. Under the vestibular fold it pouches laterally to form the laryngeal ventricle. It then turns around medially along the floor of the ventricle to cover the conus elasticus and the vocal ligament and thence inferiorly to create the true vocal fold. It then continues inferiorly to become tracheal mucosa. Superiorly, it also drapes over the lingual surface of the epiglottis, creating the valleculae.

The epithelial lining of the larynx consists of respiratory epithelium (pseudo stratified, ciliated, columnar epithelium) and stratified squamous epithelium. Areas having direct contact with saliva and food particles, and those directly involved with phonation, are lined with the latter epithelium. These include the lingual surface of the epiglottis, pyriform sinuses, superior half of the laryngeal surface of the epiglottis, superior surface of the false vocal folds, the true vocal folds and subglottic aspects of the true vocal folds.

Muscles

Intrinsic muscles of the larynx

All the intrinsic muscles of the larynx with the exception of the vocal fold tensing muscles, the cricothyroid muscles, have a common function of origin: they are all originally parts of sphincteric mechanisms for sealing the larynx and lower respiratory tract off from the digestive tract. With the exception of the cricothyroid muscles and the most lateral (and vertical) fibres of the thyroarytenoid, the thyroepiglottic muscle, which are inserted instead into the epiglottis, the rest all have attachment to the arytenoid cartilages. Fortunately, the intrinsic laryngeal muscles have descriptive names outlining their attachments:

1. posterior cricoarytenoid
2. lateral cricoarytenoid
3. oblique interarytenoid
4. aryepiglotticus
5. transverse interarytenoid
6. thyroarytenoid, functionally, subdivided into two parts:
    (i) medially, vocalis muscle fibres
    (ii) laterally, lateral thyroarytenoid or muscularis fibres.
    The thyroarytenoid muscles also send fibres almost vertically to attach not to the arytenoid but to the epiglottis. These are the:
7. thyroepiglottic fibres of the thyroarytenoid
8. cricothyroid.

Note: The cricothyroid muscles are situated outside the laryngeal cartilages and have a different innervation to that of all the other muscles, the external laryngeal nerve. All the other intrinsic muscles are innervated by the recurrent laryngeal nerve. It therefore seems probable that unlike all the other muscles, the cricothyroid muscle was never an evolutionary requirement for sealing the larynx.

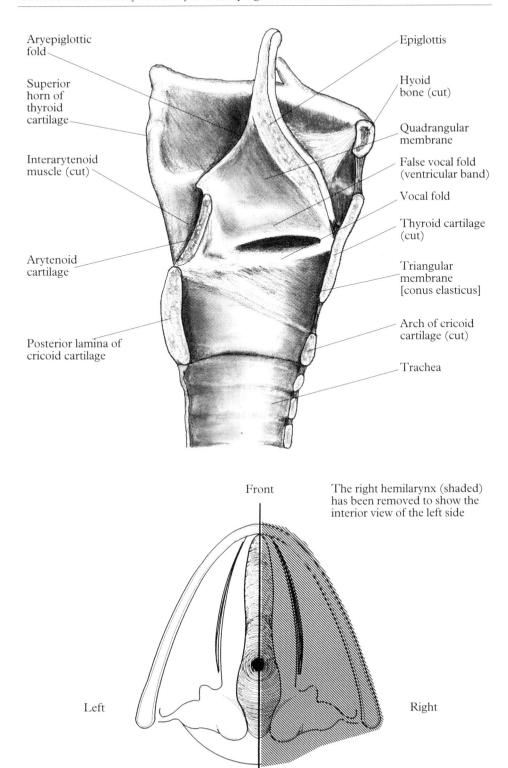

Aryepiglottic fold

Superior horn of thyroid cartilage

Interarytenoid muscle (cut)

Arytenoid cartilage

Posterior lamina of cricoid cartilage

Epiglottis

Hyoid bone (cut)

Quadrangular membrane

False vocal fold (ventricular band)

Vocal fold

Thyroid cartilage (cut)

Triangular membrane [conus elasticus]

Arch of cricoid cartilage (cut)

Trachea

Front

The right hemilarynx (shaded) has been removed to show the interior view of the left side

Left

Right

Back

Figure 1.4 Sagittal section of the larynx showing the interior of the left hemilarynx

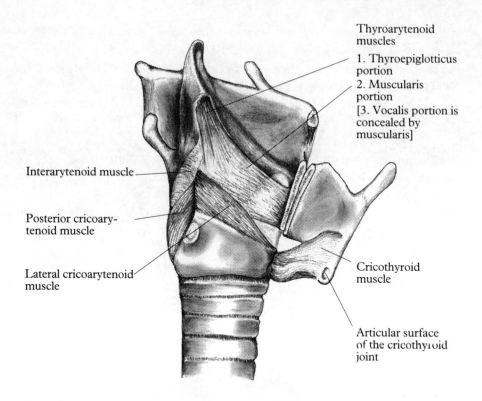

Thyroarytenoid muscles

1. Thyroepiglotticus portion
2. Muscularis portion
[3. Vocalis portion is concealed by muscularis]

Interarytenoid muscle

Posterior cricoarytenoid muscle

Lateral cricoarytenoid muscle

Cricothyroid muscle

Articular surface of the cricothyroid joint

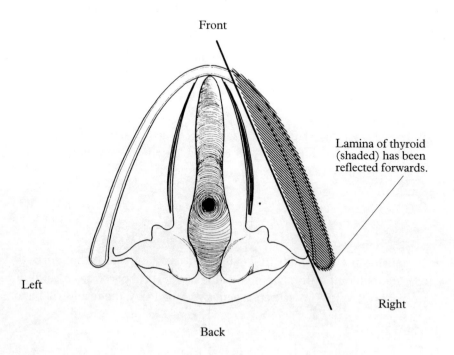

Front

Lamina of thyroid (shaded) has been reflected forwards.

Left

Right

Back

Figure 1.5 Right lateral view of laryngeal intrinsic muscles with the right thyroid lamina reflected forward

All of the intrinsic laryngeal muscles are paired in a broadly mirror-image arrangement to right and left of the midline sagittal plane. The only exceptions are the transverse fibres of the interarytenoid, which are attached to identical sites on both arytenoids at each end of the muscle. Even after a unilateral recurrent laryngeal nerve palsy, these fibres will continue to cause some abduction of the vocal fold.

The posterior cricoarytenoid (PCA) muscles

These muscles are shaped like the fanning out of two scallop shells. At their broad ends they are inserted into the back of the body of the cricoid cartilage, to left and right of the midline. The muscle fibres travel outwards and upwards converging like the ribs on the shell to form the strong musculotendinous attachment covering the whole superior surface of the muscular process of the arytenoid cartilage.

The action of the posterior cricoarytenoid is to pull the arytenoid cartilage backwards, rotating the cartilage upwards and outwards away from the glottis. This action is classically described as abduction (drawing apart) of the vocal folds. Recent observation suggests that PCA's parting of the folds may be assisted by another muscle, the lateral cricoarytenoid. More correctly, acting alone against all other muscular activity, this muscle may be described as a muscle that lengthens the vocal fold and tenses the vocal ligament. Despite all the published literature in many totally respectable sources suggesting that this muscle alone is responsible for vocal fold abduction, even simple inspection of the structural conditions operating in the larynx shows that this simplistic statement cannot be wholly correct (see below).

The lateral cricoarytenoid (LCA) muscles

These muscles are small and originate on the superior rim of the cricoid cartilage. The muscle fibres lie in a posterosuperior and medial direction crossing the top of the cricoid to attach to the lateral half of the muscular process of the cricoid cartilage. The classical description of this muscle's action is that of 'medial compression' or approximation of the tips of the arytenoid vocal processes. A more logical description is given below. It is pointless to describe the activity of this muscle in isolation, that is, a muscle that slides the arytenoid a little bit laterally along the long axis of the cricoarytenoid joint. Physiologically its activity is always in tandem with other muscles. With simultaneous activity of the oblique interarytenoid fibres and maybe even the contralateral aryepiglottic muscle then the action becomes sphincteric, causing the arytenoid to rotate anteromedially about the long axis of the cricoarytenoid joint thus bringing the tips of the vocal processes together ('medial compression'). With simultaneous activity in the PCA, the result will be to negate the adductive capacity of the most superior and medial fibres of the PCA and to alter the pull of the most lateral and oblique fibres into a more strongly abductive direction. This combined activity appears to produce a complex combination of posterior rotation about the long axis of the cricoarytenoid (although much less than by the unrestricted activity of PCA alone), plus some lateral slide along the

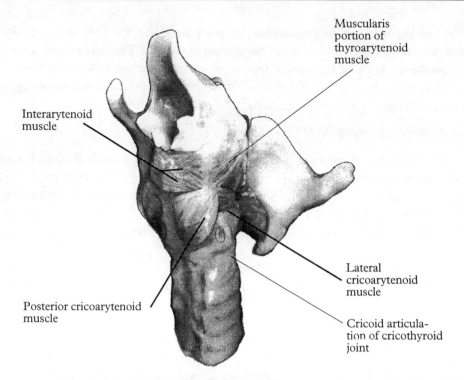

Muscularis portion of thyroarytenoid muscle

Interarytenoid muscle

Lateral cricoarytenoid muscle

Posterior cricoarytenoid muscle

Cricoid articulation of cricothyroid joint

Figure 1.6 Intrinsic muscles of the larynx: right posterolateral view with the right thyroid lamina swung forward and outward to reveal the muscles

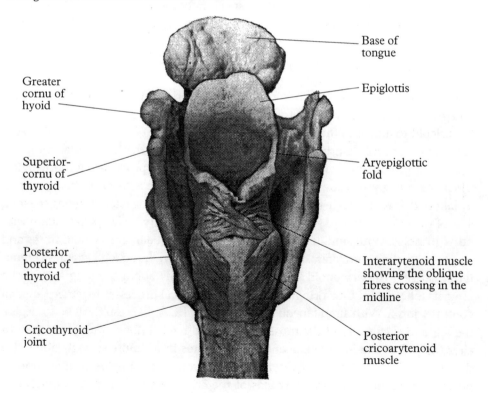

Base of tongue

Epiglottis

Greater cornu of hyoid

Superior cornu of thyroid

Aryepiglottic fold

Posterior border of thyroid

Interarytenoid muscle showing the oblique fibres crossing in the midline

Cricothyroid joint

Posterior cricoarytenoid muscle

Figure 1.7 Posterior view of the larynx

same axis together with lateral tilting. The overall effect when seen from above is abduction of the vocal fold with limited elongation of the folds (Figure 1.1). (For a more detailed explanation read the section on muscle function, pp. 67-75).

The oblique arytenoid muscles

The oblique arytenoid muscles originate on the medial half of the muscular process of the arytenoid. The muscle fibres lie in a similar plane to those of the LCA, i.e. they run upwards in the direction broadly following the circumference of the cricoid, crossing the midline to attach to the apex of the contralateral arytenoid.

The aryepiglotticus muscle

This is really the prolongation of some of the fibres of the oblique arytenoid muscle running anteriorly in the aryepiglottic fold from the arytenoid apex to attach to the epiglottis.

The transverse arytenoid or interarytenoid muscle

This muscle is attached at both ends to each arytenoid cartilage. The attachments extend over the entire length of the dorsolateral ridge and dorsomedial concave surface of the arytenoids. Despite being an unpaired muscle, there is a double innervation from both recurrent laryngeal nerves indicating a double embryological origin of the muscle. It would appear that it opposes the natural tendency for the arytenoids to separate by sliding downwards and out when the vocal folds have been adducted and tension is being applied to the vocal fold/PCA by cricothyroid activity.

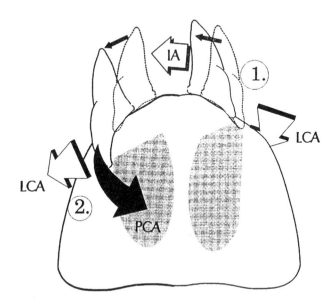

Figure 1.8 Diagram of the posterior aspect of the cricoid body and arytenoid cartilages
① Muscles involved in medial compression (IA and LCA).
② Muscles involved in abduction (PCA and LCA)

The thyroarytenoid muscle

The thyroarytenoid muscle is a complex structure with two distinct portions of differing function. It arises from the deep surface (back) of the thyroid lamina lateral to the insertion of the vocal ligament. Almost L-shaped in cross-section, the upper, lateral portion is a flat sheet lying deep to the quadrangular membrane within the aryepiglottic fold. There is a considerable increase in muscle bulk inferiorly where its medial (vocalis) fibres travel posteriorly with the vocal ligament forming the shelf-like body of the vocal fold. The posterior ends of both parts of the muscle are widely attached to the arytenoid cartilage; the fibres of vocalis (the lower, medial portion) attach to the inferior fossa and vocal process of the arytenoid cartilage, and the upper lateral thyroarytenoid fibres attach to the whole of the dorsolateral ridge of the cartilage.

That there is an evolving differentiation of function of the two parts of this muscle is borne out by recent comparative studies of the muscle fibres in human larynges and those from other species. In canine larynges both parts of the muscle appear to be innervated by a mixture of 'fast-twitch' and 'slow-twitch' fibres, such as would be suitable for a mixed function of rapid sealing of the larynx and primitive voicing. In man the lateral thyroarytenoid retains the twitch capacity in the lateral fibres but the superior vocalis portion has become expanded and is entirely populated by 'slow-twitch' fibres in very small motor pools suitable for the sustained and very accurate muscle contractions needed for voicing (Sandens, 1995).

In addition to these two principal parts of the thyroarytenoid muscle there is another condensation of muscle whose fibres run in a much more oblique line from the upper margin of the origin of the thyroarytenoid in front ascending posterosuperiorly, within the aryepiglottic fold. This is the thyroepiglottic muscle, and it is considered also to be a part of the thyroarytenoid muscle, although its insertion along with the aryepiglotticus into the lateral border of the epiglottis technically makes it a muscle of the aryepiglottic fold. These muscles function together with the muscularis portion of the thyroarytenoid to control the configuration and degree of constriction of the laryngeal inlet (aryepiglottic folds) and ventricular bands (false vocal folds). They are sometimes collectively referred to as the muscles of the quadrangular membrane.

Extrinsic muscles of the larynx

These will be outlined in functional groups.

Anterior strap muscles

The larynx is unique in the body because it is a semi-rigid articulated structure, and yet it lacks the passive support of a joint or joints that might connect it somewhere to the rest of the skeleton. As every voice user is aware it is highly (and controllably) mobile in the neck in a broadly vertical plane, and to a lesser degree in the anteroposterior plane. The control of laryngeal position is not achieved by the tugging of the pharyngeal musculature alone, but by the coordinated activity of all the extrinsic strap muscles as well. The muscles can be broadly divided into functional groups.

(i) Muscles that lower laryngeal position

Sternothyroid

This has its origin on the deep surface of the manubrium sterni and ascends to insert into the oblique line of the thyroid cartilage. It lowers the larynx.

Sternohyoid

The sternohyoid overlies the sternothyroid. This flat muscle also takes origin on the posterolateral surface of the manubrium sterni, and passes up over the thyroid cartilage to attach to the lower border of the body of the hyoid bone. It lowers the hyoid bone, and consequently, the larynx. Both the sternohyoid and the sternothyroid pull in a slightly anterior direction.

Omohyoid

This muscle originates on the superior border of the scapula. It ascends anteriorly to a position superior to the medial end of the clavicle, where the cervical fascia binds it in position. From there it turns superiorly to insert into the inferior border of the body of the hyoid, lateral to the insertion of the sternohyoid. Why the belly of this muscle is tethered in cervical fascia is not clear. The effect would seem to be to render a more anterior direction to its laryngeal depressor action.

(ii) Muscles that raise laryngeal position

Thyrohyoid

The thyrohyoid raises the thyroid cartilage with respect to the hyoid bone. This flat muscle originates at the oblique line on the thyroid lamina. It runs upwards deep to the other strap muscles to insert into the lateral part of the inferior border of the body and greater cornu of the hyoid. It maintains the stability of the thyrohyoid membranes and is the sole muscular suspension of the larynx under the hyoid bone. It can rotate the thyroid posteriorly at the cricothyroid joints if the cricoid has been prevented from passively following due to other antagonizing forces. The posterior part of the lower attachment, however, the portion arising at the oblique line, would seem to have a vector of pull running through the cricothyroid joint; in other words the posterior part of the muscle has the capacity to draw the thyroid cartilage towards the hyoid with very little rotational force at the CT joints.

Geniohyoid

The geniohyoid muscle raises the hyoid bone with respect to the mandible (jaw) with additional anterior pull on the hyoid bone. It has attachments to the front of the body of the hyoid and the lower genial tubercle at the midline inside the lower margin of the mandible. It also pulls the hyoid anteriorly, assisting in the creation of space in the hypopharynx.

Mylohyoid

The mylohyoid muscle raises the hyoid bone with respect to the mandible (jaw) and elevates the body of the hyoid. It is a flat sheet of muscle arising from the entire mylohyoid line on the inner surface of the mandible. It is attached to its opposite number in a fibrous raphe stretching between the body of the hyoid and the symphysis (midline) of the mandible. It forms the floor of the mouth. Contracting the muscle not only raises the anterior body of the tongue, it also elevates the body of the hyoid.

Digastric

The diagastric muscles raise the hyoid bone with respect to the mandible (jaw), with neutral elevation regardless of anteroposterior laryngeal position. There are two distinct muscles connected by a common tendon. The anterior belly arises from the lower border of mandible near the midline; the posterior belly arises on the skull base medial to the mastoid process. Their common tendon is bound to the body of the hyoid by a fibrous tunnel at the junction between greater horn and body. These muscles are important for laryngeal raising during swallowing.

For further details of the role of these muscles in the positioning of the larynx and its effect on fundamental frequency, see Chapter 6.

Muscles of the supraglottic vocal tract

Pharyngeal constrictors

These will be reviewed from the bottom upwards.

The inferior constrictor

This muscle is actually in two parts.
(i)   Cricopharyngeus. This arises (a) between the origin of the cricothyroid muscle and the cricothyroid joint, and (b) from the tendinous band between the inferior thyroid tubercle and the cricoid. Fibres are more or less contiguous with the muscle from the opposite side, i.e. the median raphe is minimal and they are continuous and blend with fibres of the upper oesophagus. The resting tone of this muscle is high in order to prevent the intrathoracic oesophagus inflating like the lungs with inspired air. The muscle relaxes with the approach of a swallowed bolus of food. The muscle anchors the cricoid cartilage posteriorly, and therefore assists in the closure of the cricothyroid visor if the thyroid cartilage is tilted forward above it. The upper fibres may anchor the cricoid against the tug of the trachea and oesophagus.

(ii) Thyropharyngeus. This muscle arises from the oblique line and inferiorly from the lateral border on the thyroid lamina plus a slip behind the line inferiorly. The fibres insert posteriorly into the median raphe. The muscle contracts immediately after the passage of a swallowed bolus of food, effectively 'stripping' the bolus onward towards the stomach. The lower fibres are almost horizontal while the upper fibres are set obliquely, ascending posteriorly to their insertion into the raphe behind the pharynx. Because of the oblique setting of the fibres, contraction on swallowing or voicing produces much less tendency to rotate the thyroid cartilage backwards than might be expected; indeed, if the hyoid is being held forward, then thyropharyngeus may actually tend to rotate the thyroid cartilage forwards on the cricoid.

Note: There is a weakness in the muscular coat of the pharynx between the crico- and thyropharyngeus muscles known as Killian's dehiscence. Normally, the two parts of the muscle function independently but in a coordinated manner. Should the swallow become dyscoordinate for any reason, then any resultant waves of high pressure may produce a pulsion diverticulum or pharyngeal pouch through the weak point at Killian's dehiscence.

The middle constrictor

This is also a fan-shaped muscle arising from the lesser cornu of hyoid and lower part of the styloid ligament together with the whole of the upper border of the greater cornu of the hyoid. The lower fibres, as before, insert into the median raphe to form a cone within the inferior constrictor. The upper fibres similarly overlap the superior constrictor so that the arrangement is broadly one of concentric funnels inserting into lower ones. This arrangement not only assists the smooth progress of a wave of contraction to progress down the pharynx on swallowing, but when contracted independently of the inferior constrictor, also permits an inverted U-shaped constriction in the pharynx, which is essential for the generation of a particular resonance characteristic, 'the singer's formant'. (Selective production of constrictions at different positions in the supraglottic vocal tract dictates the frequencies at which the formants of a sung or spoken vowel sound will occur. For a description of the resonance characteristics of the vocal tract, see Chapter 13.)

The superior constrictor

This is a complex more or less quadrilateral sheet arising anterior to the pterygoid hamulus and on occasion to the adjoining posterior margin of the medial pterygoid plate, to the pterygomandibular raphe, to the posterior end of the mylohyoid line of the mandible and to the side of the tongue. The fibres curve back to insert into the median raphe up as far as the pharyngeal tubercle of the occipital bone.

Unsurprisingly, the four parts are described according to their origin:

pterygopharyngeal
buccopharyngeal
mylopharyngeal
glossopharyngeal.

The constrictors are all supplied by the pharyngeal plexus; the motor and sensory fibres coming from trigeminal, glossopharyngeal and vagus (motor fibres of accessory origin). Pharyngeal rami come from the superior (jugular) ganglion. The autonomic sympathetic fibres are from the ganglion, and the parasympathetic are postganglionic, mostly via the glossopharyngeal nerve.

Note: All of the above muscles do exactly what their names suggest: they constrict the pharynx, or in the context of this book the major part of the supraglottic vocal tract. None of them is capable of actively dilating (increasing the volume of) the supraglottic vocal tract. Only the extrinsic strap muscles of the larynx, which, together with the suprahyoid muscles, are responsible for raising the larynx and drawing it forward (in the phase of swallowing immediately prior to a food bolus being squeezed from the back of the tongue into the pharynx), are capable of active pharyngeal dilatation. This is of great importance when considering the shaping of the supraglottic vocal tract to make a tube that resonates correctly for production of vowel sounds or higher resonances ('formants') that give brilliance and carrying power to the singing voice.

The stylopharyngeus

This muscle originates on the medial side of the styloid process. It is a long thin muscle that initially travels down the outside of the pharynx, then passes inside between the superior and middle constrictors to spread out beneath the mucous membrane, some of the fibres blending into the constrictors, lateral glossoepiglottic fold and, with palatopharyngeus, into the posterior border of the thyroid cartilage.

The stylopharyngeus is supplied by the glossopharyngeal nerve, it is, a pharyngeal elevator and widener.

You cannot talk about swallowing or the modification of the supraglottic vocal tract for particular resonating characteristics without including the palatal muscles.

The palatal muscles

Levator veli palatini

This muscle rises from:

1. the base of skull (petrous temporal bone) just anterior to the opening of the carotid canal
2. the fascia hanging from the tympanic temporal bone that forms the carotid sheath
3. the cartilaginous part of the Eustachian tube.

It therefore lies inferior to the Eustachian tube. It passes though the upper margin of the superior constrictor in front of salpingopharyngeus and spreads out in the soft palate between two layers of palatopharyngeus in the palatine aponeurosis. It elevates the soft palate.

Tensor veli palatini

This arises from the scaphoid fossa of the pterygoid process, the lateral lamina of the Eustachian tube and the medial side of the spine of the sphenoid. The muscle descends, becoming tendinous to turn round the pterygoid hamulus, passes through the origin of Buccinator and inserts into the anterior palate in the palatine aponeurosis and palatine crest of the horizontal part of the palatine bone. It tenses the anterior, relatively unmuscular part of the palate.

This muscle alone is innervated by the mandibular nerve; all the other palatal muscles are innervated by the pharyngeal plexus.

Palatoglossus

The palatoglossus arises from the palatine aponeurosis to the side of the tongue. It forms the anterior arch of the fauces.

Palatopharyngeus

This muscle arises in the palate from two fasciculi separated by the levator veli palatini. The posterior fasciculus arises jointly with its opposite number in the median plane on the pharyngeal side of the palate. The anterior bundle arises at the posterior margin of the hard palate from the palatine aponeurosis. It passes between the levator and tensor veli palatini and unites with the posterior bundle and also salpingopharyngeus. This conjoint flat muscle passes laterally and down-wards and is inserted into the posterior border of the thyroid cartilage together with stylopharyngeus. It forms an internal longitudinal coat for the pharynx, and it also forms the posterior arch of the fauces.

The palatopharyngeus pulls the free border of the palate down. This may be the reason that increased nasality is often noted with a persistently raised, backed laryngeal position.

Salpingopharyngeus

The salpingopharyngeus originates on the inferior part of the Eustachian tube cartilage. It travels downwards to blend with the palatopharyngeus. It may simply represent a slip of palatopharyngeus.

References

Boileau Grant JC (1972) Grants Atlas of Anatomy 6th Edition. The Williams and Wilkins Co. Baltimore.

Dickson D, Dickson W (1971) Functional anatomy of the human larynx. Proceedings of the Pennsylvanian Academy of Ophthalmology. p.29.

Dickson DR, Maue-Dickson W (1982) Anatomical and physiological bases of speech. Boston: Little, Brown and Co.

Laitman JT et al. (1995) Formation of the larynx. In Rubin JS, Sataloff RT, Korovin GS, Gould WJ (Eds) Diagnosis and Treatment of Voice Disorders. New York: Igaku-Shoin.

Maue WM (1970). Cartilages, ligaments and articulations of the adult human larynx.University of Pittsburgh PhD dissertation.

Maue WM, Dickson DR (1971). Cartilages and ligaments of the adult human larynx. Archives of Otolaryngology 94: 432.

Sanders I (1995) In Rubin JS, Sataloff RT, Korovin GS, Gould WJ (Eds) Diagnosis and Treatment of Voice Disorders: New York: Igaku-Shoin.

Vilkman E, Sonninen A, Hurme P, Körkkö P (1996) External laryngeal frame function in voice production revisited: a review. Journal of Voice 10: 78–92.

Vocal Fold: Structural and Ultrastructural Considerations for Phonosurgeons

TOM HARRIS

This chapter is intended chiefly as an 'aide-mémoire' for those who may be called upon to operate on the vocal folds, although others may also enjoy reminding themselves of the sophistication of the seemingly simple vocal folds.

The anterior, intermembranous or vibrating portion of the vocal fold extends between its attachments at the muscular process of the arytenoid cartilage posteriorly and at the anterior commissure anteriorly. The layered microstructure of the vocal fold (Figure 2.1) has been elegantly described by Hirano and Kakita (1985), amongst other publications.

The covering epithelium

From the surface inwards, it consists of a durable but flexible layer of non-keratinizing stratified squamous epithelium between 0.05 and 0.1 mm thick, similar to that of the skin covering of the body. It will permit a degree of stretching sideways but is relatively incompressible. (In physical jargon it is said to be anisotropic.) This relatively waterproof layer covers and encapsulates a complex layer that appears to be largely made up of semifluid gel-like substance, the lamina propria.

The lamina propria

This second layer is actually much more sophisticated than initial impressions suggest: there are at least three major divisions of the lamina propria, a catch-all description for all the non-muscular material between the epithelium and the fibres of the vocalis muscle.

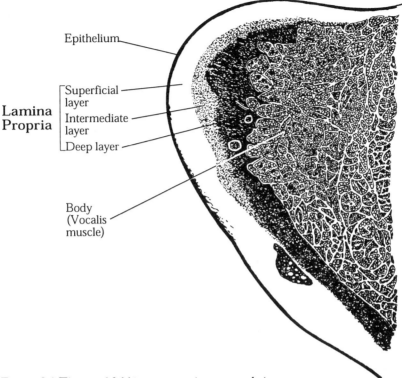

Epithelium

Lamina
Propria

Superficial
layer

Intermediate
layer

Deep layer

Body
(Vocalis
muscle)

Figure 2.1 The vocal fold in cross-section: coronal view

The superficial layer

This consists mostly of elastin fibres with a few collagen fibres embedded in an interstitial fluid and matrix composed of mucoproteins and mucopolysaccharides (Hirano et al., 1981). It is the fibroblasts of the superficial layer of the lamina propria (SLLP) that are responsible for the production and maintenance of the ground substance. This fluid-retaining material is amorphous but retains its structure as it is interspersed in the elastin/collagen framework of Reinke's space. The elastin fibres can stretch longitudinally to almost double their resting length, and because they are not longitudinally aligned, the superficial layer is readily deformable in all directions (isotropic). The SLLP in health is a resilient, thin gel, which can be very considerably deformed and yet retain its structural integrity under conditions of great physical stress, and is essential for the generation of mucosal waves on phonation. A possible reason for the traditional lack of surgical regard for this structure is that, in health, it measures only approximately 0.5 mm in thickness in the mid-section of the fold.

The intermediate layer

This is again made up chiefly of elastin fibres. This time, however, the fibres are densely packed and although they anastomose and branch freely, the majority are aligned longitudinally between the anterior and posterior attachments of the vocal fold. There are aggregations of elastin fibres at the anterior and posterior ends of the vocal ligament known as the anterior and posterior maculae flava. They appear to function as shock absorbers at points of maximum impact on phonation. Collagen fibres are also present as a minor component in this layer.

The deep layer

The deep layer immediately underneath the intermediate layer is made up principally of the relatively inextensible collagen fibres that are also aligned longitudinally in a coil-like fashion, although the alignment alters inferiorly where the layer becomes contiguous with the fibres of the triangular membrane of the conus elasticus. Together, the intermediate and deep layers of the lamina propria are between 1 and 2 mm thick and make up the vocal ligament. The main stress applied to the ligament is one of extension, and the deformation under stress is described as being anisotropic.

The body of the vocal fold

The vocalis muscle

The vocalis muscle, the medial portion of the thyroarytenoid muscle, is 7–8 mm thick and, in turn, lies deep and lateral to the lamina propria in a manner akin to muscle underlying a layer of fascia. This represents the major part of the muscle and is histochemically different from the muscularis portion. In the human larynx the innervation arrangements are significantly different from other species: there is a gradient from the most medial fibres nearest the ligament (the superior vocalis), where the densely innervated fibres are almost exclusively of the slow-twitch variety, through to the muscularis portion, where the fibres are entirely of the fast-twitch variety (Sanders, 1995). This is reflected by the human capacity to produce a very sustained phonatory tone. The fibres are gathered in small bundles, or fasciculi, and the bundles in the superior vocalis appear from observation of phonation to be capable of differential activity to change the shape of the vibrating free border to produce the variable thickness required for different registers and pitches. The inferior part of the vocalis is hypothesized to be the functional equivalent of the lower mass in the two mass model of vocal fold activity.

Although the classical description of the vocal folds' laminated epithelial, lamina propria and muscular layers satisfies the morphological requirements, it does not lend much understanding to the mechanical ability of the vocal folds' ability to vibrate at widely varying pitches and intensities without damage under normal conditions. It is the interplay between all the layers, the isotropic layers being firmly sandwiched between the anisotropic, which allows for the generation of complex mucosal waves. It is the ability to apply tension longitudinally along the intermediate and deep layers of the lamina propria that permits thinning of the fold at its free border while at the same time producing an increase in firmness of the fold. It is also the ability of the vocalis muscle to selectively stiffen in different configurations that permits a wide range of vocal timbres.

All the descriptions in Table 2.1 may therefore be regarded as valid; which one is used depends chiefly on whether the user is speaking or writing from a physical, morphological/histochemical or functional standpoint.

From the standpoint of the surgeon operating on the vocal folds the system falls nicely into the first, physical, category; the tissue planes naturally divide between the mucosa and the ligament. Unfortunately, tissue damage is no respecter of surgical planes, and the results of damage are reflected by the disruption of the normal arrangements of any of the five principal histologically discrete layers. Hirano's description of vocal fold vibration in a two-part system, the 'cover-body' theory, makes it quite obvious that any microsurgery must be designed to minimize any disruption of the vocal fold cover, while the aim of any 'framework'

Table 2.1 Description of the vocal folds		
Three layer description of physical characteristics	Five layer description of histological characteristics	Two layer 'cover-body' description of functional characteristics *(after Hirano et al., 1981)*
Mucosa	Epithelium	Cover
	Superficial layer *Lamina propria*	
Ligament	Intermediate layer *Lamina propria*	
	Deep layer *Lamina propria*	
Muscle	Muscle	Body

surgery has to be to produce as little damage as possible to the function of the vocal fold 'body'. This is why Isshiki type I thyroplasty is to be preferred from a functional point of view to injection of Teflon® paste or similar preparations. It also demonstrates clearly why any Teflon or collagen paste left between the intermediate and deep layers of the lamina propria can produce such unfortunate results when the patient attempts voicing postoperatively.

With all the stresses produced within the layers of the vocal fold cover during phonation, how is it that the epithelium does not simply strip off the superficial layer of the lamina propria? The answer appears to lie in the ultrastructure of the basement membrane zone or transitional area between the epithelium and superficial layer of the lamina propria. Underneath the basal cells of the epithelium, the electron microscope reveals that their plasma membranes contain structures known as attachment plaques. The basal cells overlie a layer known as the lamina lucida, which in turn contains aggregations corresponding to the attachment plaques known as sub-basal dense plates. These dense plates are in turn anchored by microfibrils to a layer of type IV collagen/proteoglycan, the lamina densa. It is this lamina densa of the basement membrane that maintains the structural integrity of the epithelium. Beneath it things are even more complex. There is no evidence of collagen from the lamina propria simply embedded into the lamina densa to secure adhesion; instead, there is a very subtle and flexible arrangement of type VII collagen fibres that helps to maintain the attachment of the basal cells/basement membrane to the superficial layer of the lamina propria (SLLP). **Both** ends of these fibres arise in the lamina densa and the mid-portions form loops that project into the superficial layer of the lamina propria. The thicker type III collagen fibres of that layer pass through the loops, as do other more deeply set loop fibres (Gray et al., 1994). Their appearance and position almost suggest a sort of ultramicroscopic layer of inverted staples attaching a web of fibres in the SLLP to the basal layer of the epithelium in a manner that allows for gliding, bending and compression of the layers of tissue without shearing a plane between them.

It is now thought that loss or damage to these loops allows the shearing stresses produced by phonation to damage the vocal fold cover, blistering the epithelium off the SLLP and thus inducing the inflammatory repair that produces nodules.

This hypothesis is not incompatible with the standard teaching concerning the pathogenesis of polyps and polypoid degeneration (Hirano et al., 1980): it may be that it is damage to this structure that permits unusual stresses to the microvasculature of the vocal fold cover, causing extravasation of blood and subsequent development of polypoid change if the process is repeated and becomes chronic.

References

Gray SD, Pignatari SSN, Harding P (1994) Morphologic ultrastructure of anchoring fibers in normal vocal fold basement membrane zone. Journal of Voice 8: 48–52.

Hirano M, Kakita Y (1985) Cover-body theory of vocal fold vibration. In Daniloff RG (Ed) Speech science. San Diego: College-Hill Press, pp 1–46.

Hirano M, Kurita S, Matsuo K, Nagata K (1980) Laryngeal tissue reaction to stress. In

Transcripts of the ninth symposium: care of the professional voice, part II. New York: The Voice Foundation.

Hirano M, Kurita S, Nakashima T (1981) The structure of the vocal folds. In Stevens KN, Hirano M (Eds) Vocal fold physiology. University of Tokyo Press.

Sanders I (1995) The microanatomy of the vocal folds. In Rubin JS, Sataloff RT, Korovin GS, Gould WJ (Eds) Diagnosis and treatment of voice disorders. New York: Igaku-Shoin, pp 70–85.

CHAPTER 3

Outline of Common Benign Lesions Causing Dysphonia

TOM HARRIS

Lesions within the larynx that cause dysphonia may do so for a limited number of reasons:

1. They may interfere with the contact area between the vocal folds during the closed phase of the vibratory cycle.
2. As a result, they produce air escape during the closed phase.
3. They may also cause structural alteration to the layers of the vocal fold, thus inhibiting or abolishing the generation of normal mucosal waves on phonation.

Treatment of these lesions will be dealt with in subsequent chapters of this book. When planning management of the problem, consideration should always be given as to whether the body's normal resolution/repair processes will heal a lesion faster or more effectively with or without physical intervention and whether there is any realistic possibility that conservative treatment and a 'wait and see' approach will deal with the problem in a time-frame that the patient can afford.

Acute non-specific laryngitis

This is an extremely common problem that rarely presents in the voice clinic, owing to its capacity to resolve. It is characterized by modest oedema and erythema of the mucosal cover. The pathogenesis is multifactorial: vocal abuse, local chemical irritation (smoke, etc.) are both implicated. The problem will usually resolve spontaneously but a brief period of voice rest, steam inhalations, rehydration and voice therapy may aid the process and prevent its recurrence.

Chronic laryngitis

'Acute' implies a discrete episode of damage, whereas 'chronic' implies that damage is ongoing and occurring at the same time as repair and resolution of tissue damage. Spontaneous resolution is not therefore the norm. The condition is characterized by moderate mucosal oedema and (usually) by more marked diffuse erythema of the mucosa than in acute laryngitis, and a variable degree of epithelial hyperplasia. The stiffening of the vocal fold mucosa observed on videostrobo-laryngoscopy may be much more pronounced than in the acute form. The problem is frequently associated with alcohol abuse, smoking and vocal abuse. Improvement will only be observed if there is a significant change in lifestyle, and then only slowly.

Chronic laryngitis may be associated with gastro-oesophageal acid reflux (GOR, or GERD in the USA). Reflux has been implicated in the production of 'posterior laryngitis' with the predominance of inflammation being seen over the interarytenoid region. This is not always the case. Twenty four-hour oesophageal manometry monitoring may be useful in identifying GOR as a significant causative factor, but the tests seem prone to 'false negatives' where reflux is inter-mittent. Where GOR is a factor, treatment should include elevation of the head of the bed and at least a month's course of a proton pump inhibitor or prokinetic agent (see chapter 10).

Vocal fold nodule

This is a lesion confined to the epithelium and subepithelial space of the vocal fold cover. It is not connected by fibrous tissue to the deeper layers of the lamina propria.

The lesion is first seen as an oedematous lesion that may be associated with extravasated blood under the epithelium (especially in adults) and vasodilatation. Microscopically the epithelium is hyperkeratotic and sometimes acanthotic; the lesion has been likened to a developing callus from repetitive trauma. A 'mature' nodule has abundant fibroblasts and irregular collagen fibres in the subepithelial layer, together with very variable amounts of oedema.

Although nodules may arise from a single discrete episode of trauma, a singer may tell you of the exact bar in an aria when the trouble began (see the comments above relating to the ultrastructure of the lamina propria), the lesion subsequently develops and matures as a result of repetitive episodes of damage. Children develop nodules in response to continuous shouting and yelling. Those who develop nodules seem to be relatively unskilled in the fine art of screaming at inten-sities where anyone within earshot is registering pain. In our clinic there is a marked preponderance of children with one or more older siblings.

Treatment always involves speech therapy. In the case of screaming children, they are taught not only how to modify their vocal behaviour but also how to yell more efficiently. In an adult context, although speech therapy remains the mainstay of treatment, very precise and conservative surgical removal, which does not breach the integrity of the superficial layer of the lamina propria, will greatly hasten return to normal voicing. Any wider or deeper excision than this is destined to be a disas-ter, as generations of performers who have undergone 'local stripping' will testify.

Vocal fold polyp

This lesion is removed surgically more often than any other. The pathogenesis has been associated with repetitive trauma, resulting in erythema and vasodilatation with extravasation of inflammatory material into the surrounding tissue. There is formation of multiple microscopic spaces, 'blood lakes', of (possibly) extravasated blood surrounded by endothelial cells. Polyps are associated with dilated feeder vessels. There is a complete spectrum of histological appearance ranging from polyps that are chiefly gelatinous with a loose stroma containing a few inflammatory cells and collagen, to those that contain much fibrin and eosinophilic material in the stroma and have prominent tortuous vascular spaces. Although the lesion has its base in the superficial layer of the lamina propria, it does not typically span the whole thickness to adhere to deeper layers. It may therefore be excised locally and superficially without denuding the deeper layers of the fold. It should be noted however that some polyps have deeper attachments especially at their superior margins. Preoperative stroboscopy will often warn of this potential problem.

Polypoid degeneration (syn. Reinke oedema)

This is an inflammatory condition characterized by vocal abuse and, almost invariably, smoking. The superficial layer of the lamina propria (Reinke's space) is distended by oedema fluid and inflammatory cells. To look at, it may be bilateral or unilateral, and the spreading of the swelling is limited only by the superior and inferior fibrous limits of the space. Moderate swelling may appear fusiform, although continued swelling may produce lesions that are grape-like in appearance.

Pseudocystic degeneration

Classically, polypoid degeneration is described as having a watery, thin consistency with a thin rather atrophic epithelium overlying the space. Because the process is inflammatory, however, the material in Reinke's space may be much thicker than one might expect and can even mimic a true vocal fold retention cyst. For more detailed suggestions concerning the operative and therapeutic management, see Chapters 7 and 11.

Microweb

This is a very small web situated just below the free border of the folds at the anterior commissure. It may well be invisible on initial inspection of the larynx unless the patient is specifically asked to inhale briskly. Unlike the thick fibrous webs that are usually iatrogenic in nature, these are believed by Bouchayer et al. (1994) to be congenital in origin. They consist simply of an epithelial reflection upon itself with minimal subepithelial tissue and/or fibrosis sandwiched between. Although trivial in appearance, their functional significance is clearly greater than one might expect – they can considerably affect a performer's vocal ability, and Bouchayer et al. (1994) found that 10% of vocal nodules are associated with microwebs. Treatment is surgical and consists of simple division at microlaryngoscopy.

So far the lesions that have been described involve only the epithelial cover of the lamina propria or the epithelium plus the superficial layer of the lamina. The following lesions have a much more pronounced effect on the normal functioning of the vocal folds as they involve not only the vocal fold cover, but also the deeper layers of the lamina propria. The reader is referred to Chapter 11 for further details of their surgical treatment. Surgery to excise them is both exacting and time consuming.

Vocal fold cysts

There are two types of intrafold cyst that are commonly encountered: ductal mucus retention and epidermoid cysts. Both may vary in appearance from being entirely clinically obvious, bulging out from the fold on simple laryngoscopy, to others whose presence is only suggested by an absence of mucosal waves overlying the spot where the cyst lies hidden. In the case of the epidermoid cyst, there is a variable reduction in the translucence of the cover, which may appear whiter than its surroundings. There may be a few aberrant vascular dilatations running over or converging on the cyst rather than running longitudinally as do the other vessels and this may suggest the presence of a cyst. Cysts cause major disturbance of phonation because they tether the epithelium to the deeper layers of the lamina propria. They do not 'go away given time', although dysphonia may be variable if the cyst possesses a punctum through which it may partially discharge from time to time.

Mucus retention cysts

These greyish-yellow cysts are usually situated near the mid-third of the vocal fold, just below the free border where mucus producing glands are present. They are thought to arise as a result of simple ductular obstruction of the gland, and histology of the cyst reveals that the wall is composed of columnar epithelium much as is found in normal duct tissue.

Epidermoid cysts

These cysts, if visible, tend to bulge out from the medial/superior aspect of the mid-vocal fold. As with the mucus retention cyst there is no evidence of inflammation. Histologically, the cyst wall consists of a thin keratinizing squamous epithelium and the contents are made up of squamous debris with some cholesterol crystals.

Sulcus vocalis

This condition is thought to be congenital in origin. Of the patients attending our clinic who present with a large sulcus, around 80% have ethnic origins in the Indian subcontinent. A true sulcus vocalis is an elongated pocket or furrow situated in the superficial layer of the lamina propria. It runs longitudinally along the length of the vibrating portion of the fold. The superior margin is a point where the epithelium ceases to be separated from the vocal ligament by any Reinke's space. The lining epithelium becomes intimately connected to the fibres of the vocal ligament and may actually invaginate into their substance. The inferior margin of the sulcus is demarcated by a fibrous band beneath the fold epithelium. The epithelium beneath the sulcus is recurved around this band to attach to itself forming the outer margin of a long pocket that is invaginated deep to the inferior mucosal cover, replacing Reinke's space. The histology of the lining of the elongated sulcus pocket is similar to that of an epidermoid cyst, being composed of thickened stratified squamous epithelium.

It has been suggested by Bouchayer (Bouchayer and Cornut, 1991) that a sulcus vocalis may simply be a very widely open-mouthed variety of epidermoid cyst pocket.

Voice quality where bilateral sulci are present is, of necessity, a rather breathy falsetto. A characteristic spindle-shaped bowing of the folds on phonation has been described (Lindestad and Hertegård, 1994). Our interpretation of this finding is that although there is no evidence to suggest that there is underlying pathology that producing the bowing, there is a lifetime of major laryngeal muscular effort spent maintaining very tight vocal ligaments as the folds are only capable of vibration in a pattern resembling falsetto. A falsetto voice quality is much less dependent on the production of (even a small) mucosal wave. We suggest that where bilateral sulci are present, this obligatory voice quality eventually results in stretching of the vocal ligament with the resultant glottal insufficiency as described.

Vergeture

From the French word for 'stretch-mark', this lesion, although at first glance resembling a sulcus, shows significant differences in detail. A vergeture is an atrophic area on the free border of the fold, and is characterized by an absence of any complex epithelium. The histology shows a simple low cuboidal cell lining only. There is no superficial layer of lamina propria present, and the epithelium is intimately bound to the fibres of the vocal ligament. It is suggested that the origin of this lesion is traumatic, and it should be observed that the vast majority of these lesions presenting in the clinic have a history of traumatic intubation or previous surgery. If the lesion is extensive, then patterns of dysfunction similar to those found in sulcus are usually apparent.

Scarring

Scarring is by no means always associated with atrophic notches. Every ENT surgeon has in addition encountered webs, both at the anterior and posterior commissures. They may also have noted rigid, adynamic portions of vocal folds, especially in patients with a history of previous laser surgery to the larynx. There is no characteristic appearance to identify, although absence of mucosal waves on stroboscopy will suggest that the superficial layer of the lamina propria, if it still exists, contains significant amounts of rigid collagenous scar tissue.

Laryngeal granulomas

Granuloma formation and maintenance is always a chronic process with continuing damage occuring at the same time as tissue attempts to effect repairs. Even though casual laryngeal trauma may be much commoner than previously supposed (Harris et al., 1990), chronic inflammatory processes in the larynx remain relatively rare.

Several subgroups of granuloma have been described, viz.:

(i)   arytenoid (syn. 'contact') granuloma
(ii) intubation granuloma
(iii) post-surgery (most frequently post-Teflon injection) foreign body granuloma.

The first two describe lesions that arise medially, on or slightly above the arytenoid vocal process. The granulation tissue may appear pale and polypoid, and is typically bilobed. The lesion is generally unilateral, although the same patient may develop a second contralateral lesion after the first has resolved. Surgical removal is notoriously unsuccessful.

The histology of arytenoid contact granulomas, like other lesions in the larynx, exhibits a spectrum of change: ulcerated granulation tissue at the surface, pachydermia, a core of dense connective tissue with excessive vascularity. There may be evidence of non-specific granuloma, although the inflammatory response is variable.

The histology of an intubation granuloma is similar, but there is often more erosion and fibrin deposition at the surface and the stroma tends to be more vascular than the arytenoid contact granuloma.

Arytenoid granulomas

The pathogenesis of the arytenoid contact granuloma appears multifactorial. They are more commonly found in males, especially in those who adopt a speaking voice whose pitch is right at the bottom of their vocal range. While the voice may not sound 'pressed', the vocal attack at onset of voicing is very hard (*coup de glotte*). The arytenoids are brought crashing together. This may occur despite an outwardly relaxed demeanour.

The role of gastro-oesophageal acid reflux remains controversial, different authors having found very different incidence of associated GOR (Ohman et al., 1983; Wilson. et al., 1989; Jones et al., 1990). The incidence is, however, in the author's view, generally high enough to warrant anti-reflux therapy as a standard part of the treatment regimen.

Work done with the psychological profiling of these patients shows that as a group they tend to be somewhat narcissistic and handle stress poorly (Kiese-Himmel and Kruse, 1994). They are often 'passive-aggressive' and tend to depression. In the experience of the Sidcup Voice Clinic, the patients always seem to have an underlying problem in their lives that they feel unable to deal with. It is rarely apparent at the initial consultation. The most important factor in curing this lesion is to establish exactly what this problem is, and to get the patient to deal with it appropriately. Serial observations may then demonstrate dramatic resolution of the lesion in a matter of weeks.

Intubation granulomas

Intubation granulomas, even though they have an apparently different precipitating event, show very similar characteristics. Neither the difficulty in intubation nor the length of time for which the patient is intubated show reliable parallels with the incidence of granuloma formation and maintenance. It has been shown that the incidence of damage post routine intubation for general anaesthetic is much higher than generally supposed, and yet the vast majority of damage heals (Harris et al., 1990). There is no clear consensus about treatment. Some authors still attempt surgical removal prior to medical treatment and speech therapy, others feel sure that conservative treatment is preferable and in no way delays healing. We are of the latter school and reserve surgery for partial reduction of the lesion only when the airway is compromised.

Post-injection granulomas

Prior to the popularization of the Isshiki type I thyroplasty, the most common surgical procedure for medialization of a paralysed vocal fold was injection of a supposedly inert substance such as Teflon paste. It was quick, easy to perform and, if done correctly, capable of producing excellent results. Unfortunately, all substances injected into the vocal folds seem capable of producing a chronic irritative response, and although Teflon is better than many, it too can produce granulation that will not simply 'go away', even if injected in appropriate amounts into the correct site.

Histologically, the Teflon excites a foreign-body granulomatous response, which may be delayed by months or even years before becoming apparent. Treatment is extremely unreliable and difficult. Surgical removal may be attempted, but this usually only results in debulking of the lesion with variable degrees of damage to the remaining vocal fold. It is simply not possible to remove Teflon paste and granuloma in its entirety without performing what amounts to a subtotal cordectomy.

Damage to the cricoarytenoid joints

The cricoarytenoid joint, being a structure containing a synovium, is heir to all the problems that damage joints. It is, in addition, not infrequently traumatized when subjected to forceful manipulation in directions in which it was not intended to move, for instance during endotracheal intubation at induction of general anaesthesia or emergency restoration of an airway.

Vocal fold immobility is frequently mistaken for fold paresis, and the most reliable means of differentiating the two is by electromyography .

Many inflammatory processes may damage synovial joints. In addition to rheumatoid arthritis, one should bear in mind other causes such as gout, psoriasis, tuberculosis, syphilis, lupus erythematosus, etc. Although the joint may not be entirely immobile, it is usually tender and the pain may be referred to the ipsilateral thyrohyoid membrane.

Current treatment is restricted to preservation of the airway while maintaining as much voice as possible. Effectively this means considering fold lateralizing procedures such as arytenoidopexy or arytenoidectomy, both of which will cause some deterioration in voice quality. The alternative, which permits preservation of voice, is to perform a permanent tracheostomy. This latter procedure can always be converted to one of the former if the patient wishes, but not the other way round. Although patients may be initially resistant to a permanent tracheostomy for aesthetic reasons, it remains the author's alternative of choice.

Papillomatosis

This usually presents as clinically obvious multiple red friable exophytic squamous papillomata, especially around the glottis. Observers may, however, find the appearance, especially in adults, resembles fairly gross chronic laryngitis and may not, therefore, think to check with histological evidence. They are most common in children and often disappear before the age of 11. Papillomatosis in adults carries a small risk of malignant change (Siegel et al., 1979). It is associated with human papilloma virus, especially types 6, 11, 16 and 18 (Corbitt et al., 1988; Quiney et al., 1989). The histology shows papillary fronds of well differentiated squamous cells, a thin non-keratinizing epithelium and a core of fibrovascular tissue. The more cellular atypia is present, the faster the lesions tend to recur.

Treatment is symptomatic and surgical. This is one of the few occasions in microsurgery of the larynx when the laser comes into its own. The lesions may be ablated using the laser with the single caveat that when the lesions eventually regress, the only remaining scarring in the larynx will be that due to surgical attempts to ablate the lesions. Papilloma itself leaves very little residual damage. Therefore the aim of surgery is merely to preserve the airway and permit adequate voicing – the least done, the better the eventual result.

Other laryngeal manifestations of systemic disease

Many other systemic diseases have laryngeal manifestations. They are much rarer than the lesions already outlined, but nevertheless they occur and to miss the diagnosis may have dire consequences.

The examiner should be mindful of:

1. Tuberculosis. TB can mimic a number of other laryngeal problems. Tubercles are granulomata with central caseation and surrounding zone of lymphocytes.
2. Sarcoidosis is similar to TB but on histology there is no caseation and staining for tubercle bacilli is negative.
3. Wegener's granulomatosis. Beware the subglottic stenosis with angry red granulations. Histology shows necrotizing granulation tissue with associated small vessel vasculitis.
4. Lethal midline granuloma and related histiocytic lymphomas.

If the larynx is exquisitely tender to palpation, it may even be worth considering extreme rarities such as carcinoid and glomus tumours. A fuller description may be found in Gould, Rubin and Yanagisawa (1995).

References

Bouchayer M, Cornut G (1991) Instrumental microscopy of benign lesions of the vocal folds. In CN Ford, DM Bless (Eds) Phonosurgery: assessment and surgical management of voice disorders. New York: Raven, pp 143–165.

Corbitt G, Zarod AP, Arrand JR et al. (1988) Human papillomavirus (HPV) genotypes associated with laryngeal papilloma. Journal of Clinical Pathology 41: 284–288.

Cornut G, Bouchayer M, Rugheimer G (1994) Phonosurgery for benign vocal fold lesions. Interactive video and book. London: The Three Ears Co.

Gould WJ, Rubin JS, Yanagisawa E (1995) Benign vocal fold pathology through the eyes of the laryngologist. In Rubin JS, Sataloff RT, Korovin GS, Gould WJ (Eds) Diagnosis and treatment of voice disorders. New York: Igaku-Shoin.

Harris TM, Johnston DF, Collins SRC, Heath ML (1990) General anaesthetic technique for use in singers: the brain laryngeal mask airway versus endotracheal intubation. Journal of Voice 4: 81–85.

Jones NS, Lannigan FJ, McCullagh M, Angiansah A, Owen W, Harris TM (1990) Acid reflux and hoarseness. Journal of Voice 4: 355–358.

Kiese-Himmel C, Kruse E (1994) Das laryngeale Kontaktgranulom – ein psychosomatisches Störungsbild? Folia Phoniatrica et Logopaedica 46: 288–297.

Lindestad P-Å, Hertegård S (1994) Spindle-shaped glottal insufficiency with and without sulcus vocalis – a retrospective study. Annals of Otology, Rhinology and Laryngology 103: 547–553.

Ohman L, Tibbling L, Olofsson J, Ericsson G (1983) Oesophageal dysfunction in patients with contact ulcer of the larynx. Annals of Otology, Rhinology and Laryngology 92: 228–230.

Quiney RE, Wells M, Lewis FA et al. (1989) Laryngeal papillomatosis: correlation between severity of disease and presence of HPV 6 and 11 detected by in situ DNA hybridisation. Journal of Clinical Pathology 42: 694–698.

Siegel SE, Cohen SR, Isaacs Jnr H et al. (1979) Malignant transformation of tracheobronchial juvenile papillomatosis without prior radiotherapy. Annals of Otology, Rhinology and Laryngology 88: 192–197.

Wilson JA, White N, Van Haake N et al. (1989) Gastro-oesophageal reflux and posterior laryngitis. Annals of Otology, Rhinology and Laryngology 98: 405–410.

CHAPTER 4

Mechanisms of Respiration (The Bellows)

JOHN S RUBIN

Introduction

The mechanisms of respiration act in a manner similar to bellows for a fire: they ultimately supply a steady volume of air under pressure to the vocal folds. They consist of: the lungs and pleurae, rib cage, the diaphragm and intercostal musculature, the thoracic and back musculature, and the abdominal musculature.

The most important functions of the respiratory tract are to enable oxygen to be absorbed from the atmosphere and waste carbon dioxide gas to be expelled. The air is presented to an enormous surface area of tissue, which permits the gases to exchange freely. The lungs are the spongy structures that allow this to take place. Just as a bath sponge must be squeezed to expel the water contained within it before another load can be mopped up on re-expansion of the sponge, so too the lungs must be regularly squeezed and expanded in order to exchange 'old' air for 'new'.

This is achieved by putting the lungs in a more or less rigid 'cylinder' (the rib cage), and reducing the volume within by pushing a 'piston' (the abdominal contents covered by the diaphragm). Because there is a hole at the top of the cylinder (the trachea), the reducing volume inside causes air to be blown out. The converse arrangement also is true: if the piston is withdrawn from the cylinder, then there will be a reduction of air pressure inside, and air will be sucked in through the hole to cancel out the pressure difference between the inside and outside of the cylinder. In air-breathing mammals this is achieved by tightening the domed diaphragmatic muscle that seals the chest at the bottom. Tightening this muscle flattens out the dome, thus pushing the abdominal contents out of the lower chest.

In life, however, things tend to be complex. The lungs expand and contract in association with movements of the rib cage and pleurae. The diaphragm and intercostal musculature are of particular importance as primary muscles for

49

inspiration and expiration; the thoracic and back musculature lift and stabilize the rib cage; and the abdominal musculature controls the descent of the diaphragm allowing downwards movement of the thoracic cavity and the ascent of the diaphragm with expiration.

Any problem therein, for example diastasis recti due to multiple pregnancies, an umbilical or inguinal hernia, or even muscle spasm of the shoulder girdle or paraspinous muscles, reduces the efficiency of the system and may cause problems.

Breathing seems like a simple process. Quiet respiration is generally under subconscious reflex control, predominantly driven by elastic forces and the level of CO_2. Yet during singing performance, one becomes extremely conscious of the need for efficient breath control. There seem to be almost as many techniques for breathing espoused by voice teachers as there are performers.

The phases of respiration – inspiration and expiration – occur due to the alternate increase and decrease in the size of the thoracic cavity. Quiet respiration requires little physical energy and is a reflex.

The mechanism

1. Message from brain to diaphragm to contract and thus enlarge the thorax.
2. Enlarged chest pulls on lungs causing a relative drop in lung pressure versus atmospheric pressure.
3. Air then automatically flows into the chest to counteract this partial vacuum. As lung volume increases during inspiration, alveolar pressure drops by about 1 cm H_2O and flow of air into the lungs increases to about 0.5 litres per second (Dickson and Maue-Dickson, 1982).
4. Blood is also sucked into the thoracic veins, the capillaries dilate to facilitate pulmonary circulation and any fluid in the neighbouring region is encouraged into the thorax (Boileau Grant and Basmajian, 1965).
5. At the end of inhalation, alveolar pressure returns to the same value as atmospheric pressure and flow stops.
6. During expiration the diaphragm relaxes, and the lungs and chest wall recoil.
7. During inspiration the ribs undergo rotation at the costovertebral joints, a twisting of the costal cartilages and widening of the costochondral angles. It is from this twisting and widening that the cartilages recoil at expiration (Boileau Grant and Basmajian, 1965).

The average quiet respiration airflow is 500 ml, 12–18 times per minute. Quiet respiration primarily involves nasal breathing, during which the cricothyroid muscles are relaxed, the posterior cricoarytenoid (and possibly the lateral cricoarytenoid) muscles are contracted and the vocal folds are abducted.

Gross alterations in breathing occur with speaking. During speech most airflow passes through the mouth not the nose. Inspirations are brief and rapid. Expirations are more prolonged. Airway pressures are more negative in inspiration and more positive in expiration. Much of breathing while speaking is still unconscious (Bunch, 1995). In singing, variances from ordinary breathing are even more marked, expiration is more prolonged and under more volitional control. It is possible with enough practice, however, for good breathing habits during singing to become reflex.

Lungs and pleurae

The lungs consist of a series of small air sacs, the alveoli, which are connected to the upper respiratory tract via a series of tubes, the bronchioles, which are in turn surrounded by smooth muscle. This tissue is richly perfused by the arteriovenous system. The lungs are supplied by branches of the vagus nerves and the thoracic sympathetic ganglia. Afferent vagal fibres constitute the afferent limb of the respiratory reflex arc and arrest further inspiration. Efferent vagal fibres are bronchoconstrictor and secretomotor. Efferent sympathetic fibres are bronchodilatory in nature (Boileau Grant and Basmajian, 1965).

The lungs lie within membranous sacs, which are located in the thorax and are surrounded by a bony rib cage. The right lung is slightly larger than the left due to the position of the heart (Dickson and Maue-Dickson, 1982). Enveloping the lungs is the visceral component of a serous membrane, the pleura surrounded by a parietal membrane. Intercostal nerves are sensory to the costal pleura and a broad marginal strip of diaphragmatic pleura. The visceral pleura is insensitive to mechanical stimulation having an autonomic nerve supply. The parietal pleura has a somatic nerve supply by adjacent intercostal nerves shared with the abdominal wall and diaphragm. This is of clinical importance as pleural irritation can present as abdominal pain (Boileau Grant and Basmajian, 1965, Ger et al., 1996). The pleural cavity is a fluid-filled potential space that binds the lungs to the rib cage and diaphragm such that any movements therein cause corresponding increases or decreases in lung volume.

The rest position at the end of quiet breathing is dependent on factors such as position of the diaphragm, thoracic cage, etc, and it also depends on the linkages binding them. The most critical is the pleural cavity linkage. Maue-Dickson contends that this linkage is not only a function of surface tension of the fluid within the pleural space, but also a function of the inherent elasticity of the pleura itself (Dickson and Maue-Dickson, 1982).

Inspiration

During inspiration the lungs expand by enlargement of the rib cage and thus the thorax. This may be accomplished by the prime movers of respiration, namely, the diaphragm and the intercostals, or by the accessory muscles and to some degree by the stabilizing muscles for the rib cage and by postural muscles. It is abnormal to use the accessory or stabilizers in this fashion, however, and it is always bad for singing.

The rib cage

There are 12 pairs of ribs. At birth the ribs are horizontal and are in the position of full inspiration; movement upwards or downwards is thereby an expiratory act. At this age respiration is caused by the upwards/downwards action of the diaphragm and is said to be abdominal in type. By the end of the second year the ribs are oblique, and by the seventh year respiration is considered to be largely thoracic in type (Boileau Grant and Basmajian, 1965).

Each rib articulates posteriorly with the vertebrum after which it is numbered and to a slight degree the vertebrum above it.. The costocentral articulations therein form plane synovial joints with the articular capsules, radiate ligaments and intra-articular ligaments. The costotransverse articulations are plane synovial joints with a broad superior ligament and a relatively weak posterior ligament. The ligament of the tubercle is short and weak. These ligaments prevent proximal–distal sliding but allow for superior–inferior sliding (Dickson and Maue-Dickson, 1982; Ger, Abrahams and Olson, 1996).

Anteriorly, the 1st rib is effectively fused to the manubrium sterni. The 2nd–7th ribs have a moveable synovial joint between their costal cartilages and the sternum; the 8th–10th ribs are connected with the cartilages immediately above them and thus to the 7th rib. The cartilaginous ends of the 11th and 12th ribs are free and thus form a subgroup of 'floating' or vertebral ribs. Each joint is surrounded by an articular capsule that is strongest superiorly and inferiorly. Radiate ligaments extend from anterior and posterior surfaces of the cartilages to broad attachments on adjacent anterior and posterior surfaces of the sternum.

The 1st rib is the shortest and most curved rib, the length increasing thereafter through the 7th rib and then decreasing through the 12th rib.

Their orientation gives the range through which the ribs can move. Moving from the 1st to the 7th rib, the most lateral part of each rib is located increasingly lower in relation to vertebral or sternal ends. Thus the anterior ends of the ribs and sternum move on inspiration obliquely from inferoposterior to superoanterior, increasing the antero–posterior ('A–P') diameter of the chest. This is particularly

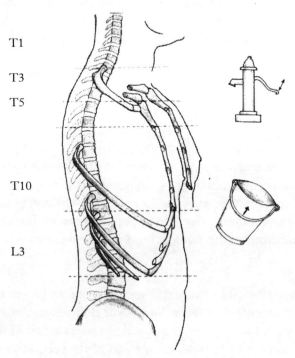

T1

T3

T5

T10

L3

Figure 4.1 Right lateral view of the spine and ribs showing the 'pump-handle' movement of the upper ribs. The movement of the lower ribs is described as 'bucket-handle'

so for the 1st–5th ribs and is referred to as a 'pump-handle' motion (Bunch, 1995; Dickson and Maue-Dickson, 1982).

Professional singers do not use this action very much as, with correct posture, the rib cage is already partially elevated. In fact, excessive movement of these ribs during inspiration is associated with accessory muscle contraction and is frowned upon by singing teachers universally (Bunch, 1995). For example, on deep inspiration the scalene muscles can raise the first and second costal arches; the sternal heads of the sternocleidomastoid can raise the manubrium etc. (Boileau Grant and Basmajian, 1965).

The 5th–7th ribs (and 8th–10th ribs), on inspiration, cause the chest wall to move in a lateral and somewhat A–P fashion. This is particularly associated with the movements of the lateral portions of the ribs and has been described as movement in a 'bucket-handle' fashion (Bunch, 1995; Dickson and Maue-Dickson, 1982). The 7th–10th ribs have flat articular facets that lie in an oblique plane allowing for sliding of the neck of the rib superoposteriorly or anteroinferiorly. The 8th–10th ribs in particular have wide excursion as they are not directly attached to the sternum. These motions are of particular importance to singers.

The muscles forming the walls and floor of the thorax play the primary role in inspiration; those attached to the rib cage a secondary role. By far the most important muscle for inspiration is the diaphragm.

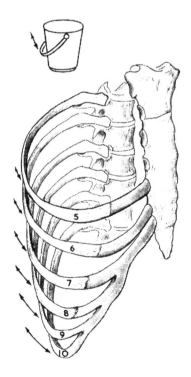

Figure 4.2 Right antero-lateral view of the lower ribs to illustrate the 'bucket-handle' motion of the ribs (after Bunch)

The diaphragm

The diaphragm is a large double-domed sheet of muscle that has a rounded cupola on each side below the lungs and a depressed median portion onto which the heart lies (Boileau Grant and Basmajian, 1965). When relaxed the right side is slightly higher than the left, the right lying at the level of the 5th rib and the left at the level of the fifth interspace. It attaches to the back of the xiphoid process, the inner surfaces of the 7th through 12th costal cartilages and to the vertebral column. The vertebral attachment on the right is to the bodies of the upper three lumbar vertebrae and is more powerful than that of the left, which is to the bodies of the upper two. The posteromedial portion is steadied by the quadratus lumborum. The central part of the diaphragm is called the central tendon, and has the shape of a trefoil. It is pierced by the inferior vena cava at the level of T8. The oesophagus pierces the decussating fibres of the right crus at T10. The aorta does not pierce the diaphragm but passes behind the median arcuate ligament at T12.

The diaphragm is supplied by the phrenic nerve (C3, 4, 5) for motor and sensory innervation. It also receives sensory innervation from lower intercostal nerves.

The diaphragm is always actively engaged in the act of inspiration, and is responsible for at least 60–80% of increased volume in deep inspiration (Bunch, 1995). When on inspiration it contracts, its fibres shorten and straighten, enlarge the costodiaphragmatic recesses and cause the domes to descend. It thereby flattens and comes forward, causing the upper abdominal viscera to descend before it, and the muscles of the abdominal wall to yield sufficiently for acceptance of the abdominal organs. This increases the length and capacity of the thoracic cavity, pushes the abdominal muscles downwards and forwards, creates a bulge in the upper abdomen (epigastrium) and allows air to rush into the lungs.

Because the muscular fibres of the diaphragm are vertical, diaphragmatic contraction could also result in the elevation of the inferior margin of the rib cage (Dickson and Maue-Dickson, 1982).

Intercostal muscles

There are three layers of intercostal muscles: external, internal and (incomplete) innermost, lying between the ribs. Their function is to maintain the stability of the chest wall, to prevent it being sucked in during inspiration.

The external intercostals

These extend from the inferior margin of one rib to insert onto the superior margin of the next. The orientation is oblique. They are found between all of the ribs and extend from the vertebral column posteriorly to the costochondral junction anteriorly. Because of their orientation they work most efficiently on the lower ribs and have greatest functional capacity to raise the lower rib. Thus the function has been considered to be rib elevation (Dickson and Maue-Dickson, 1982), although this is still controversial (Bunch, 1995). During quiet inspiration they have been said to cause the 2nd through 7th costal arches to rotate at the costovertebral and costosternal joints, causing the transverse diameter of the chest to

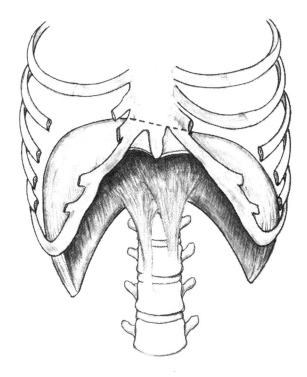

Figure 4.3 Anterior view of the diaphragm with the lower costal cartilages partially removed (after Maue-Dickson)

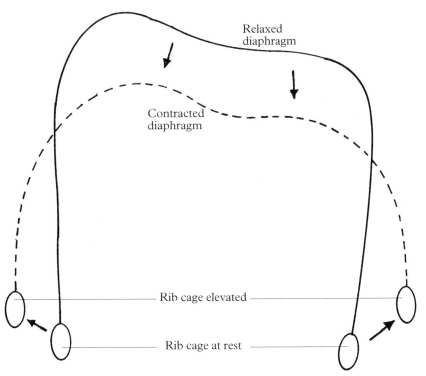

Figure 4.4 Antero-posterior view of diaphragmatic activity

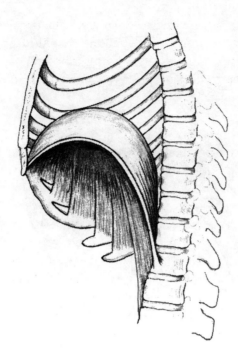

Figure 4.5 Sagittal section showing the right hemidiaphragm from the left (after Dickson and Maue-Dickson)

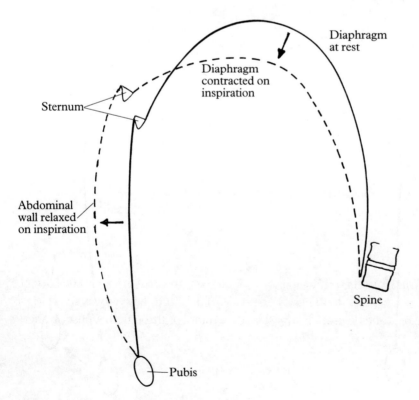

Figure 4.6 Left lateral view of diaphragmatic activity

increase and the infrasternal angle to widen. They also help to make the sternal end of the arches rise, causing the body of the sternum to be thrust forward and the A–P diameter of the chest to increase (Boileau Grant and Basmajian, 1965). Taylor (1960) has demonstrated that the external intercostals in man are electrically active during inspiration.

The internal intercostals

These lie deep to the external intercostals and extend from the rib angles posterior to the sternum anteriorly, and occupy the interchondral spaces. Their obliquity is opposite to the external intercostals. The upper attachment is more distant from the fulcrum than the lower and thus function is reversed and they are believed to lower the ribs (Dickson and Maue-Dickson, 1982) and therefore have an important role in exhalation. This will be further discussed in the section on expiration.

Campbell et al. (1970) have concluded that during phonation at high lung volumes there is contraction of the external intercostals, and during phonation at low volumes, there is contraction of the internal intercostals.

In general, the intercostal muscles are more active during phonation/singing, wherein they help maintain the subglottic pressure.

Accessory muscles

There are numerous muscles that have been implicated in inspiration as accessory respiratory muscles. These will only be listed briefly.

Sternocleidomastoid

Due to its insertion posterosuperiorly on the superior nuchal line and the mastoid process, and its origin from the medial clavicle and sternum, the sternocleidomastoid muscle could act as an accessory muscle if the head were stabilized. However, the efficiency would be poor as the direction of pull differs by 45 degrees from that of the anterior rib cage (Dickson and Maue-Dickson, 1982).

Scalenes

The direction of pull of the scalenes is almost vertical, given the course from the transverse process of the cervical vertebrae to the 1st and 2nd rib. They will elevate the rib cage but have no role in singing.

Pectoralis minor

This is a small muscle, but its axis is vertical from the 3rd–5th rib to the coracoid process. The scapula would need to be stabilized for it to have any effect, however. This could be done by grabbing hold of something, or through the muscular action of the trapezius, levator scapulae or rhomboids (Boileau Grant and Basmajian, 1965).

Serratus anterior

This muscle could potentially have a role in deep inspiration as it arises from the upper 8th–9th ribs and inserts onto the scapula, but the vector of force is lateral, and thus it would be very inefficient.

Serratus posterior inferior and quadratus lumborum

These muscles are more likely to stabilize the lower ribs than to have a direct role in inspiration, although the latter muscle, due to its relationship with the diaphragm, may have a synergistic role in 'diaphragmatic breathing' (Dickson and Maue-Dickson, 1982).

Serratus posterior superior

This muscle arises from the nuchal ligament and spinous processes of C7, T2–3, and inserts on the upper border of the 2nd–5th ribs beyond their angles. It may help to elevate the ribs in modest respiratory effort.

Levatores costarum

These arise from the transverse processes of C7 and the upper 11 thoracic verte-brae, and extend down to insert on the subjacent rib or the next lower rib. As they attach near to the fulcrum of rib motion, a small amount of pull could have signifi-cant effects. There is a possibility of elevation on inspiration (Boileau Grant and Basmajian, 1965), but Dickson feels that the muscle is working at too great a mechanical disadvantage (Dickson and Maue-Dickson, 1982).

Expiration

When the chest is fully inflated there is a natural tendency for the lungs and associ-ated chest wall structures to collapse, loosing air. This is referred to as elastic recoil. As air is expelled, the recoil diminishes until a 'neutral zone' is reached. The tidal volume of quiet breathing is found between this area of elastic neutrality and the higher volume zone of positive elastic recoil. If, however, air continues to be expelled from the lungs beyond this neutral volume, then once again elastic recoil becomes significant, only now it has become a negative force, tending to expand the chest.

During quiet respiration and speaking, the act of expiration is predominantly passive and is brought about by the elastic recoil of the lungs, transversus abdominis and the costal cartilages. As noted above, recoil of the cartilages occurs in part as a release from the twisting of the cartilages and widening of the costochondral angles that occurred with inspiration (Boileau Grant and Basmajian, 1965).

Whereas there are multiple muscle groups that can, under varying circum-stances, be brought into play for direct or accessory assistance in inspiration, there are somewhat fewer muscle groups available for expiration. There are similarities with the adduction versus abduction activity of the vocal folds; a greater number of muscle groups act to achieve the former. The qualitative and quantitative control of valving is a much more complex activity than opening the folds for inhalation.

None the less, for controlled expiration during phonation and for increasing the

intensity or duration of sound, activities that are critical in singing, more expiratory muscular activity is necessary than that obtained via recoil. This has been
recognized for over 30 years (Agostini and Mead, 1964).

Dickson and Maue-Dickson (1982) note that exhalatory muscles are required
in instances when exhalation continues below 35% vital capacity, which they
consider to be resting respiratory level, or when more alveolar pressure is required
than is provided by relaxation pressure for any respiratory level.

Clearly, the process of active expiration requires activation of muscle groups
that are either antagonists of the diaphragm or direct depressors of the rib cage.
The abdominal muscles, in particular the external and internal obliques and the
transversus abdominis, are the key muscle groups for the former activity. Together
all three act in harmony to raise intra-abdominal pressure as in lifting, breath-hold-
ing and singing, thereby pushing the abdominal contents against the diaphragm
and aiding in upwards movement of the diaphragm. It is these muscles, working
against a relaxing diaphragm, which, together with the internal intercostal muscles,
assist in maintenance of subglottic pressure.

Muscles that have been postulated to be most likely to be involved in
active/forced exhalation include the following: internal intercostals, external
abdominal oblique, rectus abdominis, transversus thoracis, transversus abdominis,
internal abdominal oblique, subcostals, sacrospinals, iliocostalis lumborum and
serratus posterior inferior. Of these, the first has been noted to have electrical
activity in conversational speech, the first four in effortful expiration, and the fifth,
sixth and seventh are likely to play some role in effortful expiration (Boileau Grant
and Basmajian, 1965; Dickson and Maue-Dickson, 1982; Bunch, 1995).

The internal intercostals have already been described anatomically.

The abdominal muscles

The contents of the abdomen are contained in a roughly cylindrical muscular bag
bounded superiorly by the diaphragm, inferiorly by the muscles of the pelvic floor
and on the sides by the abdominal muscles. The volume within this 'bag' remains
fairly constant and so tightening the diaphragmatic muscle while simultaneously
loosening the abdominal muscles will effectively shorten and widen the bag, allowing the dome of the diaphragm to flatten and descend. Conversely, tightening the
abdominal muscles and loosening the diaphragm will produce a longer thinner
sausage shape. Because the pelvic support cannot significantly alter position, this
elongation results in the abdominal contents under the diaphragm being pushed
up into the lower part of the chest thereby increasing intrathoracic pressure and/or
expelling air from the lungs.

The external abdominal oblique

This arises from the lower eight ribs and runs obliquely downwards, forwards and
medially to insert into the rectus sheath, linea alba, outer edge of the iliac crest (hip
bone) and inguinal ligament (groin). It acts like a very wide supporting sling for
the abdominal contents. (The rectus sheath is a strong fibrous sheet that spreads

from the rib cage to the pubis, covering front of the abdomen. It is split into layers medially to enclose the rectus abdominis muscle. Laterally it provides part of the attachment for the oblique and transverse musculature so their activity is roughly circumferential around the abdominal contents.)

The internal abdominal oblique

This arises from the intermediate strip of the iliac crest, inguinal ligament and posterior aponeurosis of the transversus/lumbar fascia and inserts on the cartilages of the lower four ribs, the anterior and posterior walls of the rectus abdominis sheath, linea alba and falx inguinalis. Its fibres mostly run upwards and medially, and together with its rectus sheath attachment and opposite internal oblique, form another broad, flat sling that contains the abdominal contents, especially on firm expiration.

The transversus abdominis

This originates from the iliac crest and inguinal ligament, inner surface of the lower six costal cartilages where they interdigitate with the diaphragm and the transverse processes of the lumbar vertebrae (Cutler, 1972). These fibres are generally oriented transversely to insert onto the linea alba, rather like a cummerbund.

These three muscles are important in maintenance of the intra-abdominal pressure. By contracting alternately with the diaphragm they help with expiration and are necessary for the abdominal form of respiration. By contracting simultaneously with the diaphragm they aid in micturition, defaecation, etc. They contract actively during sneezing and coughing (Boileau Grant and Basmajian, 1965).

The rectus abdominis

This muscle originates at the crest and symphysis of the pubis and, running vertically upwards, it fans out to insert into the xiphoid process and 5th, 6th and 7th costal cartilages. Its action is to diminish the capacity of the abdomen and to draw the rib cage down towards the pubis, stabilizing the anterior abdominal wall.

The transversus thoracis

This originates at the xiphoid cartilage and lower portion of the sternum and inserts on the costal cartilages of the 2nd–6th ribs. Its action is to narrow the chest (Cutler, 1972).

The subcostals (intercostales intimi)

These are thin slips of muscle that originate from the deep surface of several ribs near the vertebral column and insert into the deep surface of the 2nd or 3rd rib near the rib angles. They parallel the internal intercostals and may act like the interosseus parts of the internal intercostals thus lowering the ribs to which they attach (Dickson and Maue-Dickson, 1982).

The sacrospinals

These are powerful muscles that attach in part to the rib cage and act as a lever

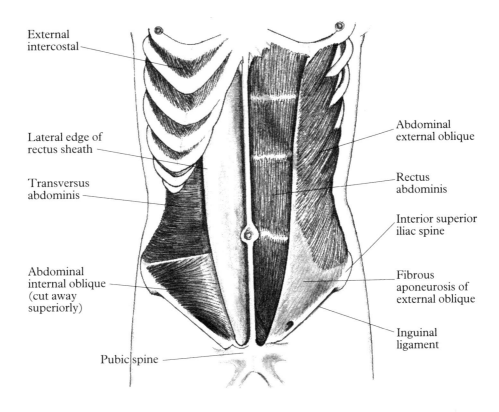

Figure 4.7 Muscles of the abdominal wall (after Hamilton and Simon, 1952)

with the vertebral column. The lumbar portion forms a lever with the lower ribs and could potentially depress them with some possibility of assistance in exhalation (Dickson and Maue-Dickson, 1982).

Subglottic pressure

Generation of subglottic pressure is the most important concept in the bellows analogy. This pressure is created by the flow of expired air against the partially closed vocal folds. It is very important in controlling airflow and in achieving a constant intensity of sound. There are mechanoreceptors in the subglottis that are extremely sensitive to changes in air pressure. They exert reflex effects on the activity of the laryngeal intrinsic muscles and are particularly important as air pressure rises during expiration.

Phonation requires close coordination between two mechanical processes:

1. Movement of the chest wall and diaphragm. This determines air flow and subglottic pressure.
2. Movement of the vocal folds and the mucosal walls of the pharynx and mouth. This determines pitch, loudness and quality of sound.

Sustaining a tone at constant air pressure and intensity and varying the pitch for the duration of the musical phrase is clearly fundamental to singing. The singer's ability to sustain steady subglottic pressure and to vary it at will results from accurate voluntary control of many muscle groups, in particular the intercostal effects at high lung volumes and the abdominal muscles working across a gradually relaxing diaphragm (Bunch, 1995). Quiet respiration is reported to use between 35 and 45% of vital capacity and normal conversational speech uses, in general, between 35 and 60% of vital capacity; very loud speech can require up to 80% of vital capacity (Hixon, 1973).

According to Proctor (1980), subglottic pressure in singing varies from 2 to 60 cm of H_2O. A moderate tone generates about 10 cm of H_2O and a very loud crescendo generates 50–60 cm H_2O. To generate these types of pressures, a coordinated effort of balancing forces between the inspiratory activities and the expiratory activities is required.

These forces and the subsequent air column developed and perpetuated is then used to activate the movements of the 'flutter-box', and to create a series of vibrations, which, when passed through the acoustic filter of the supraglottic airway, become recognizable voice sounds. The anatomical details therein are the subject of the next chapter.

Structural and pathological problems affecting breathing

Any abnormality that through either rigidity or pain reduces the ability of the chest cage to adjust its volume during respiration will be accompanied by reduced ability of the patient to produce effective and flexible breath support. Similarly, pathological processes that reduce the compliance of the lungs (make them stiffer) or that reduce the vital capacity of the lungs will also produce poor voicing.

In addition to upper airway obstruction and neurological difficulties that reduce the body's ability to squeeze and expand the lungs, there are frequently more mundane structural components to consider:

Postural problems

Examples of postural problems include scoliosis of the spine; an elevated rib cage seemingly 'stuck' in the inhalation phase of respiration; round shoulders from excessively heavy breasts; and painful 'facet locking' of the articulatory surfaces of the ribs and/or vertebrae.

Chest wall problems

Examples of chest wall problems include anatomical variants of chest cage configuration (pigeon chest/pes excavatum); rib cage injuries; contracted diaphragm; paradoxical diaphragmatic breathing; and guarding/breath holding. .

Pathological processes affecting the tissue of the lungs will also affect the way in which the lungs can be used to provide air under pressure for phonation. These diseases may affect elastic recoil (compliance of the tissue) and/or vital capacity and/or the rate at which the lungs can be inflated and deflated. A few common examples include asthma, chronic bronchitis, emphysema, fibrosing alveolitis and lung cancer.

Where there is appropriate clinical management that can improve lung function, this must be attempted where possible before any therapy for the voice is undertaken. Without the possibility of a reasonable tidal volume and adequate subglottic pressure, the results of any treatment for laryngeal dysfunction are always going to be disappointing.

References

Agostini E, Mead J (1964) Status of the respiratory system. In Fenn WO, Rahn H (Eds) Handbook of physiology, vol. 1. Washington DC: American Physiological Society.

Boileau Grant JC, Basmajian JV (1965) Grant's method of anatomy, 7th edn.Baltimore: Williams and Wilkins Co.

Bunch MA (1995) Dynamics of the singing voice, 3rd edn. Wien: Springer-Verlag.

Campbell EJM, Agostini E, Newsom Davis J (1970) The respiratory muscles: mechanics and neural control, 2nd edn. London: Lloyd-Luke.

Cutler AG (Ed) (1972) Stedman's medical dictionary, 22nd edn. Baltimore: Williams and Wilkins Co.

Dickson DR, Maue-Dickson W (1982) Anatomical and physiological bases of speech. Boston: Little, Brown and Co.

Ger R, Abrahams P, Olson TR (1996) Essentials of Clinical Anatomy 2nd Edition. New York: The Parthenon Publishing Group.

Hamilton WJ, Simon G (1958) Surface and Radiological Anatomy for Students and General Practitioners. 4th Edition. Cambridge: W. Heffer and Sons Ltd.

Hixon TJ (1973) Respiratory function in speech. In Minifie FD, Hixon TJ, Williams F (Eds) Normal aspects of speech, hearing and language. Englewood Cliffs: Prentice-Hall.

Proctor DF (1980) Breathing, speech and song. Wien: Springer Verlag.

Taylor A (1960) The contribution of the intercostal muscles to the effort of respiration in man. Journal of Physiology 200: 25–50.

CHAPTER 5

Laryngeal Mechanisms in Normal Function and Dysfunction

TOM HARRIS

Only connect!

EM Forster

Life is not so much a bowl of cherries, it is more a collection of carefully positioned sphincters. Mastery of the proper and sequential functioning of these sphincters makes life as we know it, possible.

Probably the most useful initial question a practitioner can ask is 'What were the functions for which the larynx evolved?' Complex phonatory abilities came late in the list of evolutionary imperatives and would not have been part of any initial hypothetical list of requirements. Initially, the larynx was required to provide protection for the airway, which shares an initial common pathway with the alimentary tract (gullet). It is an effective sphincteric seal of the airway, enabling the functions of swallowing and breathing to take place safely in a consecutive manner, with food and drink being passed reliably down one track (the oesophagus), while only air is permitted down the other (the trachea). Should the slightest error occur and particles of anything other than air find their way into the upper airway, then the evolutionary requirement becomes the ability to expel the potential hazard extremely rapidly by coughing before damage can take place.

In essence then, the larynx is a very sophisticated valve consisting of two main (true) folds and two accessory (false) folds of fibrous and muscular tissue that are capable of very swift opening and closure. The true vocal folds are tightly apposed by two sphincters of muscles, one for each fold, which operate via a lever system, the cricoarytenoid joint. The false folds are apposed by direct sphincteric activity of a separate group of muscles (vide infra).

While the intrinsic muscles of the larynx are charged with airway protection, the extrinsic suspensory muscles of the larynx together with those of the tongue and the sphincteric muscles of the mouth and pharynx are all originally evolved for swallowing and related activities. The additional function of the intrinsic laryngeal muscles is the production and control of a sound source. The extrinsic laryngeal muscles, oropharyngeal and tongue musculature all play a part in adjusting the resonance characteristics of the tube, now described as the vocal tract. These modifications of swallowing and airway sealing systems came much more recently in evolutionary terms. The same could be said for the ability to create efficient resonating cavities within the supraglottic vocal tract. The evolutionary imperative was the development of a swallowing mechanism; the extension of the application of this function is the ability to 'hold' one part of the swallowing gesture for a short period in order to make a suitably resonant cavity for the production of a particular sound.

The larynx and vocal tract form an astonishingly versatile system for the generation of sound. One can make a musical instrument capable of producing variable pitch by arranging that the structure of the sound source or oscillator can be altered. For instance, the pitch periodicity of a violin string may be altered simply by changing the length of the vibrator or the tension of the string from end to end. The range of frequencies possible for a particular sound source is governed by its physical attributes such as its thickness (the mass), elasticity, plasticity and shape of the vibrator. It also depends on whether or not the vibrator is homogeneous in construction or is a composite of layers of materials each with different properties.

The sound waves generated by the oscillator are not simple sine waves, but may be considered as composites made up from many smaller waves or partials of different frequencies, any of which may be suppressed or amplified. Suppression or damping of any particular partial occurs in conditions when all the wave peaks and troughs, having been added together by a resonating cavity, tend to cancel each other out. Resonance occurs at any frequency when all the wave peaks and troughs summate to produce waves of the same frequency but much greater amplitude. Changing the length or shape of the resonator will affect exactly which partials or harmonics of the fundamental frequency are to be enhanced or amplified and which will be suppressed. There are several ways in which musical instruments can alter the length of the resonator, e.g. a clarinet by opening/stopping holes or a slide trombone by lengthening/shortening the resonating tube. They are less versatile when it comes to changing the shape of the resonator to alter the resonance characteristics. Pushing a mute into the bell of a trumpet or a fist into the bell of a french horn alters the tonal characteristics of the output sound. Man-made acoustically active resonators tend to be built of rigid materials.

The human voice is subject to all the same physical rules as any other musical instrument, pendulum or system for producing controlled oscillation.

Anatomical considerations with regard to the isometric function of the intrinsic laryngeal muscles

Positioning of the vocal folds

Despite the rather daunting heading, we hope in this section to show you something of the startling simplicity and subtlety of the laryngeal muscles when they are used to move the vocal folds together (adduction) and apart (abduction). Although their closing of the airway may be described as sphincteric, most sphincters are quite simple; they produce a reduction in the internal diameter of a tube to zero by contraction of a ring of muscle rather like a purse-string. If air is blown through the pin-hole gap of such a sphincter, then poorly controlled sound production may take place, as everyone knows to their acute social embarrassment!

Control of sound quality and intensity improves greatly with the development of muscular folds with straight edges that are covered with a flexible mucosal surface, which can be brought into contact with one another to lightly seal the airway. By blowing air at a suitable pressure through the slit, a regular pattern of vibration is set up. As the folds are shaped largely by muscle, both the intensity and the quality of the sound produced can be accurately adjusted. The shapes of the folds within the larynx can be compared to two wedges of lemon with their narrow straight edges facing each other, connected at the front to form a 'V'. The back end of the 'V' can be drawn together so that the thin edges of the wedges are touching. This latter arrangement enormously increases the surface area for sound generation without making the depth of the constriction so great that air cannot easily be blown through it. Moreover, folds of tissue with straight edges can be pressed or drawn together in a manner that allows them to be thin and stretched, thin and lax, or thicker, shorter and more firm in texture. The potential for change in the character of the vocal folds is the feature that makes it possible for the laryngeal sound source not only to produce a wide range of pitch but also to vary the quality and intensity of the sound produced. The difficulty in understanding how the vocal folds may be made to do all these things arises because it is easier to study the structure and function of the vocal fold in isolation rather than attempt to understand the complete suspensory mechanism in one go.

Let us start by discussing general principles of how the shape, thickness and position of the laryngeal vocal folds may be adjusted, and not simply codify examples of any particular expression of normal function or hyperfunction. To illustrate this, we will take some very mundane examples from our own general experience and apply our understanding of them to the mechanisms seen in the larynx, viz.:

1. How about the guy-ropes that stabilize the pole(s) of a tent at opposite ends. Once you have hammered in the pegs, does changing the position or attitude of the pole change the **total** length of the supporting guy-ropes by much?
2. How many ways are there to fall off a horse?
3. Why, when you draw a bow-string to fire an arrow, does the arrow fly forwards when the bowstring is stretched in an up–down direction before it is drawn?

4. If you raise or lower a flag, does the total length of the halliard change with the height of the flag?
5. How can a body building beach-bum best show off his muscles?
6. What does (or rather, should) an athlete be doing 1 hour, 5 minutes and one second before a race?

General considerations concerning the laryngeal muscles

As far as the activity of any muscle in the body is concerned, the thing to remember at all times is that a muscle can only pull in the direction that is dictated by the attachment of its ends, and that it is only capable of moving those points of attachment closer together. Muscles cannot pull in any direction other than that dictated by the direction in which the muscle fibres run, nor can they push points apart.

Slackening of a muscle attached to a point does not in itself result in movement of the point unless some other muscle or other elastic structure is attached to the same point and already exerting pull in another direction.

As described earlier, the vocal folds are attached to a fixed point anteriorly (in front), the thyroid cartilage, and therefore the potential for repositioning depends on the movement of the structure to which they are attached posteriorly (at the back), the arytenoid cartilage. This makes a description of the forces involved in positioning the fold very much easier to understand, as only one 'point' (in this case the arytenoid cartilage) need be considered in the basic understanding of the mechanism.

The actual position of the arytenoid cartilage at any one time is always the product of the relative pulling forces of all the muscles attached to the arytenoid cartilage and the direction in which they are pulling. *It is meaningless to consider the action of any one muscle in isolation*, as the relative direction of pull is altered by the activity of all the other muscles that are attached to the arytenoid. Their collective activity dictates the position where the common point of attachment lies.

'All things being equal': the isometric activity of the intrinsic laryngeal muscles

Let us take a structure familiar to all of us, a tent whose apex is supported by a single pole. There are many similarities between the way in which a tent is pitched and the positioning of the arytenoid cartilage. The central pole is placed upon a 'fixed' point on the ground and the pole is then held upright on this spot by guy-ropes. The ropes are stretched in opposing directions between the 'moveable' tip of the pole (the common point of attachment of one end of every guy-rope), and the other fixed points of attachment for the ropes, the tent pegs. In order to change the position of the tip of the pole (the apex of the tent) in relation to the predetermined 'fixed' positions, i.e. the base of the pole and the tent pegs, one or more guy-ropes will require slackening, and others pulling in other directions will need to be tightened. Exactly how much tightening or slackening of each rope depends on two things: in which direction do you want to move the pole tip? and in what direction are the guy-ropes fixed by their tent peg attachments? You should observe that the more the pole tip moves, the more the direction of pull of any guy-ropes not in exact line with the movement is altered.

The sum of all the forces pulling in their different directions on the tent pole apex (or the arytenoid cartilage) must then cancel each other out exactly. If they did not, then the apex would move some more until the forces **did** balance in all directions. These opposing forces working in different directions that summate to give an overall effect are usually referred to as vectors.

As an example, if one guy-rope is pulling on the tip of the tent pole from the north and another guy-rope is pulling in exactly the opposite direction from the south, and if they are pulling with equal force, then the tent-pole tip will not move. If, however, there is a rope pulling from the north and a second pulling from, say, the west, then the tent pole tip will be pulled away from its original position in a north-westerly direction. Exactly which direction and how much (i.e. the vector), depends on the relative strength of the tugging of each rope.

The same rules apply to the intrinsic muscles of the larynx, which are attached to the arytenoid. It does not matter which muscles are shortened by contraction and which muscles are lengthened by paying out – whatever its position, if the arytenoid is not moving and is in a stable position, then the sum of all the pulls in different directions must be zero (Figure 5.2).

If a muscle is stretched out and thin, it does not automatically follow that it is exerting less pull than a muscle that is short and contracted.

The articular or joint surface on the cricoid cartilage, which forms the non-

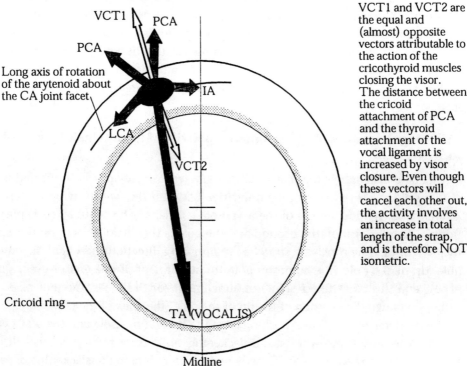

VCT1 and VCT2 are the equal and (almost) opposite vectors attributable to the action of the cricothyroid muscles closing the visor. The distance between the cricoid attachment of PCA and the thyroid attachment of the vocal ligament is increased by visor closure. Even though these vectors will cancel each other out, the activity involves an increase in total length of the strap, and is therefore NOT isometric.

Figure 5.1 Isometric muscular activity involved in positioning of the right arytenoid

moving half of the cricoarytenoid joint in the larynx, may be regarded in a similar light as the 'fixed point' on the ground where the base of the tent pole is placed. The arytenoid cartilage itself may be regarded as a sort of tent pole tip, moving about in relation to that joint surface. The muscular attachments to the arytenoid are, in a sense, like the guy-rope attachments to the apex of the tent, and the attachments of the opposite ends of the muscles may be regarded as the fixed tent pegs.

To stretch the tent analogy a little further, these rules will still apply even if you choose to park your tent on surfaces that are not flat and level. If the tent is erected on a mountain side you merely have to tilt the picture to see that nothing has changed, see Figure 1.2.

If you pitch the tent on the edge of a cliff, so that the pole is based just over the edge at the top of the cliff face while the tent pegs are driven in on the cliff face itself, to each side of the tent along the line of the cliff edge and into the ground back from the edge, then the vector of forces from all the guy-ropes that is tending to flatten the tent may be greater than when the tent was pitched on level ground, but it is met by an equal and opposite force exerted by the obligingly incompressible tent pole in exactly the same way that it did when the tent was pitched on the level. Although the site for the tent may sound unsafe, the tent pitching will be stable. Changing the position of the tip of the pole will be achieved in the same manner too.

All this is simple enough to visualize, but to complete the analogy, it must be remembered that the arytenoid is anchored over a 'cliff edge' that is not level but slopes away steeply (the articular surface is on the back/upper/outer edge or posterosuperior aspect of the cricoid lamina). Sometimes problems of misinterpretation of movements arise because generally in live patients the only angle from which the arytenoid cartilages and vocal folds can be observed is from a position directly above the larynx.

The cricoarytenoid joint

If a muscle that is attached to two bones contracts, then the bones are drawn together. If the same bones are already in contact with one another at a joint, then the only way the muscle can reduce the distance between its points of attachment is by changing the angle made by the bones at the joint in order to change their positional relationship with one another. In other words, the joint will flex, extend or rotate in response to the contraction of the muscle. The flexion of the thigh bone (femur) in relation to the shin bone (tibia) at the knee in response to contraction of the hamstrings is one such example. Both bones are vital to maintain the structure of the leg and it is therefore necessary to produce a mechanism where contraction of muscle can also **extend** the joint. Enter the concept of the 'pulley'.

Pulleys

In the anatomical context, a pulley allows a muscle and tendon to change the direction in which they pull by 'bending' their contraction force around an imaginary corner. This 'corner' is called the axis of rotation. Relative to the pull, it may be regarded as a fixed point, and because it is fixed, by definition it must produce a thrust in a direction both equal and opposite to the direction in which the muscle is pulling. The pulley forces the direction of pull of a muscle or muscles to go a longer way round, in a fixed path over the axis of rotation, and can therefore be said to be maintaining the original direction of pull for each of the attached muscles regardless of the angle of the joint.

What happens next depends on the possible movements allowed by the joint and where the contraction forces are applied in relation to the axis of the joint.

Sesamoid bones or cartilages

Sometimes a sesamoid bone or cartilage may replace muscle tendon working around a pulley arrangement. Not only is such an arrangement very strong and durable, it can also provide a common point of attachment for muscles pulling in different directions. If the sesamoid forms part of a joint 'pulley' mechanism, the final directions (vectors) of pull of all the muscles will be determined by the position and the axis of rotation of the joint. In other words it prevents the muscles from being able to pull against each other in only a single flat plane defined by their separate fixed points of attachment (viz. the tent analogy).

An example of a sesamoid forming an integral part of joint movement is the other bone that articulates at the knee joint, the patella or 'kneecap'. This bone is not essential to maintain the structure of the leg, it merely serves as a reinforcement of the pulley mechanism so that, in the case of the knee for instance, the force of contraction of the quadriceps muscle of the thigh can be turned around a corner at the knee in order to straighten the leg. Its function is to provide a strong attachment for the muscle tendon and to permit muscle to pull in one direction with the force turning the 'corner', whatever the initial degree of flexion or extension of the joint.

The arytenoid cartilage serves this function in the larynx, allowing muscles to pull around and over the superior (upper) margin of the body of the cricoid cartilage.

As described in the section on laryngeal anatomy, the cricoarytenoid joint has a saddle configuration. This limits the directions in which the arytenoid is able to move.

It is essential to understand two things about the joint: what are the movements permitted by the structure of the joint, and what are the directions in which the long (rotational) axis of the joint is lined up.

Joint movements

The considerable freedom of movement permitted by the cricoarytenoid joint is an essential requirement for activity as complex as the positioning and stretching/relaxing of the vocal folds. The easiest way to look at a saddle joint is to take the literal example of a jockey moving about on the saddle of a horse, and asking the question: 'How many ways are there to fall off a horse?'

- Rotation about the long axis of the horse, i.e. falling to either side.
- Sliding along the long axis of the horse, i.e. towards the head or the tail.
- Tilting along the long axis of the horse, i.e. burying your head in the mane or lying down on the rump.

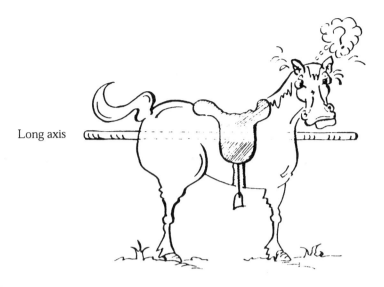

Figure 5.2 The cricoarytenoid joint is a saddle joint with movement occuring about its long axis

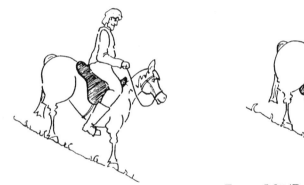

Figure 5.3i 'Saddle-joint'

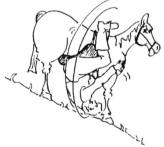

Figure 5.3ii 'Rotation'

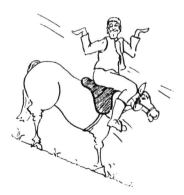

Figure 5.3iii 'Sliding'

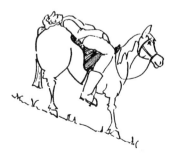

Figure 5.3iv 'Tilting'

The greatest movement in the cricoarytenoid joint is rotation; there is a lesser amount of sliding possible and the tilting is confined to activities such as closing the tips (apices) of the cartilage and is not related to pulley-like activities. Rotation permits the pulley-like action of two muscles attached to the cartilage, vocalis and posterior cricoarytenoid (PCA), both of which are attached to the cartilage, to shorten and lengthen alternately with the visible effect of moving the arytenoid about the long axis of its joint with the cricoid.

Orientation of the long axis of the joint: its alignment with the body of the cricoid cartilage

Rotation

It is not entirely correct to say that the arytenoids rotate over the top of the cricoid; it would be equally fair to say that they rotate around the sides of the cricoid body. It is entirely because of the offset of the long axis of the joint that slopes downwards and outwards behind the cricoid rim that contraction of the posterior cricoarytenoid muscle rotates the arytenoid cartilage backwards causing the vocal fold to be drawn upwards and outwards. Without this angulation, although the PCA would still stretch the fold, rotating the arytenoid backwards, the folds would not part, and breathing could not take place. Rotation of the arytenoid cartilage in the opposite direction, forwards and inwards, is also achieved by the combined sphincteric activity of a pair of muscles whose individual actions would normally be associated with sliding.

Sliding

Sliding of the arytenoid along the long axis of the joint can be achieved by pulling on the muscle most closely aligned with the axis, i.e. the lateral cricoarytenoid (LCA) muscle, which will thus pull the cartilage laterally and inferiorly (outwards and downwards). This movement is limited in its lateral extent by the posterior cricoarytenoid ligament (see Chapter 1, p. 17). The oblique fibres of the inter-arytenoid muscle are small, but they are none the less the true antagonist muscles of the LCA. Unopposed, they would slide the cartilage superiorly and medially (upwards and towards the midline). These small muscles are not strong, and are assisted by a strong cricoarytenoid ligament, but they are still significant as the opponents of LCA.

If **both** muscles are tightened equally, then because they run as part of a circle around the upper border of the cricoid cartilage, the tightening shouldl produce a partial purse-string sphincteric effect, causing the arytenoid which is suspended between them, to **rotate** towards the hollow middle of the cricoid rather than slide around its rim. A similar idea can be demonstrated by the direction of travel of an arrow when released from a drawn bow. The fibres of the bowstring above the arrow nock may be said to be pulling upwards and forwards, while the bowstring below the nock may be said to be pulling downwards and forwards with exactly the same force. The 'up' component and 'down' component cancel each other out, leaving only the 'forward' force.

Sliding medially will also be assisted by the transverse fibres of the inter-arytenoid muscles because of their size and strength. They are not attached in such a way that they should be considered primarily as muscles that rotate the arytenoid cartilage, but rather as the muscles of sliding.

Tilting of the cartilage on the joint

Tilting the tips of the arytenoids medially will bring them (but not necessarily the complete medial surfaces) together. This is seen in phonation and is thought to be effected by the **oblique** fibres of the interarytenoid muscle. The natural antagonist muscles to the interarytenoid **transverse** fibres are the lateral thyroarytenoid or 'muscularis' muscles. They too form part of a laryngeal sphincter. When tensed without opposition, they will tilt the arytenoids anteriorly (forward) and slightly laterally (outward) and the ventricular bands or false folds will be seen to be tightening. Like the other descriptions, this does not occur in total isolation in life; these two arytenoid tilting muscles pull together to form another purse-string type sphincter, rotating the tips of the arytenoids inward to constrict the laryngeal inlet.

Functional muscle groups acting about the arytenoid cartilage

The following is not necessarily 'classical' teaching on intrinsic laryngeal muscular function, it is, however, entirely consistent with our understanding of functional laryngeal physiology

[Eds.]

We are taught from early on about muscles 'paying out' while antagonist (opposing) muscles tighten; this is how the great majority of bones are moved relative to other bones at joints within the body. It is also how the difference between a thin vocal fold and a thick one is controlled.

Unfortunately very little is taught about the totality of the forces of all the muscles acting about the joint. As we showed earlier, only muscles that are pulling in exactly the opposite direction with equal force produce no movement at their common point of attachment. Other muscle pairs that are natural opponents in sphincteric activity, and that do not pull in exactly opposite directions, will produce a vector force that tends to close the space around which they are arranged. For proper phonation, it is clear that not only the length, thickness and stiffness of the vocal folds must be controlled, but also their exact positioning in relation to one another.

As a practical aid to learning this, you may find it helpful to look at the action of the laryngeal intrinsic muscles by looking at a full three-dimensional model of the larynx and considering not only the action of a muscle attached to the arytenoid cartilage if it contracts, but also the effect on the position and attitude of the cartilage if the muscle that appears to be pulling in approximately the opposite direction is also tensed.

It is clear that for a better functional understanding of the laryngeal muscles, it is always more useful to consider the function of individual muscles in conjunction with other muscles that affect the position of the arytenoid cartilage. In this way there ceases to be a paradox in statements such as: 'The lateral cricoarytenoid muscle is an adductor and abductor muscle of the vocal fold.' This statement is true if there is an understanding that in the first case it is working in conjunction with fibres of interarytenoid and in the second case with fibres of the posterior cricoarytenoid muscles.

Muscle pairs to consider (Figure 5.1)

1. Lateral cricoarytenoid (LCA) and the oblique fibres of interarytenoid/ aryepiglotticus, the lower of two supraglottic sphincteric mechanisms.
2. Lateral thyroarytenoid (muscularis) and the horizontal fibres of inter-arytenoid (IA), the upper of the two supraglottic sphincteric mechanisms.
3. Posterior cricoarytenoid (PCA) and lateral cricoarytenoid, the muscles of abduction.
4. Vocalis and posterior cricoarytenoid, the 'strap', the anterior half of which forms the body of the vocal fold.

The LCA with the oblique fibres of interarytenoid/aryepiglotticus as a unit

As described earlier, when both muscles are tightened, instead of sliding the arytenoid, they rotate it forwards so that the most anterior part of the cartilage, the vocal process, is moved downwards and inwards (inferomedially). That this is a sphincteric mechanism is often poorly appreciated, as the system is not set in a ring at right angles to the long axis of the larynx.

There are in fact two partial sphincteric mechanisms, one for each arytenoid cartilage, and they both face outwards and forwards on each side, being set broadly along the line of the long axis of the cricoarytenoid joint. The posterior muscle fibres of the sphincters for each side cross over each other in the midline behind the transverse fibres of the interarytenoid muscle and continue beyond the tip of the arytenoid into the aryepiglottic fold as the aryepiglotticus muscle.

Because the long axis of the cricoarytenoid joint is set tangentially to the sphincter, it is this mechanism that is directly responsible for forward, downward and medial rocking of the vocal process of the arytenoid cartilage producing **medial compression** of the vocal fold. This particular sphincteric activity is extremely important from a phonatory point of view, as surgeons performing injections of botulinum for spasmodic dysphonia will realize. The vocal ligament is attached to the vocal process and the vocalis to the lateral aspects of the cartilage, and hence it is this sphincteric mechanism that becomes the primary means for bringing the vibrating portion of the vocal fold into contact with its opposite number ('medial compression'). The vocalis muscles do not have the capacity to bring the folds entirely to the midline for reasons explained below, but when the vector from this muscle pair is added to the directional pull from vocalis, then the free borders of the folds can be pressed into firm contact.

The gesture is best exemplified by the appearance of Estill's 'twang' vocal quality (see Chapter 7, also Estill, 1996).

The lateral thyroarytenoid (muscularis) and transverse fibres of interarytenoid as a unit

This is the well understood and often described supraglottic sphincter. As outlined above, the joint action of these muscles is that of a closing sphincter for the laryngeal inlet. Moderate combined activity draws the tips of the arytenoids together and forwards (although the medial surfaces of the arytenoids are not necessarily in complete close contact), and increased activity of the false vocal folds is seen. It should be noted that this rather tight gesture still permits a gap between the arytenoid bodies, even if the tips are held together above the gap. More extreme combined muscular activity slides the bodies of the arytenoids together, closing the remaining intercartilaginous gap beneath the (already closed) tips and closing the false folds together to seal the laryngeal inlet.

It is a very powerful activity. In theory, if an imaginary sphincter were perfectly circular and its function was to move the arytenoid tip in a radial fashion, towards the centre, then the distance actually moved by the tip would be equal to the reduction in circumference $\div 2\pi$, i.e. a factor of approximately six. The force of the pull would be correspondingly increased by a similar amount. Clearly, in 'real life', the perfectly circular shape is not maintained by any rigid structure and the closing force is much less than the theoretical maximum. None the less it remains a very powerful gesture and is used to seal the chest prior to major muscular effort. Sealing the supraglottis is seen immediately prior to an explosive cough or forcible defaecation. Conversely, relaxing this particular sphincter while maintaining the contraction in the others results in the 'deconstriction' described by Estill.

The posterior cricoarytenoid and lateral cricoarytenoid as a unit

Traditionally, the vocal folds have been described as being abducted by the action of the PCA muscle alone, which rotates the arytenoid cartilage posterolaterally (backwards and outwards) around the long axis of its joint. The vocal folds therefore must stretch and thin a great deal to accommodate this rotation, and we would expect to see a much greater posterior movement on inhalation than is the case. The 'tent' analogy suggests that logically, lateralizing/abduction of the vocal folds for breathing would be better achieved if there were also a vector component from the lateral cricoarytenoid muscle. The resultant force of these two muscles would rotate the cricoid posterolaterally but much less than PCA alone, and there would also be a small lateral slide and tilt of the cartilage, increasing abduction and aligning the inferolateral fibres of PCA.

There is also an evident requirement to avoid the torsional element to the PCA pulling alone on the muscular process with respect to the long axis of the cricoarytenoid joint. Recent work confirms this theoretical view that, when taken in tandem with PCA rather than interarytenoid, the lateral cricoarytenoid muscle becomes a muscle of **ab**duction rather than **ad**duction.

The vocalis and posterior cricoarytenoid as a unit

When the vocalis muscle tenses and is not opposed by its antagonist, the posterior cricoarytenoid muscle, it shortens and thickens the vocal fold, pulling the arytenoid cartilage forwards and downwards, bringing the folds closer together, although they are barely touching. (Note: The vocalis cannot be said to exactly oppose the PCA as to do this would require that the vocalis was not attached to the thyroid but was instead anchored to an imaginary non-existent fixed structure in the midline of the space above the cricoid ring, which is clearly impossible. It is, however, attached in a position that is as nearly antagonist as possible.) The converse is also true. When the vocalis pays out and the PCA contracts, the vocal folds stretch and thin out, and the arytenoid cartilage are rotated upwards and outwards, causing the folds to spread apart somewhat. The net effect if only one of these muscles is contracted, whether the folds are together and thick or apart and thin, is of a minimal increase in the overall tension of these two joined muscles. Like the strength of a chain being represented by its weakest link, the overall tension exerted by these two conjoined muscles is that determined by the more relaxed of the pair.

To increase the tension in the vocal fold/posterior cricoarytenoid 'strap', it is not enough to consider tightening both components of this muscle pair, we must look at another mechanism altogether, which is described in the section below, 'Tightening the vocal folds'.

The thickness and consistency of the vibrating mass of the vocal fold

It is apparent even from a cursory inspection of a stringed instrument, that the pitch and tonal quality of the vibrating string not only depend on the tension of the string, but also depend on the thickness or vibrating mass and the consistency or stiffness of the material. Listen to the difference between a thick multilayered string and a thin simple string, or the difference between steel and gut strings.

The vocal fold, as we have seen in the section on anatomy, is a complex structure capable of mimicking all of these qualities without any great changes in the tension from end to end. In later chapters you will hear terms such as 'thin fold phonation' and 'thick fold phonation', and these terms relate to how short or long the vocal fold has been set by the positioning muscles of the larynx even before additional tension has been applied to regulate the pitch of the vibration.

Short folds: lax or stiff?

Remember that the vocal fold may be functionally thought of as a single guy-rope attached to a tent pole. Its position, how tight it is and how much washing you can hang on it depend not only on its own length and tension but also on the length and tension in all the other guy-ropes holding the tent pole in position.

As you will have gathered, it is possible to shorten the vocal fold and bring it into apposition with its opposite number with relatively little muscular effort: a slight tensing of vocalis with corresponding paying out of PCA and some accompanying contraction of LCA/oblique fibres of interarytenoid are all that is required. The vocal fold is short but not particularly thick or firm.

Although the vocal fold is not elongated, the phonation pattern is described as being 'thin fold'. There is a short closed phase to the vibratory cycle, small mucosal waves are generated, and the resultant voice has a rather breathy 'little girl' quality. The perceived pitch may be relatively low, well within the normal range for the person's age and sex.

A short fold can be made both thicker and stiffer, however, in just the same way that the body-builder mentioned earlier shows off his or her biceps muscles – the biceps are prevented from contracting further by increased activity of its antagonist muscle and as a result can pull harder and tense up without any further change in length.

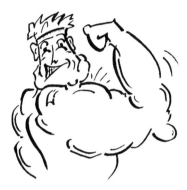

The equivalent laryngeal phonatory gesture is the short 'thick fold', which produces a much longer closed phase in the vibratory cycle. Much larger mucosal waves are generated and the vocal quality is one of 'chest register'. Both these vocal qualities are a result of change in the balance of muscular activity in the isometric mechanism of intrinsic muscles that are attached to the arytenoid cartilages.

An example of isometric activity can be seen when raising or lowering a flag on a flagstaff by pulling on the rope or halliard, the ends of which are connected to the top and bottom of the flag respectively.

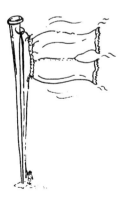

To raise the flag, one pulls down on the end of the halliard that is connected to the upper attachment of the flag, but which first passes through a pulley at the top of the flagstaff. To lower the flag, one pulls down on the end of the halliard that is directly connected to the lower attachment of the flag, while paying out (upwards) a similar quantity of rope to the upper flag attachment. There should be no dramatic increase in tension in the halliard on raising or lowering the flag, neither is there a change in overall length of the halliard; the flag has simply changed its position in response to shortening one attachment and correspondingly lengthening the opposing attachment.

Similarities with positioning the arytenoid cartilage in 'thin fold' and 'thick fold' vocal gestures may be identified.

Lengthening the vocal folds: 'falsetto' versus 'head voice'

Conversely, thinning the vocal fold by relaxing vocalis and allowing it to pay out while contracting PCA produces a thin, 'falsetto' quality to the voice, although the overall tension in the vocal fold has not risen much. In falsetto, increasing stiffness in the vocal fold is largely confined to the vocal ligament under the mucosa of the free border. There is little bulking up of the body of the fold by stiffening the vocalis muscles. This is not the same as 'head register', which is yet another voice quality demanding thin elongated folds. Although there are many other differences in the production of head and falsetto voice quality, the main physical difference between them at the level of the vocal folds (the sound source) is that in head register the muscle underlying the vocal ligament is tensed and stiffer than is required for falsetto. (We would strongly recommend any reader who is seriously interested in the physical and acoustic considerations involved in register shift to read Vilkman et al. (1995). Their concept of 'critical mass' seems utterly sensible to us. Authorities such as Baken regard this view as being compatible with chaos theory as applied to vocal fold vibration (personal communication).)

Not all laryngeal gesturing is isometric however. If a thin elongated vocal fold is required for raised pitch, then the vocal ligament under the mucosal cover of the fold will need to be forcibly put on the stretch, regardless of whether the vocalis muscle underneath it is fairly relaxed or stiffened.

Although the PCA muscle is anchoring the arytenoid cartilage attachment of vocalis, its function is merely to provide a stable anchor for the attachment of the vocal ligament so that the thyroid and arytenoid attachments of the vocal

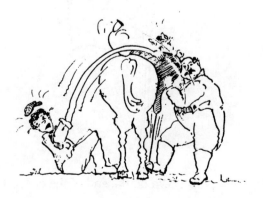

'Forcibly put on the stretch'

ligament/vocalis muscle can be forcibly moved apart by the mechanism described below.

In the context of tensioning the vocal folds, the PCA and vocalis muscles are not antagonists as described above, but work synergistically as components of a single unit, a figurative band or strap-like structure.

This notional 'strap' is tightened by effectively increasing the distance between these fixed attachments of the PCA to the cricoid and the vocalis to the thyroid. The stretching mechanism is a form of lever.

Tightening the vocal folds: the cricothyroid 'visor' mechanism

The action of the laryngeal cricothyroid muscles acting about the cricothyroid joints is to stretch the vocal folds (Figures 5.1 and 5.4). This mechanism is a normal part of the system controlling the position, thickness and tension of the vocal folds. The anatomical arrangement of the cricoid and thyroid cartilages with their connection through a pair of posterolaterally situated joints may be likened to a visor as seen in the face-plates of helmets in suits of armour. The tilting of these cartilages about the cricothyroid joints resembles the closing/opening movements of such a visor. Movement at these joints is usually in tandem, as if there was an imaginary axle running through both joints, permitting rotation with an additional small amount of antero-posterior sliding.

There has been much dispute over the years as to whether the latter, lesser movement occurs in life, and the current opinion (Vilkman et al., 1996) is that this sliding does exist and is of clinical significance.

Tilting the thyroid cartilage forward on the cricoid arch produces rotation about the axis of the cricothyroid joints, lengthening and increasing tension in the vocal folds and posterior cricoarytenoid muscles (PCA). The converse is equally true: the arch of the cricoid ring may be tilted upwards towards the lower margin of the thyroid cartilage laminae with identical effect.

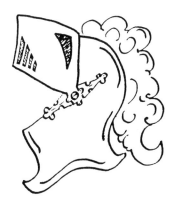

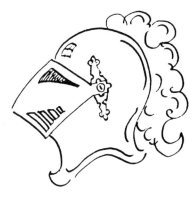

'Open visor'   'Closed visor'

To understand the mechanics of vocal fold tensioning better, it may be easier from the functional point of view to visualize a composite 'strap' whose principal component parts are: the vocal ligament and the vocalis muscle of the fold, coupled to the posterior cricothyroid muscles by their common attachments at the arytenoid cartilage. This figurative strap is firmly attached at both its ends. The 'fixed' end of the PCA muscle is attached to the back (posterior) surface of the body of the cricoid cartilage and the 'fixed' end of the vocalis muscle is its complex attachment to the thyroid cartilage. This strap may be stretched by a lever, the fulcrum of which is the cricoarytenoid joint(s). The purpose of this lever is to increase the distance between the points to which the strap ends are attached, thereby stretching it. Whether you regard the cricoid cartilage as the fixed structure and the thyroid cartilage as the lever acting about the fulcrum of the cricothyroid joint or vice versa is immaterial, the lever system will stretch the muscular attachments to the cricoid and thyroid apart.

The PCA muscles are small but extremely strong, and under most circumstances can prevent the arytenoid cartilages from slipping forwards due to increasing pull from the vocal folds. Thus anchored in position on the cricoid, the arytenoid cartilages are moved backwards in relation to the anterior attachment of the vocal folds, stretching and thinning the folds. Closure of the cricothyroid visor is achieved by the action of the (principally anterior) fibres of the cricothyroid muscles (CT).

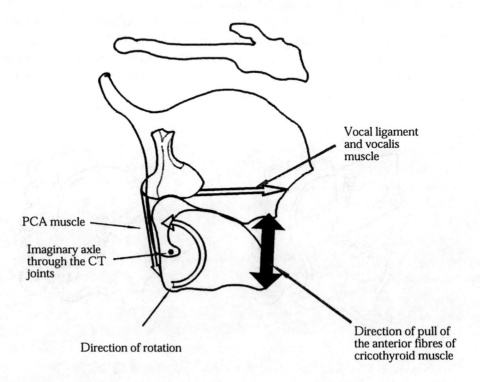

Figure 5.4 The cricothyroid visor tensioning mechanism of the vocal folds

In vivo, this action never takes place in complete isolation. For there to be any increase in tension in the vocal folds, the arytenoid cartilages to which the posterior ends of the folds are attached must be held in place by an increase in tension of the posterior cricoarytenoid muscles equal to the combined opposition of the vocalis muscle, the vocal ligament and tensioning effect of the visor mechanism.

At about this stage many people get anxious about muscles that are described both as working together (synergistically) and as working against each other (antagonistically). The answer is invariably dependent on the context of their activities, as both answers are usually correct even at the same time.

The stretching and thinning of the vocal folds is due to synergistic activity between PCA and CT muscles. They work together to oppose the vocalis. However, vocalis and CT muscles may be described as acting synergistically in other respects. In relation to the cricoarytenoid joints they both act to bring the folds towards the midline and they both tend to pull the arytenoid cartilages forward in relation to their joint facets on the cricoid. This action is in turn normally opposed by the PCA muscles.

In relation to the cricothyroid joints, however, the PCA muscles may be seen to be acting synergistically with the vocalis muscles as a sort of single strap or spring bent around the posterior border of the cricoid, with the arytenoid cartilages to which they are both attached acting as a sesamoid (a solid pulley to transfer the strain around a corner). The components of this strap are now acting together (synergistically) to oppose the activity of the cricothyroid muscles.

A note on register shifts

It is always dangerous to make generalizations, but it may be helpful here to summarize. There is a roughly inverse relationship between the stiffness of the vocal fold body (vocalis) and the vocal ligament in Western classical singing tradition. For a full 'chest' voice the body is stiff and thick and the ligament is lax. Moving into a true 'falsetto' demands slight decreased activity in the muscular body of the fold and increased tension in the ligament. 'Belting' near the top of the vocal register is necessarily fairly effortful as it involves tightening the vocal ligament and a stiff vocal fold body (the opposite of the 'little girl' voice quality).

Detailed notes on the current understanding of exactly what takes place when a singer changes register while singing a note at a particular frequency are beyond the scope of this book. Suffice it to say, it is the interaction of factors such as subglottal air pressure, the physical properties of the vocal fold cover, the medial compression of the folds, the longitudinal tension of the vocal ligaments and, depending on their stiffness, the virtual vibrating mass of the folds, which collectively dictates the resulting register. It is therefore possible to keep one or more factors relatively constant and still effect a register change by altering others. Conversely, the argument states that it should be possible to change them all and still remain in the same register. In reality however, the principal determining factor seems to be the size of the 'critical vibrating mass' of the vocal fold (Vilkman et al., 1995).

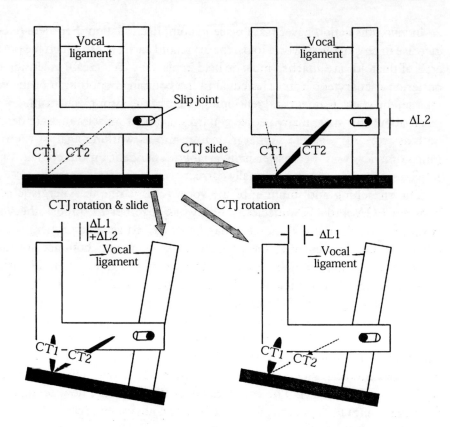

ΔLI represents the change in length of the vocal fold attributable to the rotation about the cricothyroid joints. It depends on the action of the *anterior* fibres of the cricothyroid muscles. ΔL2 represents the change in length of the vocal fold attributable to the sliding activity at the cricothyroid joints. It depends on the activity of the *posterior oblique* fibres of the cricothyroid muscles.

Top left: *Very relaxed 'normal' at rest or in full voice at low end of register.*
                      Palpation: Prominent arch of cricoid. Open visor.

Top right: *Some tension in the posterior oblique fibres of the CT muscles*
                      (CT2) may be 'normal' at rest in order to stabilize the CT joints.
                      Found in mid-register.
                      Palpation: Arch of cricoid not prominent. Neutral position of visor.

Bottom left: *Tightened CT muscles (both parts). 'Normal' for high pitch.*
                      Palpation: Arch of cricoid not prominent. Visor closed.

Bottom right: *Persistent tension of the anterior fibres of the CT muscles (CT1) even*
                      when not voicing. Not useful for voicing. Further stretching of
                      vocalis/thyroarytenoid (ΔL2) to increase pitch can only be achieved by
                      posterior sliding of the cricoid under the thyroid which is less
                      mechanically advantageous than using rotation about the joint.
                      Palpation: This common finding produces a characteristic
                      closed visor with a prominent anterior cricoid arch.

Figure 5.5 Diagram of activity in the cricothyroid muscles and its effects on the vocal folds (after Titze)

Development of dysfunctional voicing patterns

Hyperfunctional dysphonia, the 'locked visor' and its relation to vocal fatigue and vocal dysfunction

Practitioners who regularly work in voice clinics soon become aware that the biggest group of dysphonic patients is the one where no specific pathological lesion is found. Although there are a variety of factors that may precipitate the dysphonia, the most common response to these is the production of persistent patterns of vocal hyperfunction that all appear to be variants on a basic theme.

Hoarseness versus horsepower: towards a definition of vocal hyperfunction

Dysfunctional phonation is less than optimally efficient, there is too much work going on for relatively poor vocal output. This is not at all the same thing as the effortful voicing to produce the enormous vocal output necessary for vocal performance in large auditoria. Maximal or excessive muscular activity only becomes a problem in life when it is used inappropriately.

Let us use an analogy. If an athlete wishes to run the 100 metres faster than any other human being on earth, then for the duration of the time and space between the gun and the tape, maximal muscular effort is both desirable and appropriate for the occasion. Absolutely no-one in the spectators is going to accuse the athlete of 'working too hard' or 'trying too hard'. The maximal effort is appropriate to the occasion. What is more, the athlete prepares him or herself for the occasion by training the muscles to work in the most coordinated and powerful manner possible.

Outside the very closely defined conditions between the gun and the tape, however, with the sole exception of training periods, the same level of muscular activity is not appropriate: atheletes walk with a tray of glasses rather than sprint, they hand a cup of tea to someone else, they do not hurl it. The hyperactive alternative would be regarded as inappropriate if not severely disturbed to say the least.

The same criteria apply to the muscular activities demanded by voicing. There may be moments when maximal effort is called for, for example yelling 'fire', 'I'm drowning', 'help', or similar important communications. It may also be necessary (in a trained, coordinated manner) for opera, rock and roll, or strenuous pieces of theatre. Intense voicing always demands effort. The collateral is just as true: outside the limited period when the intense effort is called for, when rest is appropriate, it is not helpful to be in a constant state of readiness for the next major effort.

To use the running analogy once more: 3 hours before the race the athlete does not need to be braced against starting blocks merely to read a newspaper any more than a voice user needs to keep the cricothyroid visor closed to keep the folds under tension hours before a period of vocal exertion. Similarly, when only moderate exercise is called for (e.g. in a vocal context, voicing for normal conversation), only the most efficient use of moderate voice is appropriate. Anything more effortful than this may be regarded as hyperfunctional.

Genuine hypofunction of the phonatory apparatus seems to us to occur only as a late part of the ageing process or to be associated with a disease process. Even hysterical aphonics **hold** their vocal folds slightly apart, and one only has to look at the effortful attempts at compensation where there is a vocal fold palsy to realize that the remaining vocal activity is necessarily hyperfunctional.

It is the consideration and interpretation of what appears to be inappropriate muscular effort for a given vocal activity and inappropriate persistence of muscular effort even after voicing has finished that will form an important part of the rationale for therapeutic methods in subsequent chapters of this book.

Habitual holding of the visor in the 'closed' position: inappropriate persistence of laryngeal activity

We find that one of the most common consequences of extensive voice use, especially where the patient can be said to be 'stressed', is that the cricothyroid visor, instead of relaxing after appropriate use, remains tightly closed (Lieberman and Harris, 1993). The result is that although the patient does not believe that he or she is using the voice excessively or more than usual, the muscular effort in the larynx is maximal all day, even if the patient is not actually voicing.

The patient is perplexed if they have had a period of voice rest as the voice feels just as fatigued as it was prior to the 'rest'. There is commonly a palpable hyperlordosis of the cervical spine, usually at the level of C4–5 or C5–6. This is frequently associated with an extended head position and a kyphotic hump in the upper thoracic vertebrae. The combination of postural problems produces a characteristic cervicodorsal vertebral shelf, nicknamed the 'tea cup shelf' in the clinic.

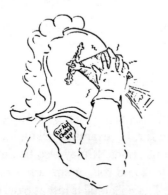 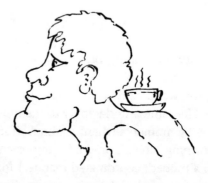

Commonly reported symptoms

Patients often present with early vocal fatigue and little vocal stamina. This is generally associated with loss of vocal range at the top and bottom. The voice may be virtually pitch-locked at the lower end of the expected range or may present as a persistent falsetto. There is generally poor intonation or lack of timbre in the voice. For those patients who are not (yet) pitch-locked, there are increasing problems with negotiating the passaggio between modal voice (e.g. chest register) and falsetto voice (e.g. head register). This may be less than essential for professional talkers but is, of course, catastrophic for singers. In addition, there may be odd notes within the normally comfortable vocal range that simply disappear.

Where the cricothyroid visor remains held or locked closed over a long period, as with every other example of inappropriate posture in the body, tissues begin to stretch, muscles to lose their resting tonus and their capacity to contract efficiently (Lieberman and Harris, 1993). In the case of the vocal fold tensioning mechanism, the part least likely to 'give' is the muscle working about the cricothyroid joints with the greatest mechanical advantage. Any muscle or ligament opposing this action is more prone to fatigue loss of tonus or actual stretching.

While we are fully aware of other variants on this basic mechanism such as the 'muscular tension dysphonia' described by Morrison et al. (1983), which possibly involves an additional element of lateral cricoarytenoid muscular 'locking' and (possibly) secondary interarytenoid failure, we propose that the following three variants of fatigue/stretching produced by persistent activity of the visor vocal fold tightening mechanism account for the vast majority of the different laryngoscopic gestures observed. These observations invariably match the mechanical problems that are suggested by the detailed descriptions of symptoms provided by the patient:

1. The posterior cricoarytenoid muscles may no longer adequately oppose the forward tension of the folds, and the arytenoid cartilages slide forward and down towards the glottis, producing the typical 'tight' vocal gesture often described as 'antero-posterior compression' (or 'Bogart-Bacall' type). This allows the vocal folds to thicken and stiffen but they can no longer be length-ened/tightened at will. There is an inevitable loss at the top of the vocal range with no falsetto voice (Figure 5.6).

2. The vocal ligaments appear to become stretched with varying degrees of bowing (glottal insufficiency). This may be due to actual stretching of the vocal ligaments or to true vocalis insufficiency. In either case it cannot be easily demonstrated directly by traditional means such as electromyography. This pattern results in poor mucosal waves, short or absent closed phase to the vibratory cycle and, more commonly (but not exclusively) in the elderly, bowing of the vocal folds. We are firmly convinced that many premature 'senile' voice changes are not simply the product of ageing, but are the result of inappropriate hyperkinetic compensatory voicing patterns. There is loss of 'chest' and 'middle' register voice quality, inability to negotiate the 'passaggio' easily and very often extremely refractory pitch instability resulting in a 'yodelling' quality to the spoken voice.

3. Anterior translocation of the cricoid (illustrated in Figure 5.6, bottom right). A frequent finding is that the cricoid arch slides forwards underneath the thyroid cartilage, even when the visor is closed. It is normal for there to be some anterior sliding of the cricoid under the arytenoid when the visor opens in full chest voice, but the posterior oblique fibres of the cricothyroid muscles are normally able to reverse this slide when the visor is closed. Where there is no evidence of associated posterior cricoarytenoid muscle insufficiency with forward tilting of the arytenoid apices, the vocal folds appear to be 'normal' in length although to the sceptical eye, the bulk may appear somewhat thinned. The vocal gesture is likewise apparently 'normal' with maybe a little additional

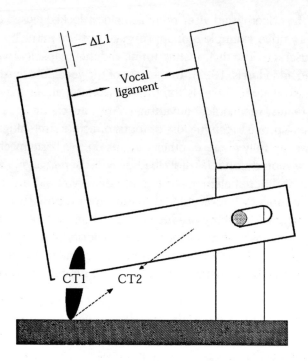

a.   *If the PCA muscles elongate under the strain imposed by the tightening of the visor there will*
     be little or no change in length ΔL1.

b.   *Despite the CT visor being closed the endoscopic appearance will show little elongation.*
     Anteroposterior collapse of the supraglottic space may occur despite little evidence of vocalis
     activity.

Figure 5.6 Effects of failure of the posterior cricoarytenoid muscles

tonus in the false folds (the ventricular bands). These findings are inevitably
accompanied by considerable tenderness in the capsule and anterior ligaments of the cricothyroid joints. We think that this occurs with insufficiency
of the posterior oblique fibres of the cricothyroid muscles that normally
oppose the anterior thrust on the joints from the combined stretched vocal
folds and PCA muscles.

It appears therefore that there is an initial common pathway for most forms of
hyperkinetic (hyperfunctional) dysphonia. There is a characteristic failure of
normal relaxation of the vocal fold tensioning mechanism even when the voice is
not being used. Differing appearances and outcomes are thought to be due to end-
stage stretching or weakening of different parts of the whole vocal fold tensioning
mechanism. The most effective treatment programme for all forms of this most
common of problems in the voice clinic is inevitably multidisciplinary. The habitual laryngeal set and patient perception of what a genuinely relaxed laryngopharynx feels like is restored by direct manipulation, either prior to or at the same time

as a course of speech therapy. The role of the therapy is to introduce more efficient, less hyperfunctional voicing patterns.

A caveat

The above is, as yet, only a working hypothesis. Much research is still needed to base these observations entirely in science. We are fully aware that there is a yawning gap where there should be measurements of work done by individual muscles. Unfortunately, simple techniques such as EMG do not give an answer. They only report on the presence of neuromuscular activity, which cannot be correlated with work done. Some techniques required are too expensive or invasive to be of practical value to a clinical team, and one of the few that seem to be promising to us is that of Cooper et al. (1993), who have been able to demonstrate a direct correlation between intramuscular pressures in the thyroarytenoid muscles of dogs with the measured isometric force of contraction. This technique is clearly some way from clinical application as yet, but we have high hopes.

References

Cooper DS, Pinczower E, Rice DH (1993) Thyroarytenoid intramuscular pressures. Annals of Otology, Rhinology and Laryngology 102: 167–175.

Estill J (1996) Primer of Compulsory Figures (Level One). Santa Rosa CA: Estill Voice Training Systems.

Lieberman J, Harris T (1993) The cricothyroid mechanism, its relation to vocal fatigue and vocal dysfunction. Voice 2: 89–96.

Morrison MD, Rammage LA, Belisle GM, Pullan CB, Nichol H (1983). Muscular tension dysphonia. Journal of Otolaryngology 12: 302–306.

Titze I (1994) Mechanics of vocal fold elongation. In Principles of voice production. Englewood Cliffs, NJ: Prentice-Hall, pp 197–200.

Vilkman E, Alku P, Laukkanen A-M (1995) Vocal-fold collision mass as a differentiator between registers in the low-pitch range. Journal of Voice 9: 66–73.

Vilkman E, Sonninen A, Hurme P, Körkkö P (1996) External laryngeal frame function in voice production revisited: a review. Journal of Voice 10: 78–92.

Part 2
Treatment Modalities

CHAPTER 6

Principles and Techniques of Manual Therapy: Applications in the Management of Dysphonia

JACOB LIEBERMAN

General considerations

This chapter is an introduction to the discipline of manual therapy and its application to voice disorders. Manual therapy examines the nature and function of the musculoskeletal system, which is comprised of the joints, ligaments, muscles and surrounding soft tissues that enable the human skeleton to be flexible and capable of meeting the body's demands for highly complex movement. The discipline provides a physiological interpretation of musculoskeletal dysfunction so that problems arising in the system can be accurately diagnosed and treated.

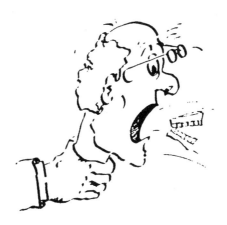

'Carpe diem, quam minimum credula postero.

Horace, Odes 1

Palpation plays an important role in the examination and diagnostic procedure. Visualization and palpation are two of the three most basic clinical tools with which to assess the mechanism of the sound source. The practitioner must be able to assess the range of movement for any joint and the tonus in the muscles and associated soft tissues that are involved in its function. Manual treatment techniques can then be applied to improve the mobility of the joint and restore the appropriate tone to the muscles and adjacent soft tissues. Osteopaths, therefore, may have a slightly different approach from chiropractors or physiotherapists, and each profession may justify their diagnoses in different ways. However, they will all treat patients using manual techniques.

This chapter will cover the following topics and their application to voice disorders: the principles underlying manual therapy, the physical examination and assessment, functional diagnosis, treatment techniques, their outcome and contraindications to treatment.

The traditional approach to dysphonia

In the past, voice patients were in general assessed by an ENT specialist and, more recently, jointly assessed with speech therapists. The aim of treatment was to remove the patient's symptoms even though the aetiology of the condition might not have been well understood. The diagnosis and management of dysphonic patients therefore reflected this tradition and was, to some extent, limited by it. Organic lesions tended to fall within the surgical domain and non-organic (functional) dysphonias were passed to the speech therapist.

Recently, as a result of the multidisciplinary approach, our understanding of the aetiology of many types of dysphonia has improved. In particular, it has become clearer that failure in one part of the vocal tract, e.g. vocal fold pathology, can arise as a result of failure in another part of the vocal apparatus, for example, a locked cricothyroid visor mechanism.

The discipline of manual therapy has a long tradition of working with dysfunction of joints and muscles that has arisen in response to the patient's posture or habitual muscle use, an example being the so called repetitive strain injury (RSI). It seems logical then, to apply this knowledge and understanding to the larynx and to see if manual therapy techniques can be used to resolve dysphonia that is secondary to musculoskeletal dysfunction.

The basic principles underlying manual therapy

For manual therapy to have meaning and validity as a treatment modality, the following principles should be borne in mind:

Structure governs function

A detailed knowledge of the anatomy, physiology, pathology and mechanical function of the structures is essential. Joints have specific axes of movement and unless these are known and fully understood, manipulating them is of limited use and may even cause damage.

Palpatory skills

The manual therapist is heavily reliant on his or her palpatory skills. These acquired skills are used to assess the range of joint movements, the quality of the surrounding soft tissue and, in particular, the muscles working across a particular joint. To be able to manipulate a joint successfully, an accurate mental picture needs to be drawn of the following:

1. the joint's plane of movement;
2. the direction of pull between muscle attachments and their state;
3. the joint capsule and related ligaments that limit joint movement.

The mechanical system as interactive functional units

Muscles and joints do not work in isolation. Any mechanical activity should be considered within the context of all other components working in concert. As a result, the manual therapist will understand the development of abnormal symptoms as a breakdown of compensation within a mechanically unbalanced system. In other words, to understand the symptoms one has to understand the system.

Compensatory systems

There may be a number of neuromuscular pathways available for human beings to perform a given mechanical task. However, if the primary system designed to perform a task fails, it is reasonable to assume that recruitment of subsidiary secondary pathways to compensate for the failure will be less efficient, and therefore more vulnerable to breakdown and failure.

Breakdown in compensation

The production of symptoms and signs may be the result of a breakdown of compensation. As a result, the weakest link in the mechanical system fails with a resultant decrease in appropriate function of that part, although increased effort persists in a different part of the mechanism. This means that the primary focus of attention for the manual therapist is not necessarily the site of the symptom or failure, but rather the site where abnormal function persists. Take, for example, vocal fold bowing that has developed as a result of long-term stretching of the folds. At assessment, one would expect to find a closed and locked cricothyroid joint. The primary aim of treatment, then, would become the release of the locked joint in order to decrease the persistent tension exerted on the vocal folds. This should take place before attempting to rehabilitate the vocalis muscles.

Patient compliance

The patient must be willing and able to allow the necessary physical contact that is involved in manual therapy.

Functional anatomy of the larynx: the manual therapist's perspective

A review of the structural anatomy and its function can be found in Chapters 1, 2, 4 and 5. This section is therefore intended simply to reiterate those principles and major functional components that form the basis of the rationale behind the application of manual therapy to the treatment of voice disorders.

Voice production, or rather noise production, is the result of three physical elements working in concert:

1. the power source: the breathing apparatus;
2. the sound source: the vocal folds and their primary tensor mechanism;
3. the resonators: the vocal tract.

The power source

The functional anatomy and the importance of the power source in voice production are described in detail elsewhere in this book and will not be discussed here; suffice it to say that manual therapy has an important role to play in improvement of rib cage mobility, direct articulation to the diaphragm, and treatment of tight external muscles of respiration and thoracic spine dysfunction.

The sound source

The production of sound may be considered to be the conversion of airflow into sound energy. This occurs at the level of the vocal folds as they resist the escape of expired air under pressure and their resistance is partially overcome by the increased subglottic pressure. This results in rapidly repeated escapes of very small quantities of air, effectively chopping up a column of subglottic air into puffs of pressure. The analogy with a DC to AC converter is commonly used to describe this effect.

Within a voice clinic, the majority of vocal symptoms and signs cluster at the level of the vocal folds. As a result, the vocal folds have attracted a great deal of research interest, which, in turn, has led to the development of diagnostic and treatment tools, together with more focused management techniques. The aim of these techniques is to improve vocal fold function to levels that are acceptable to patients.

This approach, however, often shows scant appreciation of the fact that the vocal folds do not work in isolation. They form only one component of a complex functional mechanism. This mechanism is, in turn, interlinked with other muscular systems essential to voice production. Therefore, although vocal symptoms usually manifest themselves at the vocal fold level, the vocal folds are not necessarily the main focus of attention for the manual therapist. The manual therapist will be concerned with locating the site of the mechanical failure, rather than the site of the symptoms.

Anatomically (mechanically), the sound source consists of:

1. the vocal folds/thyroarytenoid muscles and their functional anchors, the posterior cricoarytenoid muscles;

2. the cricothyroid joints, related soft tissues and cricothyroid muscles - the primary tensor mechanism;
3. the arytenoid cartilages and their soft tissue/muscle attachments, for isometric positioning of the arytenoid.

Pitch is controlled by altering the length, thickness and stiffness of the vocal folds. This is achieved through coordinated muscular control of movement of the cricothyroid visor and arytenoid cartilages, and levels of activity within the vocalis and posterior cricoarytenoid muscles. Together, these activities can either increase or decrease the tension, thickness and closure of the vocal folds (see also Chapter 5).

The resonators

For the sound generated at vocal fold level to be transformed into recognizable voicing, a resonator is required. The resonators are the walls and associated structures surrounding the air-filled spaces of the vocal tract.

For practitioners interested in assessing the musculature of the vocal apparatus and for the manual therapist, it is useful to consider the structures of the vocal tract as follows:

1. The suspensory muscles. These can be considered as inferior and superior suspensory groups and the thyrohyoid apparatus. They are concerned with the suspension of the larynx from the base of the skull and mandible, and they anchor the larynx to the rib cage, so that its position remains stable but flexible. They are also responsible for altering the length and shape of the vocal tract affecting resonance and pitch.
2. The pharyngeal musculature. This consists of:
    a. The three major constrictor muscles, which are of particular importance to resonance. They attach to their opposite numbers via a thin but tough midline band of fibrous tissue (raphe) in front of the prevertebral fascia of the spine. This provides posterosuperior anchorage for the pharynx and larynx.
    b. Multiple other small pharyngeal muscles that contribute to laryngeal positioning during swallow (such as stylo-, palato-, salpingopharyngeus) and have a lesser role as resonators in the shaping of the resonator cavity.
    (see also Chapter 1).

The larynx as a whole

If we bear these principles in mind, we can now consider laryngeal function as a whole, emphasizing the directions of pull of individual muscles and their possible functional combinations during phonation. The effects of activity in any/all of the external muscular and fibrous attachments of the larynx must be included (Vilkman et al., 1996) (see Appendix 6.1).

The resting position of the cricothyroid visor is a product of a number of pulls in different directions (Figure 6.1). Activity in posterior cricoarytenoid (PCA) and vocalis muscles tends to open the visor, activity in cricothyroid muscle and passive

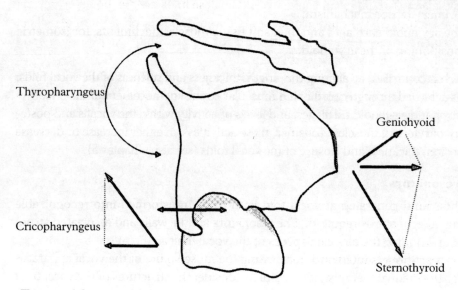

Thyropharyngeus

Geniohyoid

Cricopharyngeus

Sternothyroid

External forces which stretch the folds

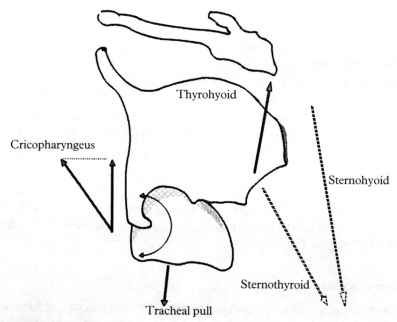

Thyrohyoid

Cricopharyngeus

Sternohyoid

Sternothyroid

Tracheal pull

External forces which shorten the folds and open the visor

The arrows indicate only the direction of the pull; they do not indicate the site of origin.

Figure 6.1 The structure of the larynx   *(After Vilkman)*

pull in the conus and median ligament tend to close it. There are, however, several external factors that should also be considered: the pull on the cricotracheal membrane inferiorly, the activity of the cricopharyngeus muscles posteriorly and the activity of the inferior suspensory muscles.

The cricotracheal attachment below gives rise to the phenomenon of 'tracheal pull'. This occurs during inhalation. This downward and slightly backward pull on the larynx is usually considered to rotate the anterior cricoid arch inferiorly. Where the thyroid cartilage remains fixed, it also opens the visor thereby shortening the vocal folds. It is difficult, however, to assess the full effect of tracheal pull during inhalation as there are many 'muscular variables' that can affect it. Because it is difficult to predict the net effect on the cricoid, it is extremely useful to assess it using palpation, both passively and dynamically (Sundberg, personal communication).

The possible effects on pitch changes caused by the action of the strap muscles namely, the sternothyroid and sternohyoid, should also be borne in mind (Sonninen, 1956; Vilkman et al., 1996).

The cricopharyngeus muscle originates on the cricoid cartilage laterally, behind the origin of the cricothyroid, and its fibres travel posteriorly around the pharyngo-oesophageal junction to attach to one another at the median raphe. This muscle is part of the 'cricopharyngeal sphincter' and as such, contracts to prevent air entering the oesophagus during respiration. It relaxes during swallowing. The horizontal orientation of its lower fibres tends to anchor the cricoid cartilage posteriorly. As the larynx rises with increasing pitch, however, the oblique fibres of the inferior constrictors tend to pull the cricoid cartilage upwards and slightly back. It is worth noting that this is the only muscle attached to the cricoid cartilage that is related to laryngeal position in the neck.

The hyoid bone and its muscular attachments, in particular the thyrohyoid muscles and membrane, are of great clinical interest to the manual therapist. Characteristically in dysphonic patients this area becomes tender to the touch. Palpation at rest reveals that the space between the thyroid and the hyoid is greatly diminished. The thyrohyoid muscles approximate the thyroid cartilage and hyoid bone; their contraction during speech is correlated with rising pitch but is not related to the slight opening activity of the visor (Vilkman et al., 1996). When these muscles fail to relax, they become chronically shortened and the patient will complain of pain or discomfort over this area. Clinical observations show that manipulation of these muscles not only reduces pain and discomfort, but also drops the vocal pitch and increases resonance.

Both the vertical position of the hyoid bone (as determined by action of the superior suspensory muscles and base of tongue) and its relative distance from the cervical spine are of great importance to the manual therapist.

The cricothyroid joint has a complex movement in both vertical-rotatory and horizontal axes. Dysphonic patients are frequently found to have difficulty controlling movements at this joint, thus compromising their ability to alter the length and tension of the vocal folds. Other muscle groups are then recruited to compensate for the inefficient use of the cricothyroid visor mechanism. Palpatory findings suggest that many patients habitually hold the visor closed, creating long-term stretching of the vocal folds. Eventually this leads to muscle fatigue, bowed vocal folds and a weak, pitch-unstable voice.

Assessment of the patient

The case history

It is tempting to resist reading yet another section on 'the case history'. However, the history and the manner in which the patient presents it can provide both mechanical and psychological information that is invaluable in deciding who to treat, how to approach treatment and what the patient's response is likely to be. In other words, taking an accurate detailed history frequently elicits the diagnosis. The examination usually confirms what the patient has already revealed.

The framework of the history-taking is important. As the patient reveals his or her story it is vitally important to observe and to listen carefully to the way in which it is told. It can be particularly helpful to pay attention to the following features:

1. the words the patient chooses;
2. the style of delivery (i.e. body language, especially laryngeal muscular effort);
3. prosody and intonation;
4. clarity and flow;
5. presence or absence of emotions;
6. what the patient **omits** to say.

From the manual therapist's perspective there are three distinct parts to the history-taking. They should be designed to elicit:

1. a framework of understanding about the patient's life and circumstances;
2. a conventional medical history;
3. the patient's exploration of the aetiology of their vocal symptoms.

The framework of the patient's life

The framework of understanding incorporates the patient's basic details about their circumstances (i.e. employment, marital status, children, leisure activities, etc.) together with the therapist's perceptions of patient's circumstances (spoken or unspoken).

Patients are asked to describe their symptoms and how they experience the problem in their own words. It is very important that patients do not simply repeat what they have been told along the way by their GP, ENT specialist, singing teacher or other involved person. Some patients, in spite of being asked their views, will persist in repeating what they have been told about their condition. This may indicate a lack of awareness of their difficulties. Patients who continue to be unable to talk about their own experience of the problem may prove to have high degrees of resistance that will impede their response to treatment.

The purpose of the open-ended section of the interview is to establish how much of the patient's complaint is mechanical and how much is related to emotional issues. Information about the onset of symptoms, whether acute or long-standing, is very important. A history of voice problems going back to early childhood is crucial information, both emotionally and mechanically.

Conventional medical history

The medical history should include the patients' perception of their general health, any known chronic illnesses and any medication. Patients are specifically asked about psychiatric history, the use of tranquillizers, sleeping pills and antidepressants. Those taking tablets of this nature are more likely to have a strong emotional component to their symptoms and may have difficulty taking responsibility for their health. Voice work tends to be a continuum, at one end of which lie the mechanical components and at the other, the emotional. The medical history should give an indication as to where on the continuum the problem lies.

Details about patients' well-being in other systems should also be sought.

Gastrointestinal tract

The patient should be questioned about changes in bowel habits, sudden weight loss, loss of appetite, swallowing difficulties, vomiting, constipation and diarrhoea in order to exclude serious pathologies. In particular, symptoms referrable to reflux oesophagitis are investigated, because of their impact on the voice. Recently it has proved useful to add specific questions about eating habits in or around adolescence, in order to exclude the possibility of anorexia/bulimia.

Cardiovascular system

Questions relating to palpitations, increased heart rate, or raised blood pressure and any treatment, will not only give a good indication as to the patients' general health, but may also provide useful clues about their levels of anxiety.

Respiratory system

It is crucial that the clinician is aware of any conditions that are likely to affect the patients' breathing. Problems such as asthma, chronic obstructive airways disease, shortness of breath, or panic attacks leading to hyperventilation or feelings of suffocation are common. They are likely to affect the patients' ability to maintain good subglottic pressure during phonation. The patients' smoking and drinking habits should be discussed, as both are irritants to the vocal tract. Spirits, particularly whisky and brandy, in addition to producing oral and pharyngeal mucosal irritation may occasionally overspill into the larynx. Furthermore, excessive alcohol intake puts patients at greater risk of acid reflux with laryngeal overspill, which may exacerbate any existing chest condition. Where patients deny smoking and/or drinking, it is important to ask whether they have ever done so in the past. Careful questioning sometimes reveals that they 'gave it up' the week before.

Central nervous system

A history of headaches, dizzy spells, fainting, double vision, weakness or tremor may indicate an underlying neurological problem.

Gynaecology (where relevant)

Important questions include the use of contraceptives (in particular the Pill), period irregularity and pain, menopause and any hormone replacement therapy (HRT). There may be a significant relationship between vocal symptoms and menses. The obstetric history may also be relevant if there is a suggestion of urinary frequency or incontinence with strong breath support.

Musculoskeletal system

Any history of chronic conditions likely to affect the head and/or torso position may be relevant to dysphonia. These include such conditions as osteo- or rheumatoid arthritis, spinal degenerative changes, and serious accidents, particularly whiplash injuries and direct blows to the larynx. A history of fractured limbs may also be relevant because of the possible effects on posture and muscle function. This is of particular importance to voice production because a dysfunction in one part of the body may affect the remainder of the skeleton and the position of the larynx. Likewise, specific conditions (e.g. ankylosing spondylitis, prolapsed disc, scoliosis) could affect the 'power source'.

Sleep patterns

The patients are asked about their sleep pattern as this is known to be a sensitive indicator of emotional disturbance and depression.

Family history

In addition to questioning patients about their own medical history, it is also important to explore the family history for such things as diabetes or any other relevant disease.

Patient's own perception of his problem

Finally the patients are asked to offer their own thoughts on and explanation for the problem and their thoughts on the possible aetiology. The patients' response to that particular question may reveal the need for reassurance, or their resentment at having to comply with the referring doctor's request for a further opinion.

Exploration of aetiology

While inquiring about the conventional medical history, insights can be obtained into the emotional aspects leading to dysphonic symptoms. For example, questions about the family medical history often reveal important and traumatic details about patients' past history e.g. an adoption, or a family split by divorce or a death. The patients may not realize that such details are important to the clinician and omit them when questioned directly about their own health. It is only when asked about siblings or the family history that half-brothers and sisters or step-parents are mentioned or an adoption is brought to light. Similarly, recent work-related or personal trauma could have an immediate bearing upon the dysphonia.

Patients are also encouraged to discuss their own feelings about how and why the voice problem has arisen. This is not an optional extra as it may be the only clue to the patient's fears or fantasies concerning his or her symptoms.

Mechanical manifestations in hyperfunctional voice production

The following section describes some of the most common clinical findings, but is by no means an exhaustive list.

Table 6.1 is arranged to show common symptoms in the left hand column and their suggested significance to the practitioner in the right hand column. As with all case histories and assessments, as the patient describes his or her symptoms the practitioner will begin to form a mental picture of the patient, and questions or hypotheses will come to mind. These will be confirmed or disconfirmed as the patient's history unfolds. These 'questions in the practitioner's mind' are triggered by the patient's comments, which are described in the left hand column. They do not necessarily relate directly to the order in which the symptoms are presented. Where appropriate, the comments are expanded below.

It is important for the practitioner to distinguish between acute and chronic difficulties, and between voice problems that are clearly audible to all, those that are only audible to a third party familiar with the patient (e.g. the singing teacher, family or friends) and those that are only apparent to the patient. If the symptoms are clearly audible to all, it is highly likely that there will be some mechanical component to the overall disorder that should be amenable to manipulative (or other) therapy (e.g. the patient presenting with vocal nodules). A complex group of patients are those presenting as a result of pressure from teachers, family or friends. A common example is the singer whose singing teacher complains about a tight quality that is audible to the teacher, but not to the patient. The patient then seeks help to satisfy the teacher rather than for their own benefit. Another example would be the patient with an irritating cough who presents because the family can no longer tolerate it. The picture becomes even more complicated when the problem is only audible to, or felt by, the patient. Professional voice-users in particular will often present with a sensation of tightness or a loss of resonance that cannot be easily heard or demonstrated.

Patient's expectations and treatment outcome

It is useful to establish what the patient's expectations are with respect to the treatment and outcome, especially in situations where neither the symptoms nor the patient's account are clear or focused. A direct but open question may enable the patient to be in touch with and express their wishes, anxieties and hopes of solving the problem. When the history is both complicated and confused it might be useful

Table 6.1 History: general description of symptoms and the therapist's formulations

Typical vocal symptoms	Questions in the practitioner's mind as he/she 'carefully listens'
	Is the date/time/reason of onset clear in the practitioner's mind?
Change in vocal quality: hoarseness/roughness/breathiness, etc. Loss of vocal range and flexibility	Are the symptoms audible to the practitioner? It makes a great deal of difference to the assessment if the complaint is only audible to the client (see below - this is particularly relevant in singers)
Difficulty with the *passaggio* Pitch breaks	Cricothyroid mechanism locked, tight vocal tract, muscle fatigue Tight inferior strap muscles (especially in baritones/basses, globus patients)
Inability to project Inability to sustain notes	Poor vocal technique, emotional issues, breath support problems, general muscle fatigue
The voice disappears after a day's work	Does the practitioner feel that she/he has a clear understanding of the onset? Is the problem acute or chronic? Mechanical or emotional? Daily pattern morning or evening? Is there a neurological component?
Total loss of voice with or without any previous history	A previous history without a clear pathogenesis may be indicative of an emotional component

to ask, for instance, 'If I had a magic wand, what condition or problem would you like me to take away?' It is equally important to establish in each session from the patient's subjective point of view whether they feel that their expectations have been met.

The practitioner's expectations

Clinical experience suggests that some objective change will take place after the first session of manipulation should the main component of the voice problem be mechanical dysfunction (see section on treatment outcome). However, 'resisting' patients who are unable to tolerate manipulation may not report changes and may even complain that the symptoms have become worse. If other physiological aspects have been reliably excluded, this is usually indicative of a strong emotional component to the voice disorder. A shift in the clinical picture and in the patient's perception of his problem is to be expected after manipulation. The reason for this is that physical therapy is very direct and interferes with existing and unconscious neuromuscular patterns. If the techniques applied are effective, it is reasonable to expect some change in the patient's awareness to a change.

Symptoms of pain/discomfort

While taking the history, it is important for the practitioner to determine whether the symptoms of pain/discomfort, as presented by the patient, stem from the musculoskeletal system. Furthermore the practitioner must consider whether these symptoms represent a mechanical dysfunction (e.g. repetitive strain) or an underlying pathological process (e.g. tumour).

In summary, from the history the practitioner should have developed a much clearer understanding of the components in the aetiology of the patient's complaint. In particular, the relative importance of vocal hyperfunction, emotional issues and/or pathological components should be distinguishable, enabling the practitioner to construct an effective management plan.

Assessment: observation

This section covers posture, breathing and the larynx. A combination of open-ended and closed questions is useful when obtaining case-history material. This process can also be applied when gathering the observational data necessary for assessment. The open-ended observational section of assessment begins during the history-taking, while the patient is actively using spontaneous speech and natural body language. During the second phase, the patient stands passively while the practitioner observes specific details of their musculoskeletal system and then confirms the findings by palpation. The third phase is active for both patient and practitioner. The patient is asked to perform specific vocal tasks while the practitioner palpates the quality and range of movement in the relevant joints and muscles.

General posture and head position

Posture may be regarded as a contributing factor to the aetiology of dysphonia when it affects the position of the larynx and the breathing apparatus. In this context the following can be regarded as true posture-related dysphonias:

1. Spinal conditions affecting breathing: conditions such as scoliosis and ankylosing spondylitis that affect rib joint mobility and spinal symmetry will limit the movement of the rib cage, thereby disturbing the efficiency of breathing.
2. Habitual posture that results in spinal asymmetry may affect the position of the larynx. Rotation of the torso in relation to the lumbar and cervical spine will pull the larynx away from the midline, through the attachment of the inferior suspensory muscles. Equally, head position also affects the position of the larynx through the attachment of the superior suspensory muscles.

3.   Head position (Table 6.2) has a direct effect on the mechanism of voice
     production in the following manner:
     a) it affects the initial resting length of the suspensory muscles;
     b) A-P displacement (e.g. C/D shelf) changes the anatomical relationship of
         the laryngeal structures to both the power source and the resonators;
     c) hyperlordosis (accompanied by C/D shelf and cervical hyperextension)
         has a negative effect on the resonators;
     d) head tilt will interfere with symmetrical activity of the suspensory
         muscles.

Table 6.2 Head position	
Observe	**Abnormal findings**
Lateral view	Anterior/posterior weight bearing C/D shelf Exaggerated spinal curves, Hyperlordosis/kyphosis Double chin
Anterior view	Marked scoliosis Shape of rib cage Head tilt Cervical spine sidebending Deviated larynx Asymmetrical SCM Asymmetric jaw

Head position, lateral view

The position of the head affects the initial resting length of the suspensory
muscles. The suspensory muscle length in turn affects the position of the larynx in
the anterior compartment of the neck. It also affects the flexibility of vertical and
lateral movement. For example, where the neck is hyperextended, the suspensory
muscles will be stretched, thereby restricting laryngeal movement, particularly
vertically. In extreme cases the patient will find it difficult to swallow. He or she will
require extra extension of the head during swallowing to provide for the necessary
elevation of the larynx.

The term 'cervicodorsal shelf' (C/D shelf), is used to describe a situation
wherein the entire cervical spine is translated forward in relation to the first
thoracic vertebra, creating the famous 'widow's hump'. The C/D shelf, accompanied by a secondary hyperlordotic segment in the cervical spine, is the characteristic end-stage of this head position.

A lateral view of the patient allows assessment of the geniohyoid pull, which tends
to move the larynx anteriorly and can sometimes be identified with a 'double chin'.

Head position, anterior view

Head tilt and side-bending of the cervical spine may interfere with functional symmetry of the suspensory muscles. The vocal tract on the dropped side may be compressed. The restriction of the internal space created by this compression can often be observed on videostrobolaryngoscopy.

Posture has long been recognized as being of importance in voice production and vocal technique (the Alexander Technique; Feldenkrais, 1949). There has been little research, however, as to which aspects of posture have direct bearing on voice production. Vilkman et al. (1996) have investigated laryngeal position and how the pull of the suspensory muscles can affect fundamental frequency; information about other factors remains anecdotal. Posture relates directly to patterns of breathing and, although beyond the scope of this chapter, it should not be forgotten.

Clinically, two important functional abnormalities of posture appear to relate directly to the vocal mechanism. The first is laryngeal deviation from the midline and the second is hyperextension of the cervical spine with anterior translocation of the head (C/D shelf).

Laryngeal deviation

The two clinical vignettes that follow relate to laryngeal deviation.

A singer presented in clinic complaining of pain in the right anterior portion of the neck and loss of vocal quality and flexibility. At assessment he was found to have a marked deviation of the larynx to the right. Palpation confirmed that the pain was due to increased activity in his right superior suspensory muscles. Further investigation showed that the condition was related to rotation of his torso to the right with side-bending of the lumbar spine to the left. While it was possible to alleviate his symptoms with soft tissue manipulation of the hypertonic musculature, without postural correction to encourage counter-rotation of his torso to the midline his symptoms would have quickly recurred. Once the postural problem had been understood, it was possible for the patient to identify his habit of facing his audience, while rotating his torso on a fixed pelvis towards the conductor. This posture had developed to allow him to address his audience, while at the same time, remaining able to respond quickly to the conductor's cues.

A young bass-baritone presented in clinic unable to sing unless his head was fixed in a certain position. On assessment he was found to have a deviated larynx and long-standing postural problems. Whenever he tried to alter his head position, he seemed to 'lose touch' with his vocal mechanism and was unable to sing. 'Losing touch' in this context refers to the loss of neuromuscular feedback owing to changes in his habitual posture. This caused acute discomfort to develop in his strap muscles unilaterally, as they became asymmetrically overused.

C/D shelf

Clinically, there appears to be a high incidence of patients presenting to our clinic with marked hyperextension of the cervical spine and anterior translation of the head. Characteristically, the anterior neck musculature becomes stretched and hypertonic, particularly the superior and inferior suspensory muscles, depriving the patient of the flexibility required to alter laryngeal position at different pitches. In some patients the cervicodorsal shelf is associated with neurological signs of numbness and pain radiating down the arm. Where this occurs, patients also suffer from chronic pain and aching in the neck and shoulders.

When the anatomical links between the head, torso and larynx are reviewed, the significance of posture to voice production becomes obvious. Related issues include temporomandibular joint dysfunction and body misalignment resulting from conditions such as short-leg syndrome or scoliosis. We are also aware of the importance of the powerful posterior neck muscles and their relationship to C/D shelf, headaches, etc. Although these are beyond the scope of this chapter, they should not be overlooked.

A degree of asymmetrical muscle activity can be regarded as 'normal' (we are all either right- or left-handed). However, in the long run it is likely that asymmetrical muscle use will contribute to mechanical dysfunction owing to the necessity for one muscle group to work harder in order to compensate for the less active group. An example of asymmetrical muscle use can be seen in patients who constantly tilt the head away from the midline. It is likely that the muscles on the opposite side, pulling the weight of the skull, will become hypertonic in their attempts to oppose the tilt and gravitational forces.

Breathing

The observational assessment would be incomplete without at least briefly considering the breathing pattern and laryngeal movement during speech. The therapist should observe the respiratory rate and quality (rapidity, shallowness, etc.), and try to identify the overall pattern of breathing (e.g. diaphragmatic, upper chest, etc). He or she should also observe for appropriate air usage during phonation. Does the patient repeatedly phonate with an inadequate breath or subglottic pressure? (A description of breathing is given in Chapter 4.)

Laryngeal movement: how much activity is observed

While taking the case history, one could observe and note:

1. the range and direction of vertical laryngeal movement;
2. any asymmetry of activity of the suspensory muscles on left and right;
3. any obliquity of laryngeal movement during speech and swallowing (This should not be confused with laryngeal deviation from the midline observed while the patient is 'at rest'. This latter finding is associated with postural asymmetry.);
4. patterns of activity in the observable suspensory muscles that anchor the larynx. In particular watch for obvious omohyoid activity;
5. the quality of active swallowing (head extension sign). Some patients appear to assist their swallow by using extra extension of the head. This may indicate tight strap muscles and an habitually raised larynx.

Assessment: palpation

It should be noted that in this section we are referring to active manoeuvres carried out either to assess muscle quality or to assess deep lying structures.

The practitioner now actively palpates the laryngeal musculature and neck extensors in order to assess the following:

1. the position of the larynx;
2. the quality of the tissues: is there a marked difference in the bulk of individual muscles between the sides; do they feel 'fibrotic', i.e. is there a limited capacity to deform or elongate on active palpation?;
3. muscle tone;
4. range of joint movement;
5. any irregular anatomical features;
6. pain and tenderness stemming from muscle tissue, joint capsules and ligaments. Particular attention is given to looking for tenderness at the tendino-osseous junction. (This is highly significant in manual therapy and where there is no pathological cause, usually indicates increased muscular activity and fatigue.)

Readers should refer to Appendix 6.2 for the full list.

Sternocleidomastoid muscles and lower anterior neck (Figure 6.11)

The practitioner should evaluate for hypertonicity, asymmetry and fibrotic changes. Particular attention should be paid to the suprasternal notch: is there reduced space between the sternal heads?; is there marked tracheal irritability/coughing?; what are the sternohyoid and sternothyroid muscles like at rest?; at what level is the larynx resting in the neck? The patient's response to the examination may be revealing. For instance, a response of a violent cough to even the lightest palpation of the thyroid notch in some patients coincides with a high degree of tension, resistance and ambivalence to treatment.

This is particularly important for male professional voice-users (e.g. bass-baritones) who anchor the larynx low in the neck to maintain resonance. Over time they may lose flexibility of vocal range. The larynx descends with age. In some elderly male patients the larynx may have dropped so low that the cricoid lies below the level of the sternal notch and is therefore difficult to palpate. The sternal notch and the state of the surrounding muscles is also one key to 'successful' physical management of the globus patient.

Larynx

Lateral laryngeal movement

Lateral laryngeal movement is defined as the amount of lateral displacement of the larynx away from the midline as the practitioner grasps the thyroid cartilage and shifts the larynx laterally.

The practitioner should evaluate the quality of 'lateral shift', looking for uni- or bilateral anchoring. A distinction should be made between diminished lateral movement due to chronically hypertonic muscles and that found in anxious patients due to 'holding' (or guarding) the larynx. A 'held' larynx can be relaxed but the chronically hypertonic larynx cannot. In some patients the larynx appears impacted against (or held very close to) the anterior vertebral column, which interferes with lateral shift.

Laryngeal rotation

Laryngeal rotation is defined by the practitioner's capacity to palpate the posterior margin of the thyroid cartilage on either side and to rotate it with the fingertips towards the opposite side. If the right margin is palpable and some rotation is possible towards the opposite side, the larynx may be said to be habitually rotated anticlockwise. Inability to rotate the larynx to either (or both) sides will give a rough indication as to the state of muscular tension. In this manoeuvre the practitioner can also assess the state of some of the perilaryngeal musculature, particularly the inferior constrictor and the posterior cricoarytenoid muscles.

Hyoid position

The hyoid bone (Figure 6.2) is the principal structure from which the larynx is suspended. The best way to feel the hyoid bone is first to find the body of the hyoid with the middle finger, and then to slide the finger and thumb back along the greater horns while waggling the bone from side to side. Doing this provides the

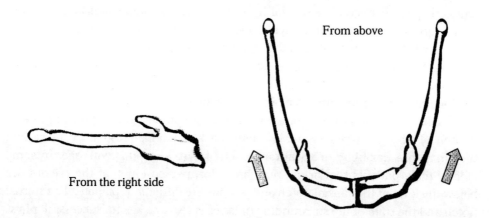

From above

From the right side

Figure 6.2 The hyoid bone

sensation of the rigid structure beneath the fingers. It also displaces the carotid sheath backwards. Practitioners with a medical background may be more accustomed to 'balloting' the bone between the fingers of both hands while standing behind the patient.

The hyoid bone has no joint connecting it to any other bone. Therefore any forces operating directly on it will affect the position of the larynx. If the superior

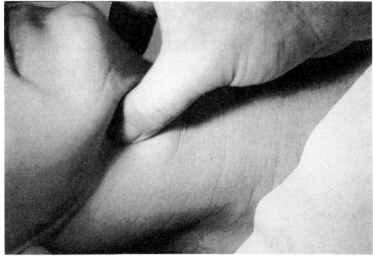

(Photo: Tom Harris)

Figure 6.3 Palpation of the hyoid bone

border of the hyoid bone is palpable the hyoid is considered to be in a neutral position. Occasionally the hyoid position is felt to be rather low. This finding may indicate lack of tonus in the superior suspensory muscles or excessive pull by the inferior suspensory strap muscles. The examiner should determine if the hyoid bone is palpable or tucked up under the mandible. Angulation and tilt of the hyoid bone are important. An acute angle with relationship to the mandible suggests tight posterior hyoglossus or stylohyoid muscles or anterior thyrohyoid ligaments. Lateral tilting of the hyoid bone may be related either to unilateral hypertonicity (tightness) of the superior suspensory muscles or to the unilateral pull of a tight thyrohyoid muscle. When the hyoid bone appears to be pulled forward anteriorly, a tight geniohyoid muscle is suspected, giving the patient the appearance of a short lower jaw.

Rotation of the hyoid bone is identified when a greater horn cannot be palpated posteriorly. Normally the posterior horns should be palpable bilaterally. Where one horn is palpable while the other is not, the hyoid is considered to be rotated towards the non-palpable side.

Note: The description of the listed palpatory findings and their significance is by no means exhaustive. The observations described above are based on the most common clinical findings but the practitioner should always bear in mind all the forces that can operate on the hyoid bone and consider each individually as well as collectively. This should apply to all the palpatory findings given in this book.

Superior suspensory muscles

The superior suspensory muscle group consists of: stylohyoid, geniohyoid, hyoglossus, mylohyoid, and anterior and posterior bellies of digastric (Figure 6.4).

Palpatory findings

Palpate the lateral surface of the hyoid bone. Assess its position in relation to the angle of the jaw (Figure 6.3). Assess lateral movement of the hyoid bone away

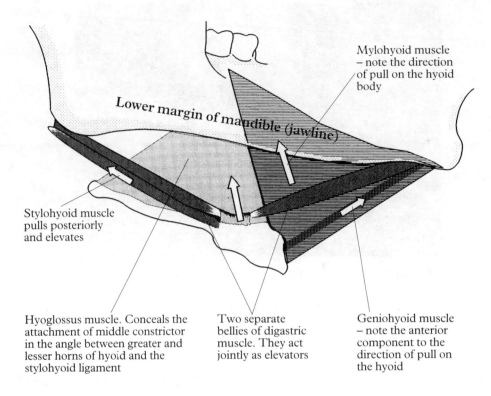

Mylohyoid muscle
– note the direction
of pull on the hyoid
body

Lower margin of mandible (jawline)

Stylohyoid muscle
pulls posteriorly
and elevates

Hyoglossus muscle. Conceals the
attachment of middle constrictor
in the angle between greater and
lesser horns of hyoid and the
stylohyoid ligament

Two separate
bellies of digastric
muscle. They act
jointly as elevators

Geniohyoid muscle
– note the anterior
component to the
direction of pull on
the hyoid

Figure 6.4 The suprahyoid muscles: superior suspensory group

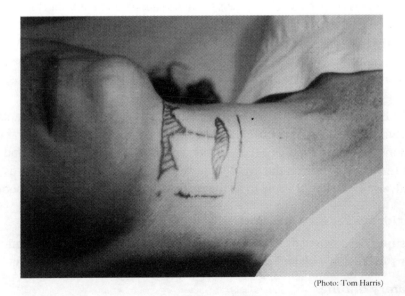

(Photo: Tom Harris)

Figure 6.5i Thyroid cartilage, anterior arch of the cricoid and thyrohyoid membrane marked
on the neck

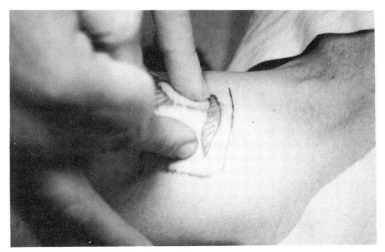

Figure 6.6 Palpation of the thyrohyoid muscles

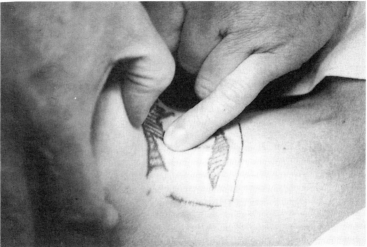

Figure 6.7 Opening the thyrohyoid gap

(Photos: Tom Harris)

from the midline. Clinically, it appears that a relaxed suprahyoid musculature will enable the hyoid bone to drop about half an inch below the angle of the jaw. A high hyoid may be tucked into the angle of the jaw. A larynx that is anchored down may depress the hyoid. Tenderness, unilateral tilting of the hyoid bone, rotation or any other combination can be found (see above).

Thyrohyoid space/gap

The relative size of the space (distance) between the hyoid bone and thyroid cartilage is assessed. It is logical to assume (although this author has not been able to identify any quantitative standards in the literature) that a reasonable space should exist between these two structures to accommodate changes in the length of the vocal tract (Aronson, 1985) (Figures 6.6, 6.9). Clinically, in patients presenting with hyperfunctional symptoms, there is a high incidence wherein the thyrohyoid gap is absent or diminished along its entire length. This finding is often combined with pain or tenderness along the thyrohyoid membrane or the thyrohyoid muscle.

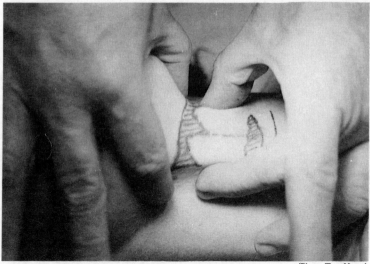

(Photo: Tom Harris)

Figure 6.8 Opening the thyrohyoid gap

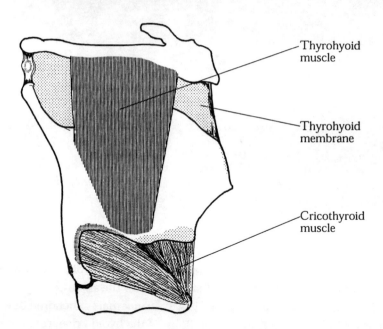

Thyrohyoid
muscle

Thyrohyoid
membrane

Cricothyroid
muscle

Figure 6.9 The thyrohyoid gap

Occasionally, the hyoid does not lie in the same anterior-posterior plane as the thyroid cartilage and can be palpated either lying in front of or behind the thyroid notch. The hyoid can also deviate laterally in relation to the superior margin of the thyroid. The reason for the deviation should be carefully analysed to identify any muscular dysfunction.

Geniohyoid muscles

For further anatomical detail concerning the geniohyoid muscles refer to Chapter 1.

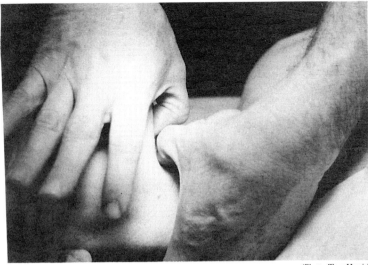

(Photo: Tom Harris)

Figure 6.10 Stretching the geniohyoid muscles

Palpatory findings (Figure 6.10)

The muscle forms part of the floor of the mouth and can be located between the symphysis menti anteriorly and the hyoid bone. A short space between the hyoid and the symphysis will indicate chronically shortened and tight geniohyoid muscles. Occasionally geniohyoid hyperfunction presents as tenderness and general rigidity, combined with an anterior larynx position well forward from the vertebral column. In the extreme situation the chin almost seems to blend with the thyroid cartilage.

The inferior suspensory muscles

These are the sternothyroid and sternohyoid muscles.

Palpatory findings

These muscles are long with thin bellies that are difficult to assess by direct palpation. None the less, their quality can be inferred by assessing the resting level of the larynx and by stretching it upwards and laterally.

Abnormal findings include a low 'anchored' larynx, particularly in professional voice-users who have been taught to sing on an habitually lowered larynx. Typically, 'globus' patients will experience some relief from their symptoms when these muscles are stretched and relaxed. An improvement in vocal range will also be noticed after relaxation of these muscles. Hyperactivity in these muscles may be related to symptoms of chronic dry cough and irritation.

Cricothyroid visor mechanism

The cricothyroid visor mechanism is of critical importance to normal laryngeal function, yet it has a relatively small range of movement and the cricothyroid muscles operating about the two joints are also relatively small (see Chapter 5). As palpatory skills improve, however, it is possible to assess the quality and range of cricoid movement in relation to the thyroid and vice versa (see Blaugrund, Taira and Isshiki, 1991).

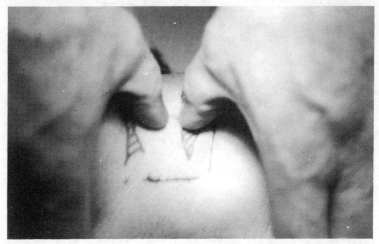

(Photo: Tom Harris)

Figure 6.11 Opening the cricothyroid visor

It is likewise possible to assess the cricothyroid muscles for tenderness, hypertonicity and difference in muscle bulk between sides. Little has been written about the resting position of the cricothyroid joint (Vilkman et al., 1996), but it is reasonable to assume that the joint is likely to 'rest' somewhere in the mid-range between maximum opening and closure. Clinically, in patients presenting with endstage hyperkinetic dysphonia there is a high incidence of an habitually closed cricothyroid visor. Other common findings associated with dysphonia and fatigue are the cricothyroid visor that is 'locked' in the mid-range position; the visor that closes normally at higher pitches, but that fails to open fully in order to produce a comfortable lower pitch range (chest voice). Clinically, it is noted that the cricothyroid visor may not only show a reduced range of movement but can also lock in any position about its main axis of movement.

Palpatory findings (Figure 6.11)

Palpate the anterior 'gap' between the cricoid arch and the thyroid cartilage with the larynx at rest. Both the gap and the anterior cricoid rim should be clearly palpable, but findings can range between full opening and closure. Tenderness will indicate tightness and fatigue. Not infrequently, a prominent anterior cricoid arch is palpable (i.e. the cricoid arch projects anteriorly beneath the lower border of the thyroid cartilage). This indicates that in addition to vertical rotation about the axis through the cricothyroid joints, there is also an element of anterior translation (gliding) of the cricoid under the thyroid. We are still uncertain whether this is a physiological or pathological movement. It may relate to a failure of joint stabilization by the posterior oblique portion of the cricothyroid muscles with consequent stretching of the joint capsules and anteroinferior ligaments, or may be due to flexion in the cartilage of the inferior horns of the thyroid cartilage. A rarer finding is a cricoid arch that is pulled back posteriorly. It is important to remember that our clinical data are based on palpatory findings that cannot always take anatomical variation into account, but can be verified at indirect laryngoscopy while the patient performs a vocal task that requires a change from mid-range to high or low pitches.

Cricothyroid muscles

These muscles have two bellies: one runs obliquely backwards to stabilize the cricothyroid joint, the other ascends more steeply and rotates the joint, closing the visor (see Chapter 1).

Palpatory findings

The examiner can palpate the cricothyroid gap anteriorly, then move both index fingers laterally around and above the anterior third of the cricoid ring, feeling for the bellies of the muscles. Significant abnormal findings include tenderness and difference in muscle bulk between the sides.

The pharyngeal constrictors

These include the inferior, middle and superior constrictors. The inferior constrictor has two bodies, the crico- and thyropharyngeus. The constrictors of both sides join with each other in a thin, firm fibrous raphe posteriorly. Despite a tissue plane that runs between this and the structures of the spine, the raphe provides a degree of fibrous connection posteriorly between the larynx and skeleton.

Palpatory findings

The quality of the constrictor muscles can be judged using a specific manoeuvre. The larynx is lifted anteriorly and rotated laterally away from the midline. This uncovers and stretches the inferior constrictor muscles on one side and they can then be palpated behind the cricoid and the posterior border of thyroid cartilage.

Abnormal findings of hypertonic musculature are identified where the specific movements of the assessment manoeuvre are not possible. Reasons for failure of this manoeuvre include a 'held' larynx, unilateral anchoring, rotation or other combination.

The posterior cricoarytenoid muscles and cricoarytenoid joints

The arytenoid cartilages are palpable and their range of movement can be assessed. It is equally possible to assess the quality of the posterior cricoarytenoid and interarytenoid muscles that attach to these cartilages posteriorly and to compare them for tenderness and hypertonicity. Manipulative techniques can also be applied to them where necessary. However, the manoeuvres necessary to examine the cricoarytenoid joints are beyond the scope of this chapter as they require highly specialized palpatory skills and techniques.

Manipulative management: aims and treatment plan

The history and assessment of dysphonic patients by the manual therapist should result in a functional diagnosis and management plan. However, treatment requires a flexible approach, guided by the patient's response, rather than a rigid plan that is devised in advance and then followed religiously over a set number of sessions. None the less, even though the actual treatment techniques are adjusted as necessary as the treatment progresses, clear aims can and should be identified prior to treatment.

For the purposes of discussion, the aetiological factors in dysphonia (which drive the aims of the treatment plan) will be divided into the factors affecting:

1.   General posture including head position.
2.   Laryngeal posture:
     (a) the suspensory muscles
         (i) suprahyoid
         (ii) infrahyoid
     (b) the thyrohyoid complex
     (c) the cricothyroid joints
     (d) the intrinsic laryngeal muscles.
3.   Other muscle groups.

It should be noted that, in reality, these factors are always inextricably interlinked.

Relaxation

Relaxation of a voluntary muscle can be defined as the achievement of the maximum resting length of that muscle after activity. In order to maintain efficient and appropriate muscle tone the concept of relaxation is important, but it is easily taken for granted. A major problem for patients is that they lack the proprioceptive ability to recognize when they continue to 'hold' muscles in their active state, i.e. contracted and bulky. This seems to be due to deeply ingrained neuromuscular habits. As a result, muscles constantly held in this state may become permanently shortened and fibrotic so that the patient is no longer able to truly relax them, even if they knew how. Passive techniques of postural correction, such as the Alexander technique, often fail to take into account that these patients may be unable to correct their posture owing to areas in the spine that are rigid and stiff with shortened and fibrotic muscles. It will require direct manipulation to restore the joint mobility so that postural correction can take place without compensatory movement elsewhere in the system.

Clinical observation suggests that muscles rarely return to their original resting length following activity unless external measures are applied, such as massage or stretching. A common mistake when working with patients is to draw attention to a tight muscle group and ask the patient to relax. Frequently they will respond with an apologetic 'I'm trying to relax', but the more they try the less likely they are to release tension and any useful experience is lost. Learning cannot take place when patients are feeling anxious and accused or while they are actively 'trying to please' the practitioner. It is paradoxical to expect a patient who is 'trying' so hard to be able to relax.

As a failure to relax muscles after activity is tantamount to hyperfunction, and voice production requires constant complex muscular activity, it is easy to see why the application of the manual therapist's approach and techniques have so much to offer in the overall evaluation and treatment of dysphonia. Voice production is a deeply unconscious activity for most patients, the patterns of which were laid down very early in life and are frequently affected or altered by emotion. Conscious awareness of sensation in the laryngeal area is likewise limited and the combination of these factors produces fertile ground for the development of hyperfunctional or dysfunctional muscle activity.

Provided simple and sensible guidelines are followed, manipulation is a safe, non-invasive and reliable form of treatment. Never take chances. The following points should always be considered prior to manipulative treatment to ensure the safety of both patient and practitioner.

Postural correction

Although there is considerable debate as to whether lasting postural changes can be effected, clinical experience suggests that patients can increase their 'body awareness' and effect lasting improvement in their symptoms. They are also able to develop some understanding of the way in which their emotional patterns can contribute to their physical symptoms.

Initially, the manual therapist alters postural patterns through passive manipulation, thereby interfering with the established neuromuscular patterns that had determined the patient's habitual posture and body language. The patient can then experience the new posture and the increased freedom of movement it allows. Usually pain and tenderness will decrease as posture, muscle length and tone alter with manipulation. The problem is that the patient has to find some way of 'holding on to' or repeating the new posture for treatment to be successful. Similar problems occur when altering breathing patterns and this topic is dealt with in Chapter 8.

As changes are introduced into the system of habitual neuromuscular patterns through the passive manipulative techniques, the practitioner will begin to introduce 'muscle energy techniques' (see Appendix 6.3 of this chapter) The practitioner is aiming to stretch or to strengthen a specific muscle working in the plane of its action while the patient either assists or resists according to the practitioner's instructions.

Once the practitioner is satisfied that the patient has internalized the new neuromuscular pattern (habits) for the new posture or muscle activity, a set of exercises to reinforce it can be commenced. The success of treatment is dependent, to some extent, on the ability of the practitioner to communicate what is required to the patient.

Techniques

Some of the most useful specific techniques will now be described. However, the reader is advised to follow the assessment protocol given in Appendix 6.2 (Lieberman protocol) and bear in mind the principles that form the basis of manual therapy. The techniques will be described in the order that they have been presented in

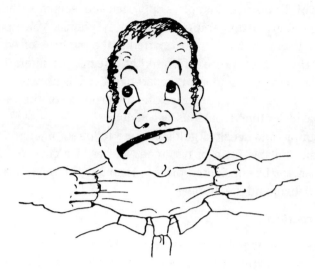

'...active techniques where these are applicable'

the treatment plan, with passive techniques described first, followed by active techniques where these are applicable. Finally, exercises are described that help to establish the new neuromuscular patterns.

Caveat. Any manual therapy technique applied to the anterior compartment of the neck should avoid deep pressure and keep anterior to the neurovascular bundle and carotid body. Energetic posterior displacement of the sheath or inadvertent compression of major vessels can cause precipitous loss of blood pressure, or even loosen atheromatous plaques in the elderly. The hyoid bone and the laryngeal cartilages are delicate structures. The practitioner needs to be entirely familiar with their shape and function and carry out the treatment techniques with care.

General posture

The patient's general posture is assessed using the concept of an imaginary 'plumb line' that runs through the patient's ear, shoulder and hip so that the weight is carried between the ball and middle of the foot. Where the weight is carried anterior or posterior to this line the spinal curves will become exaggerated. With prolonged muscular imbalance the lumbar spine can become hyperlordotic and the thoracic spine hyperkyphotic. There is anterior translation of the head position, leading to a CD shelf, hyperlordotic cervical spine and hyperextension of the atlanto-occipital joint (Figure 6.12).

The aim of manual therapy here is to reduce excessive curvature. Because of the way in which the spine is structured, the thoracic spine has relatively little mobility. As a result, it is the area most likely to become stiff or fixed, partly because of its inherent structure and partly because of the habitual postural patterns developed by patients. These two features seem to be inextricably linked and often prove to be the key to many postural problems.

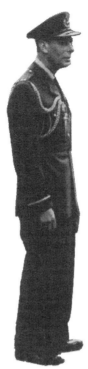

Figure 6.12 An example of posterior weight-bearing with a resultant kyphosis and an hyperlordotic cervical spine

Correction of the CD shelf usually depends on improving mobility in the upper thoracic segments. The most effective techniques for achieving this increased mobility are:

1. high velocity thrust (HVT);
2. soft tissue techniques;
3. springing of specific segments.

HVT is a technique designed to achieve relative movement between two adjacent spinal segments that are stuck together. As the stiffness is released there is a characteristic click such as would be heard when people crack their finger joints. This is known as 'gapping'. This technique should only be attempted by experienced professional manual therapists.

Soft tissue techniques include stretching, kneading, inhibition and rhythmic traction.

Springing aims to improve mobility between two adjacent segments, but uses different levers and does not necessarily aim to 'click' or 'gap' the joint.

The choice of technique is a function of the patient's age, state of the spine and the underlying pathologies. Soft tissue techniques such as stretching are considered to be the safest.

To achieve improvement of thoracic mobility, chest muscles, such as pectoralis major and minor, will need to be stretched to accommodate thoracic extension. Once the mechanics of the thoracic spine have been improved, posterior translation of the whole cervical spine becomes possible. This translation can be achieved

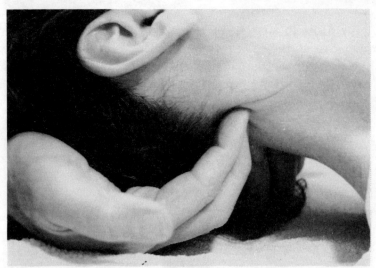

Figure 6.13 Position of the fingers under the occiput for stretching the suboccipital muscles

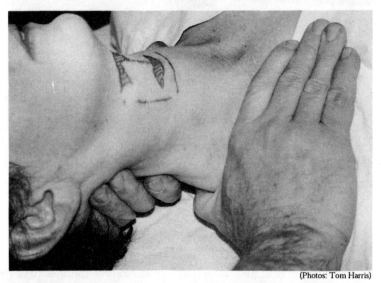

(Photos: Tom Harris)

Figure 6.14 Position of the hands for neck traction with lowering of the right shoulder

by stretching the anterior cervical flexor group of muscles, particularly the sterno-cleidomastoid. Flexion movement at the atlanto-occipital joint can be improved by intensive stretching of the suboccipital group of muscles (Figure 6.13). Another important part of this work is the need to improve rib cage mobility, as stiffness developing here can exacerbate related postural problems.

Many of these techniques require expert knowledge and training and are best done by a professional. However, improving the patient's awareness of postural problems together with advice on stretching exercises can still be helpful.

The following exercise is useful: the patient lies supine on the floor with knees flexed and feet apart. The chin should be tucked in and the hands linked and stretched back above the head. The patient is advised to breathe deeply and to make certain that the lower back does not arch while the arms are stretched up and back above the head. Gravity stretches and relaxes the muscles allowing the weight of the arms to stretch the rib cage through the attachment of the pectoralis muscles, thus extending the dorsal spine. To improve this technique one can put a small rolled towel under the occiput to ensure full flexion at the atlanto-occipital joint.

Deviation of the larynx from the midline, associated with thoracic rotation, responds to postural correction. Derotation of the torso may involve correction of thoracic scoliosis and should only be done by an expert.

Laryngeal posture

Within this group, special attention is given to the assessment, diagnosis and treatment of dysfunction of specific elements of the larynx and the vocal tract.

Aims of treatment

The overall treatment aim is the improvement in joint mobility, restoration of symmetry to muscle function and, most important, bringing to the conscious level the habitual abnormal postural patterns that need to be corrected.

Specific treatment aims include:

1. stretching and relaxing of hypertonic muscles;
2. improving CT joint movement by direct joint articulation as well as soft tissue techniques to surrounding musculature;
3. improving the function of the thyrohyoid mechanism by specific soft tissue work on associated musculature.

(a) Suspensory muscles

(i) Suprahyoid suspensory group

The suprahyoid suspensory musculature includes the geniohyoid, genioglossus, hyoglossus, mylohyoid, styloglossus and stylohyoid muscles. They are important in positioning the tongue and in swallowing. When these muscles become tight and shortened they need to be stretched in order to allow the larynx freedom of movement in the antero-posterior plane (Figures 6.7, 6.8 and 6.10).

The patient lies comfortably supine, with the head gently stabilized by the practitioner's hand. The tissues between the angle of the jaw and the superior border of the hyoid bone are pushed downwards and towards the contralateral side, gently stretching the suprahyoid muscles unilaterally. The same technique is then applied in the same way to the muscle group on the opposite side. As the suprahyoid muscles relax, it should be possible to feel the entire superior surface of the hyoid bone. Once this is possible, the hyoid bone itself can be used as a lever, and the stretching process continued using the thumb of one hand to push the superior border of the hyoid bone downwards and laterally, while the other hand continues to support the patient's head. The same process is repeated for the contralateral side.

Active resistance manoeuvre for the suprahyoid muscles

An example of an active resistance manoeuvre for the suprahyoid muscle group would be where the patient is asked to swallow while the practitioner presses gently down on the superior border of the hyoid bone, resisting the upward hyoid movement.

(ii) Infrahyoid suspensory muscles

The infrahyoid suspensory musculature includes the sternohyoid and sternothyroid muscles.

To stretch the sternothyroid muscles, they are stabilized with the thumb of one hand, while the other exerts an upward and lateral pressure on the thyroid cartilage (Figure 6.15). The same manoeuvre is repeated for the contralateral side. Bilateral stretching of these muscles can be achieved using the anterior cricoid arch as a lever and lifting it upwards. A similar technique is used for the thyrohyoid muscle, when the hyoid bone is stabilized with one hand and the muscle is gently stretched with the other. Unilateral stretching applied individually to the sternohyoid or sternothyroid can be particularly helpful where asymmetry is detected.

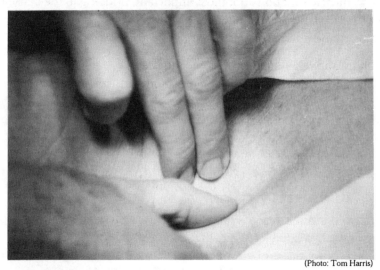

(Photo: Tom Harris)

Figure 6.15 Position of the fingers for stretching the right sternomastoid muscles

Posterior translocation of the neck, reduction of excessive lordosis of the cervical spine and hyperextension of the atlanto-occipital joint all help to achieve relaxation of these muscles.

Non-specific stretching of the entire strap muscle system can be applied by using the whole larynx as a lever, pushing it laterally from side to side, while the patient's head is stabilized or rotated to the contralateral side. Equally, an anterior stretch can be applied if the larynx is not held in a retracted position.

(b) The thyrohyoid complex (Figures 6.6, 6.7, 6.8 and 6.9)

Special attention should be given to the thyrohyoid muscle complex, which has an important role in controlling the length of the vocal tract and in altering pitch.

Place the thumb and first finger of one hand on the inferior border of the hyoid bone and the thumb and first finger of the other hand on the superior border of the thyroid cartilage. The thyrohyoid muscles can than be directly stretched by gently pulling these two structures apart.

Another useful technique is to shear the hyoid bone away from the thyroid carti-lage by exerting gentle pressure on the hyoid bone to shift it laterally, while exerting gentle pressure on the thyroid cartilage laterally in the opposite direction. Direct soft tissue techniques can also be applied to the belly of the thyrohyoid muscle.

(c) Cricothyroid joint and muscles (Figures 6.9 and 6.11)

The cricothyroid joint (CT joint) is the principal joint in the tensor mechanism. It can become restricted in its range of movements. It may be held constantly closed, causing the vocal folds to be permanently stretched and lengthened (assuming that the arytenoids maintain some opposition and do not collapse anteriorly), or in a mid-open position, from which it can close but not open further. Rarely it can be held open, thus preventing the vocal folds from lengthening and seriously reducing the higher pitch range.

Because the CT joint is the fulcrum of the main lever, it is mandatory to improve its function if it is damaged or limited. This is best achieved by direct articulation of the joint, using the thumb of one hand to pull down on the anterior aspect of the cricoid arch inferiorly, while stabilizing the laryngeal cartilage at the level of the insertion of the cricothyroid muscle with the thumb of the other hand. Gentle pressure can be applied to both cartilages, gradually increasing the gap between them to articulate the joint into its open position.

During inspiration it is also possible to combine the opening effect of tracheal pull on the joint to assist the opening of the visor, which is held in a closed position. Another useful direct technique involves cupping the thyroid cartilage between the thumb and second finger and the cricoid arch in a similar grip with the other hand, and rotating each cartilage about the vertical axis of the larynx. The patient can often assist in the manoeuvres by producing a low pitched yawn or vocal creak, either of which will tend to shorten the vocal folds and open the CT joint.

The cricothyroid muscles are the principal muscles of the tensor mechanism. They can be accessed directly for soft tissue techniques. These techniques can be applied specifically to both the oblique and vertical bellies of the cricothyroid muscle bilaterally or unilaterally.

(d) The intrinsic laryngeal musculature

Palpable muscles to be considered in this domain include the muscles anchoring the vocal folds posteriorly, the posterior cricoarytenoid (PCA) muscles and some of the muscles involved in isometric positioning of the arytenoid cartilage/cricoary-tenoid joint movement, PCA, and indirectly, lateral cricoarytenoid (LCA) and interarytenoid.

In addition, although they are not classified as 'intrinsic' laryngeal muscles, for treatment purposes we include the pharyngeal constrictor muscles in this group.

In general, these muscle groups are far less accessible than those described previously. They can be treated specifically using manual techniques, but these necessarily involve working on the posterior aspect of the larynx, which has to be palpated across the lateral pharyngeal wall. Accessing the intrinsic muscles and applying the techniques requires a great deal of palpatory skill to identify and differentiate these small structures and to assess muscle tone and the quality of the cricoarytenoid joint movement. It also requires sensitivity and skill to introduce the patient to these techniques as they are likely to feel anxious and protective of their airway. These factors make discussion of specific treatment for the intrinsic muscles beyond the scope of this chapter.

Other muscles groups

Musculature related to the temporomandibular joint (TMJ)

TMJ-related symptoms may be part of the complex of vocal dysfunction. Patients who hold the jaw habitually clenched, suffer from painful asymmetrical jaw opening or report nocturnal grinding of the teeth are all likely to benefit from manipulative techniques applied to the TMJ system. The muscles associated with TMJ function (and dysfunction) are all powerful and include the masseter, temporalis and pterygoid (medial and lateral). Specific treatment involves articulation of the TMJ joint and the application of soft tissue techniques to the associated muscles listed above.

Sternocleidomastoid muscle (SCM)

It is usually necessary to relax the SCM before the strap muscles become accessible. Soft tissue stretching techniques to these muscles should only be applied unilaterally. The stretch should be applied superficially and laterally only because of the close proximity of this muscle to the carotid body and the carotid sheath and its inclusions. The location of the carotid sinus and the effects of manipulation thereon must be constantly kept in mind by the practitioner during this procedure.

Palatal muscles

Soft tissue techniques can be applied directly to the palatal musculature intraorally. Intraoral work is, however, invasive for the patient and is best carried out by a well qualified and experienced practitioner.

Treatment outcome following specific laryngeal manipulation: pitch control mechanism and vocal tract

The following list summarizes the potential benefits of specific manipulation to the larynx, pitch mechanism and vocal tract. Obviously the practitioner will concentrate on the presenting symptoms during treatment so not all patients will report all of these benefits.

1. An immediate drop in pitch.
2. Decrease in hoarseness (when present and not due to pathology of the vocal folds).

3. Ease of swallowing and feeling of 'openness'. Disappearance of sensation of lump in the throat.
4. Decrease in pain and discomfort.
5. Increase in vocal stamina and flexibility (improvement in range and better negotiation of the *passaggio*).
6. Improved control of vibrato.
7. Increase in resonance.
8. Decrease in associated symptoms (e.g. catarrh, sore throats, etc.).
9. Specific reduction of tenderness over the thyrohyoid muscles and membranes.
10. Elimination of laryngeal 'click' during swallowing and reduction of laryngeal crepitus.
11. Decrease in visible muscular activity in the anterior neck compartment during speech and singing.

Some of the above treatment benefits correlate well with improved vocal function that is observable during follow-up laryngoscopy. The following changes in laryngeal 'set' or posture may be seen:

• reduction in lateral compression of supraglottic structures;
• reduction in excessive interarytenoid compression with overlapping of the apices and/or anterior collapse of the arytenoids;
• improved symmetry of arytenoid adduction with greater phase symmetry of the mucosal wave generation;
• reduction in false fold constriction (medialization and lateral compression);
• improved vocal fold apposition;
• elongation of the vocal tract representing a greater range of cricothyroid joint movement.

Sometimes the aims of therapy are not simply restricted to resolving the physical symptoms. Some of the broader benefits of manipulative therapy are described below:

1. Improved control over specific muscle groups. People are rarely aware of the way in which they perform mechanical tasks. As a result, muscular activity tends to spread outside the group of muscles that are required for a specific task, giving rise to a more global muscular response. For example, when learning new physical activities, such as playing the piano, tension can not only be observed locally in the fingers, hands and lower arm, but throughout the body. Manipulation helps to develop an increased awareness of the individual muscle groups, allowing physical activity to become more efficient and less exhausting.
2. Improved healing/recovery time following injury. Although patients can always relapse or damage themselves, clinical observation suggests that recovery from injury is faster following manipulation. It has been suggested that relaxation of the tissues leads to an increase in blood flow and lymphatic drainage, which may be responsible for the improvements in healing and/or recovery time.

3.   The somatizing patient begins to acknowledge emotional difficulties as being an integral part of the voice problem. The patient may then be able to accept counselling, or a full course of psychotherapy as being the most appropriate form of treatment.

Caveat: Some patients report a 'cure' following one session of manipulation. These 'miracles', while very flattering, should be treated with caution by the practitioner as they may well be indicative of strong emotional factors in the aetiology of the condition. Real injuries, or habitual patterns of muscular misuse, always take time to heal or alter, so it is important to determine why the patient has had such a speedy resolution of their symptoms. Sometimes patients are not really 'much better' but are either afraid of losing hope, or are unable to tolerate their own disappointment at their failure to improve. Sometimes they are simply anxious to please their therapist. Other patients are genuinely better because their symptoms were largely psychosomatic and they have responded to the care and attention offered by their therapist. Occasionally patients with psychosomatic conditions become anxious with good care and attention, in case the therapist should uncover the real emotional reasons for their condition. These patients may take a 'flight into health' to protect themselves from getting in touch with painful feelings or facing up to difficult situations in their lives. There may be many other reasons, but they all tend to be emotionally based and form a part of the patient/practitioner relationship.

Contraindications and side effects: physical and emotional considerations

Physical considerations

1.   Local organic pathologies that might affect bones and soft tissue (e.g. painful scars).
2.   Anatomy that deviates from the normal, e.g. enlarged/prominent carotid bodies, ossified stylohyoid ligaments.
3.   Systemic conditions, e.g. heart failure, known carotid arteriopathy, diabetes, rheumatoid arthritis, osteoporosis, severe cervical osteoarthritis and cervical spine instability.
4.   Patients who bruise easily (e.g. those on anticoagulants) can undergo manipulation but will require a particularly gentle approach as well as reassurance.
5.   Patients with eye conditions (such as detached retina) must be treated with care. Patients who experience excessive pain and discomfort during manipulation may tense up rather than communicate their discomfort to the practitioner and increase their intra-abdominal pressure. The increase in pressure may, in turn, trigger detachment of the retina in patients who are vulnerable. While not directly a result of manipulation, the detached retina may occur indirectly in response to it.
6.   Neurological diseases. Musculoskeletal dysfunction resulting from neurological damage or disease may also respond to manipulation, but the aims of treat-

ment can no longer be regarded as 'curative'. Instead the practitioner works to alleviate pain and discomfort and to help the patient maintain some level of fine control for as long as possible.

Emotional considerations and contraindications: absolute or relative

1. The 'held' or guarded larynx (see section on diagnosis). These patients should not begin manipulation until they are aware of their tendency to tighten or 'clench' the laryngeal muscles, regardless of their conscious or unconscious reason for doing so. Attempts to manipulate the larynx before the patient has released the resistance may result in physical damage.
2. Abuse. A past history of abuse, whether sexual, physical or emotional and regardless of whether the knowledge of abuse is conscious or unconscious, is an absolute contraindication for manipulative therapy.
3. Hypersensitivity/low pain threshold. Patients who are hypersensitive to touch or who have a very low pain threshold are frequently unable to tolerate manipulation. These patients may have a need to hold on to their symptoms as a defence against deep-seated anxiety. This need should always be respected by the practitioner.
4. Personality disorders (e.g. borderline psychotics). Sometimes patients will disclose a psychiatric history or, during the course of the case history and treatment, display inappropriate responses that suggest that a psychiatric condition may be present. These patients will usually be unsuitable for manipulative therapy.
5. Patients who are ambivalent towards treatment. Some patients are unclear as to the nature of their problem and ambivalent towards receiving treatment. These patients may fall into any of the following categories, and represent relative contraindications to proceeding with manipulative therapy:
   (a) Those who have instigated treatment at the request or suggestion of a medical practitioner, singing teacher or family member. These patients, when asked, are unaware of any problem and may be responding to the needs of others rather than their own need for treatment.
   (b) Those needing reassurance and advice, but who do not regard treatment as necessary.
   (c) Those who clearly present with vocal dysfunction that is secondary to an emotional state.
6. The 'guarded' patient (without known history of abuse). These patients have a need to defend themselves that should be understood where possible and always respected.
7. The projecting patient. Patients who are unable to express their feelings may fail to grieve following a painful emotional experience. Unaware of their feelings of sadness and their need to cry they rarely seek appropriate treatment, but will often somatize their emotional state into throat and voice symptoms and seek help for these instead. When working with these patients practitioners will often begin to experience what the patient cannot, and feel irrationally sad and tearful. Unless these patients can gain some insight into their feelings

and learn to express them, they are unlikely to be able to respond to manipulative treatment, and may even be highly resistant. If the treatment continues there is a risk that the practitioner may be unwittingly drawn into a relationship where they become 'the abuser' and the patient 'the abused'. This collusion is likely to be representative of the patient's habitual and unconscious way of relating to others and his anticipation of the way others will relate to him/her. The opposite can also happen, that oversympathetic practitioners will develop dependent relationships.

8.   Patients who are overly focused on the larynx. Some patients, particularly those who are professional voice-users, seem to focus inappropriate attention onto their larynges. The practitioner needs to develop a clear idea of how much of the patient's complaint is related to organic or mechanical components from overuse and fatigue, and how much of the problem is a result of increased levels of anxiety. A fine line should be drawn between attending to the physical problem and deflecting excessive attention away from the larynx, reminding the patient that the larynx and voice production is only a product of the rest of the personality. Unless these patients are made aware that their voices do not have lives of their own, laryngeal manipulation only colludes with the patients' unrealistic state of mind.

Side effects

A major advantage of manipulative treatment is that there are relatively few side effects. However, patients should be warned that they may experience slight discomfort in the area treated for approximately 24–48 hours. If the patient reports soreness and discomfort over a longer period, emotional factors should be considered. Sometimes patients will report a drop in vocal pitch. This is particularly common in professional voice-users or when the larynx is released to a lower position in the neck. A rise in pitch may be reported in patients who habitually lower the larynx as it releases upwards in the neck. Occasionally an increase in catarrh is reported, which is usually beneficial but puzzling for the patient.

Additional considerations for manual therapy

The concept of 'normal'

Comments concerning 'normal findings' in the examination and assessment of the musculoskeletal system are frequently made. In particular, the concept of 'normal asymmetry' arises as it is such a common finding in both the vocally healthy and dysphonic populations. Clinical experience suggests that this confusion between 'normal findings' and 'common findings' may hinder our understanding of dysfunction, its diagnosis and treatment. It is important to remember that we do not usually see 'normal' phenomena in the voice clinic, but patients with a vocal complaint. Asymmetry, in our opinion, is very much part of the aetiology. The fact that it can be observed in the normal population does not mean that these people are not 'en route' to developing voice problems; it may be just that they have not yet reached the point where muscular and mechanical compensation breaks down. It might be useful to reverse the argument and to ask the following question: 'How many patients who develop hyperfunctional voice problems present with "normal" or expected laryngeal use on overall examination?'

Differences in individual patients' physiognomy, tissue suppleness and comprehension

During the course of manipulative treatment, the exercises and advice that are given to patients, the existence of reasonable muscular strength, the presence of neuromuscular patterns, the patient's body awareness and the patient's knowledge of anatomy is implied and often assumed. This may not necessarily be the case. The following things are often taken for granted.

(a) The existence of good abdominal musculature

As a baby learns to move from the prone to the erect position it is mainly the extensor muscles that become active while the whole neuromuscular system is geared towards extension. The abdominal muscles are not part of this development. A good abdominal musculature will exist where patients have acquired it through exercise and sporting activities during the course of their development. The lack of a good abdominal musculature is a particular problem in Western society where a large part of our time is spent sitting.

As the diaphragm is reported to be the major muscle of inspiration (Hixon and collaborators, 1991), diaphragmatic breathing is therefore likely to be both an efficient and natural way to breathe. However, many patients use upper chest or clavicular patterns of breathing or sometimes even paradoxical breathing, where the diaphragm remains relaxed on inhalation. When diaphragmatic breathing is introduced as part of the voice therapy regime the work needs to be closely monitored. Some patients are unable to release the diaphragm without specific manipulative help to enable them to gain voluntary control over the muscle and to identify sensations (feedback) associated with its use. This aspect of the work is complementary to that of the speech therapist where patients are resistant or have difficulty in carrying out the breathing exercises described in Chapter 7.

Exercises and advice

There are times when it is appropriate to introduce the patient to exercises to help them stabilize or maintain new neuromuscular habits. These may include vocal exercises. It is important to remember that these will be practised away from the practitioner and may be open to misinterpretation. Our clinical experience shows that patients can be very 'creative' and enthusiastic in their performance of the exercises we advise. However, when called upon to demonstrate what they understood of our advice or to perform the exercises suggested, patients may produce results that bear no resemblance to the exercises we had in mind. The patients' difficulties in carrying out suggested exercises may be associated with their lack of

knowledge and awareness of their own anatomy or it may relate to their unwilling-
ness to participate in and take responsibility for their own health.

Conflicting demands on muscle groups

It is important to bear in mind that posture and breathing may create conflicting
demands on the same group of muscles. Balanced posture is achieved by the
extensor and flexor group of muscles. In the erect position that means that the
abdominal muscles maintain increased tone synergistic with the extensors (back
muscles). For diaphragmatic breathing, relaxation of abdominal muscles is necessary to accommodate the descent of the diaphragm, creating a conflicting demand.
A balance has to be found between maintaining postural support and allowing
abdominal release for diaphragmatic breathing.

Patients whose emotional make-up prevents them from 'taking in' new experiences

Some patients find it very difficult to participate actively in the treatment plan.
These patients can either be physically or emotionally restricted. Just as some
patients are physically rigid and unable to respond to manipulation, so others can
be emotionally rigid or so fragile that they are resistant to change. These patients
will need modifications to their treatment plan and prognosis.

'The show must go on'

This phrase is much used by performers and reflects the omnipotent state of mind
that is present in the show business industry from management to the last member
of the chorus. It produces great and at times unrealistic pressure on young singers
in particular. In their distress and inability to deflect the pressure, young singers
may project it into their therapist or practitioner, expecting the level of support that
will enable them to fulfil the expectation associated with the phrase. An interesting
dynamic may take place as the therapist is asked to demonstrate and provide
therapeutic skills that will 'save the day'. Because nobody likes to admit failure the
therapist will try to comply with the patient's expectations. However, there is a
danger that the therapist may lose touch with reality, which, in this context, is the
limitation imposed on both patient and practitioner by the physiology and rate of
healing in the tissues. In our clinic we generally feel it is unwise to administer anti-
inflammatory drugs just to 'help' patients through a performance while their
tissues and mechanical system are not in a fit state to perform. In our experience,
this only increases the damage in the long run.

Stress

One important note about stress. We often suggest to our patients that their problems are stress-related. Most people consider stress to be related to marital problems, breakdown of relationship or bereavement. Many events are stressful;
attempting to define them would be irrelevant, as stressors vary from person to
person. In fact, we deal with stress all of our lives. It is therefore not surprising that
many patients respond with anger to the suggestion that their voice problem is

stress-related. Many will respond 'But I do not feel stressed' with genuine feeling. However, the stress itself is not the problem, it is the incapacity to deal with an extra stress that is at issue here.

Patients usually respond better to the idea that it is the accumulation of stress factors in their lives at that particular moment and their incapacity to handle this extra stress that is causing them the problems. Earlier in the chapter the concept of a breakdown in compensation of a mechanical system was discussed and the same concept of an emotional breakdown of compensation can be seen as applicable here.

Summary

In summary, the role of manipulation within the context of the multidisciplinary clinic is a somewhat heterogeneous yet uniquely valuable one. The manual therapist offers a different viewpoint for both the history and the physical examination. His/her role is thereby complementary to the process through:

(a) development of a comprehensive understanding of the patient's complaint;
(b) provision of a functional diagnosis;
(c) assistance in determination of the aetiology of the complaint;
(d) deeper understanding of the patient's expectations;
(e) development of a treatment plan, which, where appropriate, can fully utilize his or her skills.

References

The Alexander Technique (The Society of Teachers of), 20 London House, 266 Fulham Road, London SW10 9EL.

Aronson AE (1985) Management of specific voice disorders: musculoskeletal tension (vocal hyperfunction). In Clinical Voice Disorders. Stuttgart and New York: Georg Thieme Verlag, pp 339-342.

Blaugrund SM, Taira T, Isshiki N (1991) Laryngeal manual compression in the evaluation of patients for laryngeal framework surgery. In Gauffin J, Hammarberg B (Eds) Vocal Fold Physiology. London: Whurr and Co., pp 207-212.

Feldenkrais M (1949) Body and mature behaviour. New York: International University.

Hixon TJ and collaborators (1991) Respiratory Function in Speech and Song. San Diego: Singular Publishing Group Inc.

Sonninen A (1956) The role of the external laryngeal muscles in length-adjustment of the vocal cords in singing. Acta Otolaryngologica 118: 218-31.

Vilkman E, Sonninen A, Hurme P, Körkkö P (1996) External laryngeal frame function in voice production revisited: a review. Journal of Voice 10: 78-92.

Appendix 6.1

Patient's Symptomatic Complaints (Aches and Pains) and the Practitioner's Considerations

Patient's complaints	Questions in the practitioner's mind
General non-specific pain in the throat that is unrelated to voice production or swallowing	Leaves the practitioner puzzled and in need of further information
When is the voice worst (a.m., p.m., before or after use, etc.)?	a.m. suggests the possibility of acid reflux, congestion, or emotion; p.m. with voice use usually indicates muscular dysfunction, p.m. without voice use is likely to be emotional in origin
Pain or aching around the margin of the thyrohyoid muscle, or the thyro-hyoid membrane and ligaments	Very typical of long-term hyperfunctional voice use
Discomfort during or after performance of a vocal task, recovering with rest	Strap musculature, thyrohyoid mechanism, or pharyngeal constrictor hyper-tonicity
Voice slow to warm up in the morning	Reflux, congestion, muscle fatigue, emotional or overuse the previous day without proper rest
Pain and discomfort in the anterior aspect of the neck	When specific, the tissue of origin should be identifiable with palpation
Globus Pharyngeus/hystericus (lump in the throat)	Very tight inferior strap and sternoclei-domastoid muscles

Recurrent sore throat	Tonsillitis, reflux, vocal fatigue, or emotional origin. On palpation, characteristically the anterior neck muscles are hypertonic
Difficulty swallowing (initiation, noisy with laryngeal 'click')	Neurological, postural suprahyoid muscle hypertonicity; hypertonic geniohyoid, omohyoid tightness or thyrohyoid muscles
Dryness	May be indicative of chronic anxiety state
Cough	May be associated with a deep underlying emotional component
Heartburn (acid reflux) with associated oesophageal discomfort, sore throats, globus and throat tightness	May be associated with hiatus hernia/stomach problems, stress/emotional issues or both combined (often responds well to manipulation)
Unilateral muscle ache with the larynx deviated from the midline	The larynx moves with the torso so this condition may be associated with a rotation of the torso
Head and neck postural problems, such as neck ache, headaches, 'sinus' pain, earache, especially around the mastoid process	May be associated with an hyperlordotic segment of the cervical spine
Emotional components	***As felt by the practitioner***
As disclosed voluntarily by the patient	What is it all about? What is the communication?

Appendix 6.2

Lieberman Postural Assessment for Hyperfunctional Dysphonia

This protocol is intended to accompany the instructional course on the interdisciplinary assessment and treatment of hyperfunctional voice disorder in
order to achieve satisfactory practitioner agreement

* Tick positive findings only in the shaded boxes. Rate by single mark on analogue scale where indicated ♦

Accurate assessment of the laryngeal musculature and cricothyroid joints is considered esential

General Considerations 1. Observation

A. Observations while the patient is sitting and giving the history of the
problem etc.

Sitting			
	Is the anterior neck compartment smooth or are the muscles very conspicuous?	Smooth	Conspicuous
	Is activity in the anterior neck compartment visible? (e.g. obvious omohyoid activity)	Yes?	
	Habitual head tilting?	Left	Right
	Habitual head gestures (e.g. 'yes' or 'no' by nodding)	Yes?	

B. Observations when the patient has been asked to stand passively. Frontal and
lateral viewing required.

Standing				
	Knee locking	Left	Right	Both
	Weight distribution	Left	Right	Central
	Pelvic rotation	Forwards		
	Raised shoulders (rest)	Left	Right	Both
	Weight bearing (centre of gravity)	Posterior ♦ ⊢--------⊣	Anterior	

General Considerations 2. Palpation

Palpate	Pelvic Tilt	Left	Right	
patient standing	Lumbar spine lordosis	Exaggerated		
	Lumbar spine scoliosis	Left	Right	
	Anterior head translocation	A. Normal posture	1–2 cms	≥ 3 cms
		B. Occipital contact with vertical surface without chin raising	Contact Yes?	
patient required to lie down	Thoracic/ cervical spine	Contact of C7 with horizontal surface?		
(Osteopathic)	Thoracic spine fixed segment	Indicate level. Vertebrae		

Cervical & Laryngeal Considerations 3. Palpation

Neck Vertebrae	Cervicodorsal vertebral shelf (Level of hyperlordotic segment)	C2–3 (4)	C4–5	Other
Posterior Musculature	Paravertebral muscular tenderness lateral to the hyperlordotic segment	Left	Right	Both
	Occipital/Submastoid tenderness (delete if N/A)	Left	Right	Both
	TMJ tenderness	Left	Right	Both
Anterior Musculature	Sternomastoid muscles while standing erect	Lax ◆ ├------------┤ Hyperactive L ◆ ├------------┤ R ◆ ├------------┤		
	Suprahyoid tension	Slight ◆ ├------------┤ Great		
	Larynx in midline	Left of midline	Right of midline	
	Infralaryngeal strap ms.	Hyperactive	Underactive or absent	
Laryngeal Musculature	Overall tension of laryngeal suspensory muscles	Tightly held ◆ ├------------┤ Loosely Held		
(For experienced practitioners only)	Possible to palpate structures medial to the posterior margins of the Thyroid Laminae?	Left	Right	Neither
(For all practitioners)	Thyrohyoid Membranes held/reduced in area	Left	Right	Both
	Tender/guarded cricothyroid muscles	Left	Right	Both
Cricothyroid joints	Cricoid arch position (When visor is closed)	Neutral ◆ ├------------┤ Anterior translocation		
If arch is translocated	Does it change: A. On full head flexion B. On full head extension?	More so ◆ ├------------┤ Same Less so ◆ ├------------┤		
	Individual joint laxity	Greater on Left ◆ ├------------┤ Greater on Right		
Visor position	Position at rest	Widely open Neutral ◆ ├------------┤ Closed		

Cervical and Laryngeal Considerations 4. Palpation of Patient Manoevres (Standing Position)

Ask the patient to 'siren' up and down through their entire vocal range	Palpation of the C-T visor shows:	No Movement Excellent Range		
	From its 'rest' position, the visor:	Opens	Closes	Both
Ask the patient to swallow twice. During the swallow, is there	Head extention?	Yes		
	Can the patient raise the larynx freely?	Yes		
	Decrease in any anterior position of cricoid arch?	Yes		

Appendix 6.3

Classification of Osteopathic Techniques: The Technical Vocabulary

Passive (the patient in the supine position and relaxed)

1. Articulation
2. Stretching
3. Kneading
4. Inhibition
5. Rhythmic traction
6. Springing

Semi-active (the patient is supine performing controlled breathing or a controlled action which involves a specific muscle or joint)

Muscle energy

1. Isometric contraction
2. Isotonic contraction
3. Isolytic contraction

Low velocity stress

1. Sustained leverage
2. Sustained pressure
3. Sustained traction
4. Sustained articulation

Relaxation techniques

1. Functional
2. Cranial holds

High velocity thrust

1. Combined leverage and thrust
2. Momentum induced
3. Minimal leverage modification
4. Non-leverage thrust using springing
5. Momentum induced

Notes
The differences in the techniques lie in the modification of the following factors:

1. Force of application
2. Amplitude
3. Velocity
4. Plane in relation to the direction of muscle fibres or joint axis of movement
5. Tension
6. Type of leverage used
7. Contact point pressure
8. Hand and fingers position

Speech Therapy for Dysphonia

SARA HARRIS

I see a voice: now will I to the chink....

William Shakespeare, *A Midsummer Night's Dream*,

Introduction

This chapter is aimed primarily at speech and language therapists who are working in the field of voice and particularly those who do not have the advantages of working in a multidisciplinary voice clinic. It is hoped that it will also be of interest to ENT surgeons, as the majority of voice patients are referred to speech therapy by ENT surgeons. It is therefore important that they know which patients are most appropriate to refer and how these patients are likely to be treated. Other professionals working in the field of voice, such as singing and voice teachers, are also likely to find the chapter useful. It may help to throw light on how speech therapy techniques relate to singing and voice techniques, and also when to refer clients on for investigations. Of course, many of the therapeutic exercises developed to improve voice production came originally from singing and voice teaching and have either been adapted or simply borrowed wholesale.

The chapter is divided into two main sections. The first aims to cover the therapeutic process employed by speech and language therapists working in a voice clinic team, and includes the assessment and the general management of patients in a voice clinic setting. The second main section covers the treatment of voice disorders. It begins with general topics and exercises traditionally used in voice therapy and goes on to discuss two very useful systems of exercises that have been designed specifically to teach control over the vocal mechanism: the Accent Method and Jo Estill's Compulsory Figures. There are many other systems (e.g. Coblenzer, Pahn's Nasalization, Boone's Voice Program for Adults, etc.) that will not be specifically discussed but are referenced at the end of the chapter for further information. The different muscular mechanisms used during phonation are also discussed, together with the common patterns of functional breakdown. Although no dramatic new exercises for voice therapy are presented, the 'tried and proved' ones will be described and the most useful 'prescriptions' for each disorder pattern will be suggested with an explanation as to why they should work. To some extent, for the patient at least, correcting voice production does involve trial and error. The therapist will have a clear idea of what aspects of the patient's voice production they wish to alter and what vocal changes they wish to hear. However, patients may find particular techniques hard to follow and errors can easily creep into vocal exercises. The skill of the therapist is in identifying the errors, introducing alternative techniques and helping the patient develop ways to monitor new vocal patterns until they are able to produce them reliably in spontaneous speech.

The therapeutic process

Speech and language therapists specializing in voice problems usually begin by addressing the following issues:

(a) What symptoms does the patient describe?
(b) What physical evidence is there of damage or disease that might create the symptoms?
(c) What is occurring mechanically to create the symptoms?
(d) How and why do patients become dysphonic?
(e) What underlying psychological processes might be present that may have been either causal or contributory to the patient's condition?
(f) What techniques/retraining can help restore healthy phonation patterns or compensate for the effects of the vocal condition?

In this section we will try to move through some aspects of the process in a practical way.

The case history: 'If you want to know what's wrong, ask the patient'

Vocal symptoms

The first question it seems wise to address is the nature of the voice disorder. As with most 'things medical', if you want to know what is wrong, ask the patient.

First let us consider **how** the patient describes the symptoms. It is worth paying attention to what is **not** described and **not** said, as this often gives insight into aspects of the disorder of which the patient is perhaps unaware. Patients will usually focus on one or two key areas of their voice problem depending on their vocal awareness and experience. While singers may complain of a 'crack' over two notes at the *passaggio**, most patients are vocally untrained and will

---

* (Passaggio is the Italian word for passage, i.e. the transition between two voice registers. It is most commonly applied to the transition between modal and 'head' voicing - thick to thin fold and vice versa.)

complain about more general vocal attributes such as hoarseness or discomfort.

Broadly speaking, patients will divide their symptoms into areas of vocal quality, comfort, stamina, volume and pitch, in roughly that order (Harris et al., 1986).

Voice quality patients often use terms such as 'hoarse', 'rough', 'husky' and 'gravelly' to describe voice problems that may be associated with vocal fold mucosal changes, vocal abuse/misuse or certain changes in vocal gesture/posture. The words 'weak', 'breathy', 'fading' or 'cutting out into a whisper' tend to suggest vocal fold palsies, neurological conditions and more commonly, psychogenic conversions with incomplete or absent glottic closure. Although of course it is not possible to use the patient's description as diagnostic, research does show that voice quality can be reliably recognized, categorized and graded by listeners. Most of our perceptual assessments are based on similar terms (Isshiki, 1966; Laver, 1980).

Comfort is often a major component of voice disorders (Mathieson, 1993). Unfortunately it is difficult to assess objectively, nor is it necessarily related to other symptoms that can be measured accurately. It is not unusual for patients to congratulate therapists for 'curing' them, leaving the therapist dumbfounded as the vocal quality appears not to have altered significantly! The patient, however, was only concerned with removing the pain or discomfort from the act of speaking.

Patients use many terms to describe their vocal tract discomfort. Descriptions of pain may include such terms as 'burning', 'stabbing', 'sharp' and 'raw', while less severe discomfort might be described as 'hot', 'stinging' or 'rough'. These descriptions often relate to particular areas within the vocal tract. They may be very specific so that the patient can actually point to the site of the pain, or they may be more diffuse. The most common places that can be isolated into 'spots' are the areas defined by the thyrohyoid muscles and membranes, the cricothyroid visor (both the joints and the muscles) and the oropharynx (the back of the mouth) (see Chapter 1). These 'spots' to which pain is being referred are often very specific to a particular structure. For instance, a unilateral ache over the posterior border of the thyrohyoid membrane may lead the clinician to suspect an arytenoid granuloma, particularly if the pain is sharp and associated with yawning, sneezing or shouting.

The extrinsic musculature in which the larynx is cradled and suspended may also create discomfort. Descriptions tend to be less severe and include terms like 'aching', 'tired', 'swollen', 'tight' and 'effortful'. The areas of discomfort described are usually much less well defined.

No discussion of vocal tract discomfort would be complete without the dreaded 'lump in the throat'. Clinical observation suggests that this syndrome is on the increase and involves the cricopharyngeus and constrictor muscles. It is usually referred to as 'globus pharyngeus' or, less kindly in the past, as 'globus hystericus'. In the absence of any swallowing difficulty, globus is frequently attributed to 'stress'. While often there are emotional elements to the problem (and there are any number of very apt English colloquialisms such as 'I feel all choked up', 'It brings a lump to my throat', 'I can't swallow that!', etc.), there can be many other contributing factors, such as gastro-oesophageal reflux and cervical spine problems. The mechano-emotional factors are better dealt with in Chapters 6 and 9.

Stamina is another vocal attribute that troubles patients greatly. Stamina can be loosely described as the length of time patients can speak or sing before they begin to observe deterioration in one or more of the other vocal attributes, e.g. the vocal quality may change, the pitch may alter, volume may reduce or discomfort may be felt. Recently vocal stamina has been the subject of interesting research using vocal loading or stress testing. The results have implications for monitoring the effectiveness of voice therapy, particularly for professional voice users (Gelfer et al., 1991; Stemple et al., 1995; Lauri et al., 1997).

The case history: related questions

In addition to the description the patient gives of their vocal symptoms, many clues come from the case history. Each clinician has his or her own style in taking a case history, but most start with the presenting symptoms as outlined above. They will also ask about when the symptoms were first noticed, what circumstances surrounded their onset (for example, infections or stress) or whether the problem seemed to the patient to have come out of the blue. Who first noticed the symptoms may also be of interest. Quite often patients are unaware of vocal changes and it is relatives or friends who suggest that medical advice is necessary. It is also important to know whether the symptoms are constant, variable or episodic. If they fluctuate, under what circumstances do they appear better or worse?

The intention behind taking a case history is to learn about the patient's past and present physical and emotional well-being and to determine whether other medical conditions are likely to contribute to the voice problem. On the basis of the information given, the clinician must decide whether or not to seek medical help for the patient. Most prefer to eliminate the possibility that the voice disorder is related to a disease process before turning their attention to voice production patterns and stress factors. The case history interview also allows the patient and clinician time to relate to one another. This is probably the most important part of the therapeutic process, as it usually dictates just how successfully they can learn to share information and whether the patient can 'receive' help and support from the clinician in whatever form is appropriate.

The case history should cover a number of different general areas. Some therapists may prefer a checklist, especially when they first start working in the field of voice, but others prefer to write their own at the time they first see the patient, relying on memory and experience to elicit the information they require. Both methods work well, but it should be remembered that valuable information can be lost when the therapist becomes more concerned about completing a checklist in the correct order, than attending to the way in which the patient tells their story.

There are many good books that cover the case history and provide excellent checklists (Green and Mathieson, 1989; Colton and Casper, 1990; Morrison et al, 1995). The case history of singers/performers is dealt with in Chapter 8.

A useful question, which is not always included in the case history, is 'Why did you seek help?' The most common answers relate to fears about cancer or some serious disease process. Performers may be more concerned about immediate decisions such as whether or not it is safe to sing tonight's concert. Either way, these patients may improve considerably with simple reassurance if the larynx is intrinsically healthy. As a result, advice in the clinic or a follow-up session from the speech therapist may be all that the patient needs (or wants) for the symptoms to resolve. Sometimes, however, the patient has sought help because their spouse/work colleagues/friends have pushed them into it. They may be unaware of the problem, or the symptoms may not cause them any trouble in their daily lives. Although this presentation may cover up a very real anxiety, where patients are genuinely unconcerned, they are unlikely to comply with or respond well to therapy. Their lack of awareness may mean that they have very poor auditory and kinaesthetic feedback so that they are unable to hear or feel the changes that exercises make to their voices. They may simply be unmotivated and happy to live with their symptoms. Again, advice, reassurance and clear information on how and when to be re-referred often saves time, energy and frustration on both sides.

What physical evidence is there of damage or disease that might create the symptoms?

The case history information will give valuable clues as to whether there is likely to be vocal damage or more general disease at work. It is easy to assume that because a patient has seen their GP they will have discussed their health problems and that the GP will have excluded any active disease. Unfortunately this is not necessarily the case. Frequently patients do not recognize the relevance of their symptoms and fail to tell their doctors important facts. One patient who came to the voice clinic with recurrent sore throats had completely omitted to tell the GP about the indigestion he had been having, with pain radiating to the back and right shoulder. When this information came up in the speech therapy interview and was discussed with the GP it did not take long for the relevant tests to be carried out and the hiatus hernia and gallstones to be diagnosed. When asked why he had not thought to mention this, the patient explained that he had experienced indigestion 'for years', and although it had become worse, he had not been worried about it. The sore throats, however, were more recent and he found them far more difficult to tolerate as they affected his voice production. It had never occurred to him that the two things could be connected. Needless to say the troublesome sore throats resolved with the appropriate treatment.

This story is not uncommon, so therapists should note down any material from the history that they feel may be significant and discuss it with the surgeon or the patient's GP. The surgeon or GP can then decide whether to investigate the patient's symptoms further or refer on to another specialist.

Evidence of damage or disease within the larynx will be determined at the voice clinic examination and an overview of common lesions causing dysphonia can be found in Chapter 3. In addition to their conventional role in exclusion of damage and disease, rigid videostrobolaryngoscopy and fibre endoscopy of the larynx are also essential for assessment of the habitual muscular patterns responsible for both vocal damage and the patient's symptoms. Muscle groups that over- or underwork can be identified, allowing the therapist to choose those vocal techniques most likely to restore the balance and reduce hyperfunction. A detailed study of the muscle groups in question is found in Chapter 1, and the most common patterns of hyper-function are discussed in the second section of this chapter and also in Chapter 5.

How and why do patients become dysphonic?

Perhaps the most common question asked by patients is 'I have talked like this for years, why has my voice gone wrong now?' Actually, it is an extremely pertinent question and it may prove difficult to give the patient an accurate answer.

Voice problems are like jigsaw puzzles: first the pieces have to be found and only then can they be assembled into a picture. The pieces of a voice problem are gleaned from the case history and the examination of the voice in clinic. Fitting them together takes place slowly as part of the process of voice therapy. It may not be complete until the end of the therapy period.

In the past, the problems of patients presenting with damage to the vocal folds, for example polypoid vocal 'nodules', were considered to be straightforward. The reason for the patients' hoarseness was obvious and the usual remedy was to remove the offending lesions surgically. More recently, with the advent of multi-disciplinary work, it has become apparent that damage to the vocal fold cover is a process that can produce various responses. Recurrent episodes of acute localized bleeding, for example, eventually develop into classical firm nodules, and the polypoid degenerative changes of chronic inflammation are usually produced by persistent vocal abuse and/or chemical irritants. The nature of the process for each individual patient has to be understood in order for its effects to be reversed or minimized. If the mechanical stresses engendered by the patient's voice production are carefully examined, it is usually possible to identify how recurrent episodes of abuse/misuse have created the nodules, polyps or vergetures/scars observed at laryngoscopy. In a way these lesions can be looked on as the product of repetitive strain injury to the vocal folds.

Understanding the muscular patterns involved in vocal strain or abuse usually gives an indication of which techniques are most likely to help improve the voice production. However, understanding muscle misuse alone may not go far enough back through the layers of causality to produce improvements that will last. To do this, we need to understand the reasons behind the changes in voice use. These reasons may be physical, environmental, emotional or, more commonly, a combination of all three. For example, patients suffering from oesophageal reflux have an excellent reason for persistently tight laryngeal muscles because of the need to guard the airway against possible inhalation of acid. Equally, patients with chest or abdominal problems affecting their breathing and support will also have good reason to alter their phonatory patterns (see Glossary in Chapter 8 for a definition of support). Vocally untrained patients working in high levels of noise, or those whose work requires constant shouting (e.g. swimming/aerobic instructors, stock market traders, etc.) repeatedly put the vocal folds under levels of mechanical stress that can only rarely be sustained without damage. Finally, the patient's emotional life may have changed. Situations leading to anger and frustration may develop at work, conflicts or a bereavement can occur and these factors may be the final straw that pushes the patient over the edge into vocal pathology. (Psychological factors are discussed in greater depth in Chapter 9.)

Patients are rarely able to assimilate all the factors involved in the development of their voice disorder immediately. During the course of therapy they begin to pay more attention to new aspects of their problem. For example, many patients who initially deny the presence of reflux in clinic may, after a few therapy sessions, report that they have experienced the symptoms of reflux, sometimes for many years, without realizing it. Subsequent treatment of the reflux will frequently resolve the patients' vocal symptoms without the necessity for any voice therapy at all.

Some patients are reticent to raise emotional issues in clinic for all sorts of reasons. During the course of therapy, however, a good relationship will hopefully develop with the therapist that allows painful emotional experiences to be expressed. As a result, both patient and therapist gain new insight into the nature of the voice disorder and changes in management can be discussed as it becomes clear that psychotherapy or counselling may be more appropriate and fruitful. The patient can then be referred to a psychotherapist, counsellor or a speech and language therapist who has specialized in counselling.

The role of the speech therapist in the voice clinic

The role the speech therapist plays in the voice clinic depends on experience, confidence and the working relationship between the individual therapist and the voice clinic surgeon. It would seem that the most effective clinics are those where the therapist and surgeon have an equal relationship. Both should respect each other's areas of expertise and feel confident to question each other about their clinical observations. Unless both feel free to discuss the work and confident about explaining how they arrived at their particular management decisions, no multidisciplinary learning can take place.

In many clinics now the speech therapist has been taught to carry out videostrobolaryngoscopy of the larynx. This can be particularly useful where the voice clinic therapist works with other surgeons who do not have access to the sophisticated equipment necessary for this procedure. Provided the video examinations carried out by speech therapists are assessed jointly with an ENT surgeon to ensure accurate diagnosis, it seems appropriate for therapists to carry out videostroboscopy during voice therapy sessions to monitor the effects of therapy techniques and to demonstrate the nature of the problem to the patient.

Perhaps the most important role of the speech therapist in the voice clinic is to observe the voice production patterns of patients as they give their history at the initial interview. As the patient is speaking, members of the clinic team will be observing from their different perspectives how the patient communicates. There will, of course be a considerable overlap. The speech therapist is looking out for:

- difficulty on rising from the waiting room chair or while walking into the clinic;
- habitual posture and overall physical tension during speech;
- facial movement (or lack of it) and any sign of dribbling or dysarthria;
- disorders of articulation or fluency;
- difficulties in comprehension or expressive language;
- habitual breathing patterns at rest and in speech;
- prosody and intonation patterns;
- non-verbal communication patterns that relate to social/emotional behaviour.

The observations that are made then dictate the questions the therapist puts to the patient during the case history. For example, where a patient presents with a rather expressionless face, poor articulatory movement and a monotonous, slightly hypernasal voice, the therapist will be asking questions that will help differentiate patients suffering from Parkinsonism or other neurological disorders, from those suffering from hearing loss, cleft palate, poorly fitting false teeth or emotional problems. The clinic surgeon will also wish to ask questions that help identify any contributing disease factors in case the patient needs further investigations or referral to other specialists.

Many clinics now ask patients to complete a case history form prior to their clinic visit or while they are waiting to be seen (Sataloff, 1984; Harris et al., 1986; Donnelly and Kellow, 1989). Although these questionnaires save time and ensure that no important questions are left unanswered, they have drawbacks unless the material is reviewed or expanded upon in the clinic. The way in which the patients present themselves in clinic 'leads' case history questioning in a way that can provide much valuable information. This can easily be lost if questionnaires are relied upon, producing a 'mental set' among the clinicians. It should be noted that in these days of medicolegal vigilance yet another advantage of patients filling in their own history questionnaires is that the negative findings are recorded. It is easy to overlook the documentation of negative findings during a busy multidisciplinary interview.

More detailed assessment of the patient's voice production is rarely possible in clinic. There is much to be said for the therapist interviewing and assessing new patients prior to their voice clinic appointment. For example, where the clinic can be held in the afternoon, patients may be seen in the morning. This allows for voice recordings, phonetograms, laryngography, spectrography, airflow studies, etc. to be carried out so that the results are then available for the rest of the team at the afternoon voice clinic. The speech therapist could carry out such testing while the clinic is running, but the disadvantage is that he or she is then unavailable for the initial examination of some patients while others are assessed. This problem could be overcome if a volunteer/technician was trained to carry out the assessment procedures in a separate room, supplying the clinic with the results for new patients and reassessments for follow-up patients.

Unfortunately, voice clinics require extra paper work and it usually falls to the speech therapist to carry out the general organisation, e.g. keeping up-to-date clinic lists with all the relevant details, together with diagnoses and management plans, while the surgeon is usually responsible for writing up the medical notes and completing the waiting list forms, etc. The extra administration that falls to the speech therapist should be borne in mind by his or her manager when planning and setting up a voice clinic service. Alternatively, outpatient management may be able to organize proper ancillary staffing in some hospital trusts (see Introduction).

The general management of dysphonia

So far we have discussed general principles relating to voice patients in a voice clinic setting. Sooner or later though, the assessment phase is over (or at least ongoing) and the practical management of the patient becomes the main focus of attention. The multidisciplinary nature of the voice clinic facilitates flexible management of the patient who may see one or several of the clinicians, serially or concurrently. For example:

1. Where the voice clinic personnel includes an osteopath or physiotherapist who specializes in manipulative therapy, patients may receive manipulation prior to or concurrently with speech therapy. Laryngeal manipulation is designed to articulate laryngeal joints, muscles and the adjacent soft tissue (see Chapter 6), and is particularly effective in releasing tension associated with voice disorders. While many patients will release laryngeal tension with simple massage to the neck and shoulder area others may require specific laryngeal manipulation before they are able to make the best use of voice therapy techniques. Manipulation allows the patient to develop kinaesthetic awareness of appropriate muscle use, which can then be reinforced by vocal exercises.
2. The same scenario occurs when singers discover new ways of developing their vocal range, voice quality or resonance through speech therapy exercises, but would benefit from the help of a singing teacher in order to apply these discoveries to their singing technique.
3. The benefits of surgical intervention may be enhanced when voice therapy and/or manipulation is carried out before and after surgery. Medical treatment of any concomitant condition will also need to be carried out and monitored concurrently with the treatment modalities described above.

Therapy choice: group versus individual

Traditionally, most speech and language therapists considered that voice work should be individually tailored to the patient's needs and that group work was best reserved for sessions on vocal hygiene and more general topics like relaxation. The advantages of working with patients individually are easy to see:

1. The patient and the therapist are able to build a good working relationship which can be a major factor in the success or failure of therapy.

2.   The therapist can respond immediately to the effects of particular techniques on the patient's voice, trying new ones or incorporating others into the therapy regime.
3.   There is room to deal with gaps in the patient's understanding or emotional problems that arise during the course of therapy.

Recently, however, this concept has been challenged and many therapists are applying voice work to groups (Morris, 1992; Harris et al., 1995; Bunker et al., 1996). The change in practice may well have to do with increasing numbers of referrals and pressure on therapists to produce cost-effective management packages that reach the maximum number of patients. It may also reflect a change in attitude away from the concept that a voice disorder is specific to an individual, towards the idea that the principles of efficient voice use are universal and are applicable to all. Looked at in this light, group therapy provides an excellent forum to introduce a number of topics. These include:

1.   normal voice production versus the development of vocal pathology;
2.   vocal hygiene;
3.   case history factors;
4.   postural correction and relaxation/release exercises;
5.   breathing exercises and the coordination of breath and voice;
6.   structured vocal techniques (for example Accent Method, Pahn's nasalization, Froeschel's chewing exercises);
7.   psychosomatics.

Discussion of case history factors provides patients with the opportunity to ask questions about their general health or specific symptoms. While the group situation may make this daunting for some, there are patients who will only explore areas of concern because others have had the courage to do so. Many patients report that they feel less alone with their voice problems after talking with other group members. Patients also report feeling less inhibited about trying vocal exercises in unison with others.

Where the speech and language therapist running the group has been trained in counselling, or where a trained psychotherapist/psychologist could be included, it is very valuable to discuss the way in which emotional issues can relate to the development of voice problems. Although the topics of psychosomatics and emotion need to be handled carefully, patients usually report that work in these areas is fascinating, rewarding and helpful (see Chapter 9).

Usually the whole group works through a particular therapy technique. However, there are occasions when some members would benefit more from other techniques. Within limits, the group will tolerate and be interested in the selection of techniques that suit individual group members. It is wise, however, to suggest that the whole group tries them, because frequently they are found to be of broader value than the therapist had realized. The introduction of different techniques also provides further opportunities to extend the work on perceptual feedback across the group as a whole.

Although the therapists and group members start the sessions with fear and trepidation, it is amazing how quickly anxiety disappears and positive, reassuring relationships are established. Even 'difficult' patients can benefit from a group, because other group members provide support and constructive feedback, in addition to that already provided by the therapist(s).

Selection and planning of a group

It is important to select patients carefully for a group to ensure that they have the best chance of receiving appropriate therapy without undue stress or embarrassment. It is also important to the therapists so that they can manage the group effectively and deliver care at the right level. The following are useful principles to bear in mind, but each therapist should be free to make his or her own criteria based on experience.

1. It is suggested that numbers be limited to between four and six if only one therapist is to run the group, or if the helper is totally inexperienced, for example, a new student. It is also wise in this case to choose a homogeneous group of patients, such as those with vocal fold pareses or spasmodic dysphonics.

2. Where two experienced therapists can work together, the group can include between eight and ten patients suffering from broader categories of dysphonia, such as vocal nodules, Reinke's oedema or hyperkinetic dysphonia.

3. Group sessions usually last approximately 2–3 hours, and sessions are spread over 6–8 weeks, depending on whether assessments are to be included and the amount of work to be covered. A refreshment break is important both as a rest and for socializing.

4. Great care should be taken if patients with differing degrees of dysphonia are to be included in the same group. Although it is best to include patients who sound roughly similar, more severely dysphonic patients can be mixed in a less severe group, provided there are several of them. One severely hoarse patient in a mild to moderately hoarse group can feel marginalized.

5. It is essential to have met and assessed each patient prior to the group starting to make sure that no seriously disturbed or disruptive patients are included who would destroy the cohesion of the group and create anxiety for the therapists.

6. Where possible it is helpful to assess patients prior to the group, as, once the group sessions have started, assessments are time-consuming and disruptive to the therapy. However, time constraints sometimes make pre-group assessment impractical. Where this is the case, assessment is best carried out either in the second session, or the latter part of the first session, to allow patients time to relax in the group. The assessments should be on an individual basis, with one therapist taking patients from the group while the other continues to work with the remainder of the group.

7. It is very important that patients understand that they must take responsibility for their treatment by attending regularly and practising the work given. It needs to be made clear that the therapist's role is to provide information, education, support and voice exercises to help patients to change their voice production. It is not possible to perform miracle cures. A clear outline of the

work to be covered on the course can be given to patients prior to the start date or during the first session. It is important to provide worksheets or, best of all, a tape for home practice every session.

8.   At the end of the course, patients are given a group follow-up appointment. The follow-up usually takes place some time later, after a review period for practice and consolidation. The review period is flexible, and can be anywhere between 6 weeks and 3 months, although experience suggests 6–8 weeks is most effective. By 3 months, practice is likely to have dropped off and the patient's life has moved on. As a result they often fail to attend review appointments, either because they forget or because they have improved and feel review is no longer necessary. If they are still having trouble, longer gaps can reduce motivation, leaving patients feeling depressed about the effectiveness of therapy and less inclined to try a different approach.

It is important to give patients a clear idea of what should have been achieved by the review session and to reassure them that decisions concerning further management, assessment and intervention will be made at that time. It is also wise to ensure that follow-up voice clinic or ENT appointments are arranged at the end of the course or after the follow-up session.

Advantages of group work

1.   Patients learn from one another and provide each other with ongoing support. The latter is especially valuable for those who feel isolated and alone.
2.   Group pressure persuades patients to practise much more than they usually do in individual therapy.
3.   Patients often hear vocal change better in one another than they can in themselves. This acts as an excellent boost to motivation.
4.   Patients who would normally blame their failure to progress on the technique and the therapist find this harder to do when others around them are responding well.
5.   Groups can be enormous fun and keep patients motivated and attending regularly.
6.   Patients can sometimes turn out to be quite difficult, for example, those who constantly question the therapist, who have difficulty grasping the work, or who are generally attention seeking. Provided the therapist handles the situation carefully, these patients can often benefit more from a group than from individual therapy as the group situation provides a structure and feedback system that can provide a wider reassurance and security.
7.   Patients who fail to attend therapy do not waste therapist time.

Disadvantages of group work

The main disadvantages of group work are that:

1.   Patients sometimes require individual attention either in learning techniques

or because emotional problems emerge during sessions or in their daily lives. It may be appropriate to move these patients to individual therapy, or to make some time before or after a group session to handle problems.

2. The techniques used may be difficult for some patients to grasp. Sometimes there is room to explore other techniques in group time; at other times, patients need individual help within the session. This is usually possible where two therapists run the group; otherwise careful advice and structuring of the home practice can be given and progress reviewed the following week. If all else fails, the patient can transfer to individual therapy.

3. Patients find the group situation difficult to handle for emotional reasons, or because they feel that they need different management. Usually these patients drop out of the group within the first 2 weeks, and may well have failed individual therapy as well. It is important to contact non-attenders to offer alternative management and to make sure that they are followed-up in the voice clinic (or ENT clinic).

Aims of voice therapy

Before considering vocal techniques it is important to be sure of the aims of voice work. Let us briefly return to the concepts of vocal quality, comfort, stamina, pitch and volume, as some or all of these are the vocal features that therapy will aim to affect. During the assessment process the therapist will be deciding which aspects of the patient's voice production need attention and how the work should be structured, i.e. the aims of therapy. These may be both short-term and long-term depending on the time available to carry out the treatment. They must also take into account the patient's objectives in coming for voice therapy. For example, the therapist's main aim may be a referral to psychotherapy, while the patient's main aim may be to speak without pain. Here, a flexible management plan will be needed that takes into account the patient's practical needs, while at the same time retaining the long-term goals most likely to guarantee the successful outcome of therapy. To take the former example, the therapist may then grade his/her aims in the following way:

1. Explain the nature of vocal pain and its relationship with excessive muscular effort.
2. Identify the muscle groups responsible for the discomfort.
3. Provide exercises to help reduce excess muscular effort and pain during speech.
4. Discussion/counselling to help the patient achieve insight into their symptoms and facilitate acceptance of psychological help.

The therapist's short-term aims are usually related to altering very specific aspects of voice production and do usually correspond to the patient's aims, e.g. where the patient's aim is to be able to speak against noise without the voice deteriorating, the therapist's aims might read:

1. reduce laryngeal constriction;
2. increase airflow;

3.   tune the vocal tract resonators to produce a bright resonance (at approximately 2.5 kHz) using 'twang' quality to increase intensity. Pahn's nasalization programme is also designed to achieve this (Pahn, 1964; Estill, 1996).

Outcome measures

It is becoming increasingly important for therapists to evaluate the effectiveness of their work. It is also necessary to decide on the number of sessions patients should be offered before investigating those who fail to improve. Time limits for improvement can only be decided by individual therapists based on their knowledge of each patient's case. However, most agree that if the patient fails to respond after two (or three) sessions, the therapist should try alternative techniques and recheck the case history.

It is important to choose measures that will not only quantify the therapy outcome but also suit the needs of individual patients. The best course seems to be a combination of instrumental and perceptual measures taken before and after treatment.

The instrumentation measures selected depend largely on what is available to the clinician in terms of hardware (e.g. video recording of the laryngeal examination, EGG, spectrographic analysis, airflow measures, etc.) and the amount of time available for assessment. Perceptual analysis (e.g. Laver's Vocal Profile Analysis) is easier to carry out nowadays as almost all clinicians have access to a tape recorder. Patients can also chart their different symptoms on a simple rating scale. Their pre- and post-therapy scores can be compared showing their subjective impression of the therapy outcome.

Instrumental measures might include:

1.   observable physical or mechanical changes at laryngoscopy;
2.   changes in acoustic measures of the patient's voice (acoustic analysis, spectrography, etc.);
3.   changes in vocal fold contact measured by EGG (for details of 2 and 3, see Chapter 13).
4.   Airflow derived measures.

Perceptual measures might include:

1.   the patient's perception of various aspects of vocal change;
2.   perceptual (psychoacoustic) analysis of voice recordings, for example the Vocal Profile Analysis (Laver, 1980).

It should be remembered, however, that all measures are subject to some level of inaccuracy. Voices fluctuate in quality for many reasons over a short space of time, clouding the picture of what has, or has not, been achieved during therapy. Vocal quality can be affected by hormonal changes, physical changes (such as nocturnal reflux), emotional responses or combinations of any or all of the above. Measurements of Fo and aperiodicity are subject to variability depending on the particular algorithm used in the analysis (Bielamowicz et al., 1996; for further explanation see chapter 13). The patient's subjective assessments of change can be affected either because they have under- or overestimated their response to therapy, and/or because they are anxious to please the therapist.

In the long run it is important to keep in mind the aims of voice therapy for each patient and to assess whether or not these have been achieved. They are mostly concerned with restoring vocal health, as assessed by laryngeal examination, and the patient's own perception of whether the presenting symptoms have resolved.

Unfortunately, some patients do not improve with voice therapy. The reasons for failure may be because:

1.   the diagnosis is inaccurate;
2.   inappropriate therapy techniques are being used;
3.   there are underlying medical factors that have not been addressed;
4.   unrevealed emotional factors are affecting therapy;
5.   the patient has not understood the work given or is unmotivated to practise.

In these cases it is vital to reassess the patient carefully and alter management accordingly.

An excellent summary of the recent research carried out on the efficacy of voice therapy can be found in Enderby and Emerson, 1995.

Classification of dysphonia

It is customary to categorize dysphonia according to the presumed aetiology, for example, misuse/abuse, hyperfunctional, hypofunctional or psychogenic. However, another equally valid approach is to classify dysphonia much more specifically into patterns of inappropriate activity within the different laryngeal muscle groups. When looked at in this way, conditions previously considered to be results of hypofunction may well, in fact, turn out to be the 'end states' of different types of hyperfunction (Hillman et al., 1989; Colton and Casper, 1990). Therapy is at its most effective when it is directed precisely at the dysfunctional group of laryngeal muscles. Just as it is more effective to release tight muscles with manipulation than to ask the patient to relax, so is it more efficient to use techniques directed at specific muscular misuse rather than follow a general regime of exercises (Colton and Casper, 1990).

Remember that the position of the vocal folds depends on the isometric function of the group of muscles attached to the arytenoid, that is, a balanced set of muscular 'guy-ropes'. The arytenoid position is changed for each phonatory gesture by tightening some 'guy-ropes' and allowing antagonist muscles to slacken. Remember also that the sum of all the pulls in all the directions (the vectors) will be zero when the movement is complete, irrespective of the final length of the muscles or position of the arytenoid.

Intrinsic muscles only begin to fail when constant external tension is applied to the system by muscles that are **not** attached to the arytenoid, i.e. the cricothyroid tensioning mechanism. Persistent and inappropriate stretching of the vocal folds and their attachments can be reduced or removed by working to release the cricothyroid mechanism. Once this has been accomplished, inappropriate vocal fold positioning can be dealt with more efficiently. For example, suppose the posterior cricoarytenoid muscle (PCA) is failing to oppose vocal fold tension sufficiently. Therapy exercises could be aimed at either strengthening the PCA or reducing the vocal fold stretching by opening the cricothyroid (CT) visor. If tension is removed from the vocal folds, the PCA can recover and rebalance in relation to vocalis and the vocal ligament, restoring efficient phonation.

The principles of efficient voice production are potentially the same for all patients. It is true that some of our patients have specific restrictions on their ability to use the vocal mechanism, particularly where there is permanent damage to the larynx and/or paralysis. Even where there is no apparent damage, it would seem that certain patients are vocally limited either because they are less adept at controlling the laryngeal mechanism, or because their tissues seem less robust than normal. Although these patients may require help in learning how to compensate effectively for disability, the main aim of therapy is still to re-establish the most efficient laryngeal function possible for any particular patient.

Before moving on to discuss the treatment of dysphonia in more detail, two groups of dysphonic patients whose problems will not be discussed in detail should be mentioned: children with dysphonia and the dysarthrophonias.

Children with voice disorders

The subject of voice disorders in children is broad and, apart from some general comments given below, is beyond the scope of this chapter. More detailed information can be found in the reference section (Boone, 1980; Wilson, 1987; Hodkinson, 1990; Andrews, 1991).

Children's voice problems largely fall into the category of vocal misuse and abuse. Nevertheless, careful diagnosis is essential to exclude papilloma, congenital webs, haemangioma, stenosis, vocal fold cysts, sulci and, although very rare in children, cancer. Most children can tolerate stroboscopy using a rigid laryngoscope and where the facilities exist, a 70° narrow rigid telescope makes the examination easiest for the child. However, even today, when all else has failed, there are still rare occasions when a child requires examination under general anaesthetic to exclude vocal pathology.

Once the diagnosis has been made and explained to the parents (and the child if he or she is old enough), vocal hyperfunction can be treated. The therapy approach is decided on the basis of what is most likely to be appropriate for the individual child and his or her family. It may involve individual therapy, group therapy or indirect help through parental advice and support. Sometimes a combination of approaches is necessary. The aetiology of the voice disorder needs to be carefully explored through the case history, observation of the child and discussion with the parents. The same medical factors that have been discussed above do apply to children and need to be identified and treated if the voice disorder is to resolve with therapy.

In the majority of cases emotional factors play an important part in the aetiology of voice disorders in children (Sederholm et al., 1995). This can be difficult to tackle as parents may prefer to focus their attention on the voice problem, rather than see their child as having any emotional difficulties. Raising the possibility of emotional problems in children can arouse guilt and implied criticism of their parents. It is wise to include a psychologist, family therapist or a speech and language therapist experienced in counselling at interviews with parents if psychological factors are to be addressed.

Although voice therapy with children needs to be approached differently from work with adults, the basic aims remain the same and the interpretation of the laryngeal examination will also be similar. Muscular tension dysphonias (Morrison et al., 1983) and anterior third nodules abound among children with dysphonia (McAllister et al., 1994). The same therapy aims and techniques used for adults with these conditions can be applied, even if they need to be presented very differently. It is particularly useful to teach children who are constantly shouting to do so economically by tuning in the 'singer's formant'. Alison Bagnall has produced a helpful video entitled 'Yell Well', which gives practical suggestions as to how this can be achieved. She has done much valuable work in applying Estill's Compulsory Figures to the field of voice pathology.

Group voice therapy can be useful with children and their parents. Much of the ear and kinaesthetic training lends itself well to group work and children will readily explore their vocal potential together in games. The parents are also seen in a group so that the work carried out on the course can be explained and observations about the children's behaviour can be discussed. These group meetings often provide greater insights about the children, their home situation, and the views and fears of their parents than would usually emerge during individual interviews. The very fact that they share their experiences as parents is often enough to reduce anxiety allowing them to begin to explore their feelings about their children and how they communicate. Practical advice can be given on how to help the children at home and follow-up meetings can be arranged if parents wish, either individually or in the group.

Dysarthrophonias

Voice problems often occur in conjunction with dysarthria following a cerebrovascular accident (CVA), head injury or as part of a degenerative process, such as motor neurone disease or Parkinsonism. The treatment of these problems is beyond the scope of this chapter as they are usually part of a much wider picture of speech and language disturbance and are rarely the main focus of attention in rehabilitation. Dealing with dysarthrophonia requires considerable expertise in working with neurological problems and is probably best dealt with by a speech and language therapist specializing in the field of neurological disorders. Excellent chapters on neurological voice problems can be found in all the recent major text books (e.g. Green and Mathieson, 1989; Fawcus, 1990; Case, 1991; Rubin et al., 1995).

Dysarthrophonia can and should, however, be assessed in the voice clinic in order to understand the nature and extent of the problem. Ideally, of course, the treating therapist should attend the clinic and take part in the assessment procedure. However, life is rarely ideal and where this is not possible it is essential that the treating therapist has access to accurate information about the voice clinic diagnosis and liaison, where this is appropriate.

The treatment of voice disorders

General topics and traditional exercises

Posture and relaxation

Traditionally, voice therapy tended to follow a pattern of postural and relaxation techniques, followed by breathing exercises, voicing and resonance work, with a final period of consolidation and review. As we begin to understand the nature of the muscular patterns we are trying to alter, so our techniques can become more specific. This is not to say that there is no place for following the pattern described as there are certainly times when it is helpful to do so. It is more, perhaps, that the exercises we choose from our repertoire are better designed to make the changes we want.

Inappropriate muscular tension is frequently generated by poor posture. Our sedentary life style and our reliance on machines such as cars and computers has increased our chances of misusing our bodies and allowing poor posture to develop (see Chapter 6). It is therefore especially important that speech and language therapists continue to help patients develop an awareness of their postural habits and to give them simple guidelines to achieve and maintain good posture. Unfortunately, some patients lose flexibility of movement in the spine and are unable to alter their posture without compensating somewhere else in the body, creating different and sometimes worse difficulties. These cases need to be recognized and referred for assessment by other colleagues, such as osteopaths and physiotherapists, who are able to mobilize the spine and enable postural change. Good advice and patient monitoring then has a better chance of success, as do more specialized techniques, such as the Alexander, Feldenkrais or Pilates techniques (Alexander, 1932; Feldenkrais, 1949; Barlow, 1973). (The Pilates technique addresses body awareness through exercises directed towards specific muscle groups. It can be valuable in helping to correct patients' postural problems by systematically strengthening weak muscle groups while persistently hypertonic groups are relaxed and lengthened. Exercises are mainly carried out from a lying position on specially designed plinths. There is little in the literature relating to this technique, but further information on where to seek help can be found in the Useful Addresses section at the end of this chapter.)

A short worksheet of useful exercises that can be given to patients to work through is given in Appendix 7.1.

Working on both posture and relaxation requires patients to develop their proprioceptive skills allowing them to tune into physical sensations that they can later use to develop a monitoring system. The ability to self-monitor will enable the self-correction necessary to alter poor posture and decrease associated muscular tension. Some practical ideas to help patients develop these skills also appear in Appendix 7.1.

Relaxation, palpation and manipulation

Patients often use inappropriate and/or excessive muscular effort in conversational speech. This is easily observed by watching the activity in their faces and necks together with general head and body movements. Without actually touching the patient, however, it is less easy to distinguish between a lively conversational style and excessive muscular tension.

Until relatively recently speech therapists have tended to be reticent about touching patients. This is largely because their training does not include guidance as to what to palpate, how this should be done or what to make of the findings. A further factor is the nature of the relationship between the therapist and patient. Counselling can so often become part of the therapeutic work. When it does, the way in which touch is interpreted may be altered, leaving both patient and therapist vulnerable. In the past, therefore, assessments of tension have tended to describe only gross observations. Similarly, relaxation work mostly concentrated on specific head and neck movements, clenching and releasing different muscle groups (Jacobsen, 1938) and various imaging and biofeedback techniques that induced global physical and mental relaxation. Although these exercises are still useful, palpation and manipulation provide a more direct and effective way to assess and release tight muscles.

Surprisingly little research appears to have been carried out on the effects of laryngeal palpation and manipulation, despite good clinical evidence of its value (Aronson, 1985; Boone and McFarlane, 1988; Mathieson, 1993; Roy and Leeper, 1993). With guidance and practice it is not difficult for speech and language therapists to learn how to identify differences in muscle tone and to locate areas of habitual hyperfunction. Learning palpatory skills from an experienced osteopath or physiotherapist is invaluable and allows therapists a clearer understanding of their professional boundaries.

Although it is appropriate that palpation becomes a part of the assessment and treatment, it is essential that speech and language therapists recognize their limitations and when to seek expert help from a trained colleague. For example, there is a great difference between reducing strap muscle tension by gentle massage and manipulation of the posterior cricoarytenoid muscles behind the larynx. The latter should not be attempted without careful training and supervision from an expert. At present there are relatively few osteopaths or physiotherapists who have applied their manipulative skills to the larynx, and this makes further training and research difficult to acquire. However, much good experience can be gained by making palpation a regular part of the assessment procedure, along with careful study of the relevant anatomy and physiology (Dickson and Maue-Dickson, 1982; Harris and Lieberman, 1993; Vilkman et al., 1996).

A protocol for palpatory assessment designed for speech and language therapists is provided in Appendix 7.2 of this chapter, and some suggestions for treatment are discussed later in this chapter. The whole topic is covered in more detail in Chapter 6.

Breathing

To breathe or not to breathe? Traditionally voice therapy has been based on the premise that voice disorders resulted largely from faulty breathing patterns. Voice therapy, therefore, has tended to focus on breathing exercises aimed at improving these faulty patterns. Much controversy exists today concerning the role of breathing in voice therapy. Some authorities feel it is unnecessary to work on breathing at all (Fawcus, 1990). The truth usually lies somewhere in between the two extremes, so those who feel 'if you adjust the vocal folds correctly the breathing will take care of itself' will be no more or less right than those who say 'if you get the breathing right the voice will take care of itself'. It seems sensible then to:

1. Review the role of breathing in voice production from first principles and decide whether it is logical to work on breathing to improve voice production (see Chapter 4).
2. If that decision is 'yes' then what exercises are likely to be the most effective? (if 'no', this need only be a very short paragraph).

No one can deny that breath is important to voice production, as it is generally recognized to be the initiator of vocal fold vibration. If a larynx is removed from a recently deceased person and warm wet air is blown through the glottis at an appropriate rate, vocal fold vibration is initiated. This vibration will be sustained for the duration of the airflow. It is true that only a very basic 'quack' is possible without the control of the airstream normally provided by vocal fold adjustments and the presence of supraglottic resonators. However, although the recently removed larynx can be manipulated in every possible way, without airflow it will never achieve sound, primitive or otherwise.

It would seem then, that phonation and airflow remain inextricably interlinked. It is therefore logical to suppose that if you alter one, the other will also alter as the relationship between them has changed. The inverse relationship between the velocity of the airflow and the resistance created to it by the vocal folds is well understood. Furthermore as Titze (1994) notes: 'by varying the glottis continually (more closure for higher pressures and less closure for lower pressures) the pulmonary system can regulate the flow of air to be more constant. This regulation, which is accomplished automatically by the nervous system, applies to both inspiration and expiration. *The important message is that laryngeal action and thoracic action are not independent. There are reflexes that tie them together as a functional unit.*'

During breathing at rest, inspiration and expiration are usually perceived as being approximately equal in length, although recently objective evidence suggests that expiration lasts slightly longer (Hoit and Hixon, 1991). If there is little need to exchange carbon dioxide for more oxygen, this is followed by what is perceived as a short pause before the cycle begins again. However, as soon as the mechanism is used for speech or singing, the ratio between inspiration and expiration changes dramatically to approximately 1:8 in speech, with expiration controlled to last approximately 8 times longer than inspiration. This change creates a problem for the respiratory system as tidal volume is no longer moved in and out at the same rate. The rate of inspiratory airflow is now much greater than expiratory airflow and as a result the motor system governing breathing has to be reorganized in order to maintain efficient gaseous exchange. The increase in the rate of inspiration means that it is essential to keep the airway free of any constriction, so the vocal folds open (abduct) widely, although, even then, it is still common to hear turbulence on fast inspiration.

A description of breathing and how it takes place can be found in Chapter 4 and also in Proctor (1980) and, more recently, Hixon (Hoit and Hixon, 1991). It is more important from the point of view of clinical management to ask the question: 'Is there a right way to breathe? And if so, what is it?' Hixon's studies seem to show that people use a number of different habitual breathing patterns and as they do not drop dead instantly, each is successful in achieving the main aim of maintaining good gaseous exchange. However, observation of small babies suggests that, initially at least, diaphragmatic movement forms the major component of inspiration (Boliek et al., 1996). Most authorities continue to view the diaphragm as the major muscle of inspiration in adults as well (Hoit and Hixon, 1991).

While this does not mean that diaphragmatic breathing can be considered as the 'right' way to breathe, it is perhaps possible to consider it to be an economical way to breathe, i.e. economical of muscular effort. Abdominal breathing requires displacement of soft tissue, while upper chest or clavicular breathing is achieved by altering the shape of a semi-rigid bony box. The former also produces a greater change in lung volume than the latter (see Chapter 4).

Clearly, provided the breathing pattern used is equal to the demands made upon it, it probably does not matter what type is used. If, however, there is evidence that it is **not** meeting an individual's requirements, it is important to consider whether altering the pattern might improve the effectiveness.

What alters breathing patterns?

The most common factors affecting habitual breathing patterns are chest conditions such as asthma or chronic obstructive airways disease, which reduce vital capacity or the compliance of the lungs. Upper airway problems, for example nasal blockage, can also affect breathing patterns.

Posture can affect breathing in a number of ways (see Chapter 6). One particular aspect that is often overlooked is the effect of a tightly held in abdominal musculature. For example, dancers, athletes and gymnasts, among others, have learned to maintain tight abdominal muscles in order to protect their lower backs or to look slim. As a result, they may have difficulty in releasing the abdominal muscles in order to make space for the abdominal contents, displaced by the descending diaphragm. The postural effects of pregnancy together with the reduction in abdominal space both tend to alter the breathing towards an upper chest pattern in women.

It is also important to consider the emotional tendencies of the patient. Those who have high levels of anxiety or anger may tend to lock the abdomen and restrict their breathing. Both these emotional states involve the secretion of adrenalin. Adrenalin increases the rate of respiration and adds accessory muscle activity (upper chest and clavicular area) to the normal abdominal pattern in preparation for the respiratory requirements of 'fight or flight'. It also diverts blood flow to the muscles and increases their resting tone. Although there does not appear to be much literature relating the effects of habitual emotional states to long-term changes in breathing patterns, it is well documented in the psychosomatic litera-ture that anxiety and hostility/anger have serious effects on body tissues and general health (Levy and Heiden, 1990; Everson et al., 1996).

Finally, Hixon's research suggests that people of differing body types may tend to adopt different breathing patterns, the endomorphs relying more on abdominal breathing and ectomorphs tending towards chest breathing (Hoit and Hixon, 1991).

Given that abdominal breathing appears to be both natural and economical of muscular effort, it seems logical to encourage patients to adopt it. Where they do, they are likely to reduce unnecessary muscular tension in the accessory muscles of respiration, including the shoulders, neck and the suspensory muscles of the larynx. Improvements in the control of both airflow and subglottic pressure tend to reduce hyperadduction (overly tight vocal fold closure), which is associated with what Johan Sundberg describes as 'pressed phonation'. Sundberg further refers to 'efficient phonation without undue hyperadduction' as 'flow phonation'. These terms seem useful and appropriate as they describe the perceptual quality of the physical events extremely well (Smith and Thyme, 1981; Sundberg, 1987).

How can breathing patterns be improved?

Altering the breathing pattern at rest alone is unlikely to improve phonation. It is the combination of improved airflow and the coordination of this with gentle vocal fold closure that seems to reduce vocal hyperadduction and constriction, restoring healthy vocal folds and efficient phonation. Clinically, the aims are to:

1.   improve the patient's awareness of their breathing pattern;
2.   establish easy abdominal breathing at rest;
3.   coordinate voiceless sounds with abdominal exhalation;
4.   coordinate phonation with abdominal exhalation;
5.   coordinate breath and voice for simple words, phrases and sentences;
6.   develop control over the abdominal muscles to assist stressing and vocal volume.

Other exercises that improve resonance balance, alter tongue position and increase vocal range can be easily incorporated into the general scheme outlined above to condition abdominal breathing into conversational speech.

Working on awareness can be approached through watching, listening and feeling. The easiest to begin with perhaps is watching.

Watching

Patients can watch themselves in a mirror or simply look down at the chest/torso area and observe the movements that occur during breathing. If the patients are working in a group it is easier to pair them so each can observe the other's breathing pattern. The following are useful observations:

1. What movement occurs in your chest when you breathe in?
2. What movement occurs in your lower abdomen (tummy) when you breathe in?
3. What does your chest do when you breathe out?
4. What does your tummy do when you breathe out?
5. How does your chest move when you speak?
6. How does your tummy move when you speak?
7. What movement do you see when you take a sharp breath in? (this breath is like a quiet gasp).
8. When you are breathing at rest which is longer, the breath in or the breath out, or are they the same?
9. When you speak, do you speak on the breath in or the breath out?
10. What happens to the length of the breath in and the breath out when you speak?

The answers to these questions seem obvious, but it is amazing how many people have never given any thought to the process of breathing. They are even less aware of what happens to their breathing when they speak. It is very important for patients to develop observational skills during therapy as they are all that will be available to them later to monitor changes in everyday life when there is no therapist to remind them what **should** occur.

Listening

Developing auditory awareness is essential when working with voice-disordered patients. It is extremely difficult to alter voice quality when patients are totally unable to hear the vocal changes that occur during voice exercises and vocal play. Developing auditory skills for voice will be discussed later, but the work starts when dealing with the breathing.

The following exercises and questions are useful to get patients thinking.

(a) Cover your ears and breathe through your mouth - listen to the breath and notice which is louder, the breath in or the breath out?
(b) Breathe through your nose at rest. Is it quieter, louder or the same as mouth breathing? Can you think of a reason for your findings?
(c) Listen to yourself speak. Can you hear your breathing?
(d) Listen to others speaking. Do you hear their breathing?
(e) Can you think of any reasons why some people breathe noisily while others do not?

(f)   Can you think of anything that might affect how noisy your breathing is?
(g)   Cover your ears and breathe through your mouth. Can you breathe quietly so
      that you cannot hear yourself? (See section on releasing laryngeal constriction
      p. 177)

Feeling (kinaesthetic feedback)

Feeling, or kinaesthetic feedback, is a far more important element in voice therapy
than is usually recognized. Although most therapists would consider kinaesthetic
feedback to be important, there seems to be relatively little practical work given to
patients to improve their kinaesthetic skills. Unfortunately, many of our patients
seem to have very little awareness of the state of their bodies, never mind awareness
of the state of muscular tension in, say, the cricothyroid visor (see Chapter 5).
However, if vocal re-education is to be successful, then the patient needs to develop
the ability to monitor whether they are producing their voice well or returning to
their former habits. Without outside reminders from therapists and technology (for
example, the laryngograph) the only modalities left are listening, watching and feeling. Watching becomes extremely difficult in a social or work situation, which leaves
listening and feeling. It is interesting that the patients who use a varied vocabulary to
describe the sensations associated with their voice disorder usually do much better
than those who simply describe the voice as being 'hoarse'.

Learning to develop 'feeling' as a skill is perhaps best introduced in combination with 'watching'. If the patient has already been working on posture and relaxation then some of the concepts should already have been introduced. If not, then
it may be useful to adapt some of the ideas given in Appendix 7.1 to develop more
general kinaesthetic awareness before applying these ideas to breathing.

When working on the breathing pattern, ask the patient to place one hand on their
lower abdomen and the other on the upper chest, so that they can watch and feel the
breathing pattern at rest and in speech as described above. Once the patient has identified their habitual pattern they can try to alter it to the target pattern. It may be helpful to alternate between the two patterns, to see and feel how the movement changes.
Once the target pattern is established the patient repeats the exercises with his or her
eyes closed to cut out extraneous information and to tune into the sensation. Singers
and dancers are particularly good at this type of monitoring, which may be a major
reason they respond so well to therapy. With a little practice though, most patients
can begin to feel the slight pressure changes against their hands as they monitor their
inspiration and expiration. They may also describe a feeling in the stomach/abdomen
of downward pressure on inspiration as the abdominal contents are displaced, or
alternatively a pressure in the upper chest as they produce upper chest expiration.
Ask them to describe what they feel. It may be necessary to give them some suggestions at first until they get the idea of talking about physical sensations.

Once abdominal breathing has been established in the clinic session and the
patient can reproduce it accurately, they can begin to monitor themselves during their
everyday life. Useful moments might be on the bus or train, while they are waiting to
be seen for appointments, in the commercial breaks on TV, in fact, any 'dead' time

during the day when they have a moment to think 'How am I breathing?', and 'Can I correct it?'. Little and often is much better than an hour's practice once a week. Some patients teach it to their spouses or children. There is no better way to be sure you have understood the principles than to have to teach it yourself, as therapists know.

All this sounds as if it takes the first six sessions of therapy, but surprisingly it is usually successfully accomplished in the first session together with coordination of breath and phonation. It may be necessary to recap during the second session to troubleshoot any problems, and again on each subsequent session to check that no errors have arisen.

The role of the abdominal muscles

The most accessible abdominal muscles involved in assisting controlled expiration are the rectus abdominis and the internal and external obliques (see Chapter 4). These muscles are related to respiration, as they can be recruited to assist the ascent of the diaphragm and the descent of the rib cage, acting rather like a piston. They do this by shifting the abdominal contents upwards under the relaxing diaphragm, thus increasing intrathoracic pressure and accelerating the airflow out.

In practical terms patients need first to learn where these muscles run, from pictures and by feeling them on their own bodies. They need to experience their effect on respiration. This can be done by placing their hands on the abdomen and asking them to laugh or to cough. They will feel the abdominal muscles 'kick' increasing the rate of exhalation. To gain further control of these muscles patients can try the following exercises.

1. Pulling the lower abdomen in and out. Place one hand on the lower abdomen so it covers from the pubic area up to the navel (i.e. the lower tummy bump). The other hand should cover the area from the navel to just under the lower end of the sternum (the upper tummy bump). The patient is then asked to pull their tummy towards the back so that the lower abdomen seems to curl up and under the upper tummy bump, which curves slightly down and over it. The movement is a little like opening a can of sardines with a key, and work can be felt on either side in the groin area. The lower ribs will kick very slightly outwards as the abdomen is pulled in. The patient can practise this movement on its own to develop kinaesthetic awareness of abdominal muscles, not only in their contracted state, but also when that contraction is released and the tummy jumps back out again. Control of this 'release phase' is extremely important in order to make space for the abdominal contents on inspiration and to enable further abdominal muscle contractions that may be required for stressing speech.

2. Placing both hands either side of the lower abdomen, pretend to blow out three dinner candles extremely quickly. Feel the abdominal muscles 'kick in' on the forced blowing.

3. With hands either side of the lower abdomen, imagine you are blowing up a lilo (airbed or swimming arm bands). Feel the strong, smooth contraction of

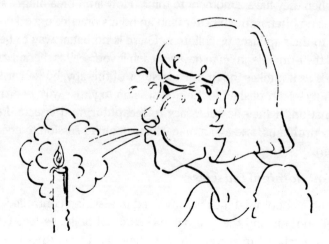

the abdominal muscles as you blow up the imaginary lilo/air bed.

4.   To demonstrate the effect of the stronger, controlled airflow on sound production, ask the patient to produce a sustained fricative (for example /s/ or /z/) and pull the tummy in and out as they do so. It is immediately noticeable that the sound can no longer be kept steady and that the volume of the sound fluctuates, becoming louder and a little higher in pitch as the abdominal muscles are pulled in, then softer and lower in pitch as they are released.

Some patients find this hard to do in phonation and the therapist may feel that they are still 'overcontrolling' the airflow on /z/ with excess adductory effort. To help their kinaesthetic awareness, it may be useful to give them the experience of allowing increased airflow to alter the sound artificially. The patient is asked to produce a long steady fricative while the therapist applies abdominal pressure externally by pushing the abdomen in and releasing it again rhythmically. Because of the problems some patients have with being touched, it is worth explaining the task first, asking their permission and checking that they have no abdominal pain. The therapist can put his or her hand over the patient's hand on the abdomen to prevent direct contact with the body that could feel threatening or suggestive to the patient.

Patients soon discover that an increase in airflow tends to increase the perceived loudness of the sound without any vocal effort on their part. The abdominal muscles can also be used to stress words as well as increase the general volume of their voices. It is important, however, to ensure that patients do not hyperadduct the vocal folds and constrict during these exercises.

Although a little simplistic, these exercises still provide a useful, practical demonstration of the effects of the abdominal muscles that can shortcut confusing technical explanations. They also form an excellent basis for introducing the Accent Method (AM), which is described later in this section, and condition abdominal muscle control for expiration in spontaneous speech.

Coordinating breath and voice

When working to coordinate breath and voice, breathing and vocal techniques can no longer be separated. From the moment voicing is added to controlled expiration we have to begin to consider the role of the glottal resistance to the airstream and to refine our work to achieve specific aims for each patient.

The coordination of breath and voicing requires control over the initiation of phonation. This can be carried out in three ways:

1. Glottal onset (often referred to as glottal attack), where glottal closure precedes the onset of expiration and phonation. It should not be confused with 'hard glottal attack', which implies hyperadduction and constriction.
2. Simultaneous onset, where the glottal closure is synchronized with the onset of the expiratory airflow and phonation.
3. Breath before tone (also known as 'aspirate onset'; Estill, 1996), where the expiratory airflow precedes glottal closure and the onset of phonation.

These glottal onsets can be applied to any different voice quality, but are usually associated with characteristic vocal sets (Estill, 1996). Glottal onset, which requires short, relaxed vocal folds and increased bulk in the vocalis muscles, is usually associated with speech quality. Simultaneous onset, which requires rather longer, thinned vocal folds, is often associated with 'head register'. Breath before tone with long, thinned and stiffened vocal folds is associated with falsetto quality.

Learning to produce and apply different glottal onsets marks the beginning of an ability to differentiate between laryngeal muscle groups and thus to develop control over the vocal mechanism (Estill, 1996). Work on vocal onset can be particularly valuable when therapy is aimed towards altering a specific voice quality or vocal set, e.g. trying to eradicate the habitually thinned folds associated with the 'little girl voice', which is commonly used by women in the UK.

The voice pattern of the patient will dictate which type of onset will be most useful to concentrate on in therapy with each patient. Patients with habitual hyperadduction often respond well to work either on simultaneous onset or 'breath before tone'. Although Estill associates 'breath before tone' with falsetto quality in singing, it can be adapted for use with modal voice to decrease glottal resistance. The easiest way to introduce it is by preceding the phonation onset with a gentle voiceless fricative, for example, fffvvvfff. Once patients can reliably produce voice with decreased glottal resistance and a stronger airflow, simultaneous onset can be introduced by removing the voiceless fricative so that the patient produces its voiced counterpart (vvv). The simultaneous onset can then be trained into spontaneous speech (see the Accent Method, page 167).

Traditionally, glottal onset has been shunned by speech therapists because of its associations with hard glottal attack, which is common among dysphonic patients and known to be abusive and irritating to vocal fold mucosa. However, where patients are unable to achieve or maintain glottal closure, glottal onsets are appropriate and helpful. Patients are asked to close the glottis gently but firmly and to feel the pressure of air build up below the vocal folds. They then release the airstream (subglottic pressure) in tiny voiceless 'pops'. These are produced very lightly, but are clearly audible, and it is important not to allow any constriction/hyperadduction to creep into their production. Once established, the glottal pops are voiced and then prolonged, producing and maintaining good closure. The technique is usually continued by working through words, phrases and sentences that include a preponderance of vowels, especially at the beginning of utterances. Once full vocal fold closure has been established, it is maintained by flowing the end of each word into the beginning of the next, supporting phonation with smooth, steadily controlled contraction of the abdominal muscles. The technique is closely akin to the prolonged speech technique sometimes used with stammerers. Prosody needs to be addressed, together with 'stressing', much of which can be carried out by the abdominal musculature (see section on Accent Method, page 167).

Maintaining breath control during speech

Work that maintains the coordination and control of breathing and voice during speech and singing is part and parcel of some vocal techniques, such as the Accent Method. Where it is not built into a technique it should be addressed anyway, as it may well be important to the patient's ability to maintain successful vocal change over time.

To produce relaxed, fluent speech, the speaker must know exactly when the subglottic pressure begins to fail and undue strain falls on the voice. It is then possible to '**top up**' the breath at appropriate moments to prevent fatigue and constriction.

The top-up breath is a short sharp inspiration, through the mouth, like the quiet gasp that occurs with a delightful surprise. It is not at all the same as the constricted gasp that occurs when an unpleasant shock is experienced. Patients can practise this breath in isolation initially, monitoring the sudden descent of the diaphragm with a hand on their stomach. It is important not to do too many consecutive top-ups or patients will hyperventilate and feel giddy. If this happens, reassure them that this is normal and restrict the number of top-ups they repeat at any one time. The top-up breath can then be practised in automatic speech, either (a) between groups of numbers, days, months, etc., or (b) by starting with three and increasing each count by one until the patient feels they are using residual air. The lower abdomen should move smoothly in as each group of numbers is spoken and each word should be run into the next to prevent hard attack and maintain the vocal set.

(a)
1 2 3 4 (top up)
5 6 7 8 (top up)
9 10 11 12 (top up)
13 14 15 16 (top up)
17 18 19 20

(b)
1 2 3 (top up)
1 2 3 4 (top up)
1 2 3 4 5 (top up)
1 2 3 4 5 6

Reading passages to practise breath control, topping up, stressing and prosody in continuous speech are useful, as are rhymes and poems. The longer sentences can be divided up into sense units that are easy for the patient to manage and pave the way for moving into spontaneous speech.

Voice therapy techniques

This section highlights treatment techniques and their application to specific patterns of laryngeal muscle misuse. The range of techniques described is by no means exhaustive but covers the most popular and effective methods currently used in speech and language therapy. Some have already been synthesized into systems designed to start patients at single sound level and gradually work through more complex patterns to spontaneous speech. Others focus only at the single sound or syllable level and require the therapist to build the new pattern into speech.

Let us begin by exploring two of the most useful systems and then move on to the more familiar techniques.

The Accent Method

This useful technique to coordinate breath and voice was devised by Svend Smith, a Danish phonetician. One evening, probably in a spirit of scientific endeavour, he was attending a night club, and his attention was rivetted by the rhythms being played by the jazz singer Josephine Baker's bongo drummer. Smith arranged a meeting with the drummer, and together they devised a series of rhythms that could be used for his voice exercises. The voice exercises were based on the prosody of speech and were called the Accent Method. The Accent Method is well described in other references so only a brief description of the technique will be given here (Smith and Thyme, 1981; Kotby, 1995).

Initially, abdominal breathing is established with the patient lying supine. A strong airflow should be developed using elastic recoil of the lungs. The airstream is then interrupted by the lips or tongue to produce voiceless fricatives, such as /ɸ/ (bilabial) /s/, /ʃ/('shh') /f/. The patient's attention is drawn to the strength of the sounds compared with the small amount of effort required to produce them. The therapist provides the modelled sound and the patient repeats it, feeling with his or her hand the inward movement of the abdominal wall as the sounds are produced.

Gradually the voiceless fricatives are replaced by their voiced counterparts. Blowing through closed lips, /ɸ/ becomes /β/, /s/ becomes /z/, /ʃ/ becomes /ʒ/, and /f/ becomes /v/ (see also Laukkanen et al., 1996). The voiced fricatives are produced in low modal voice with high airflow and a relatively low glottal resis-

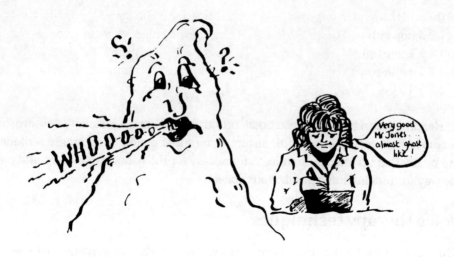

tance so that phonation is breathy. Patients are encouraged to feel the pressure of the air pushing behind the oral constriction provided by the lips and tongue during the early stage of production. They notice how this quickly falls as the pressure drops and the respiratory musculature returns to its rest position. In this way, patients become aware of how it feels to displace the ribs, diaphragm and abdominal contents on inspiration and how they return to a reliable 'rest position' following expiration.

Although not directly part of the Accent Method, it is useful at this stage to draw attention to the feeling of effort created in the respiratory musculature and vocal tract as the breath is pushed past the normal rest position of quiet breathing on to residual air. In this way the sensations can be learned for full inspiration, rest position for quiet breathing and the use of residual air. The patient can then learn how to produce voice on a higher airflow controlled between adequate inspiration and just past the rest position, thus avoiding habitual voicing on residual air that is so common.

Once the patient has established easy, relaxed phonation on a higher airflow, the abdominal muscles are introduced to begin to control the speed of expiration (see above for practical exercises on how to do this). The patient is asked to allow a breathy vowel to start on elastic recoil, then to 'pull in', kick, or squeeze the abdominal muscles to accelerate the airflow before letting the sound die away as the abdominal muscles are released. The effect on the sound is one of increased loudness, together with a very slight increase in pitch. It is a little like being in the car with a foot on the accelerator pedal listening to the engine note. As the accelerator pedal is depressed, the note of the engine becomes louder and a little higher in pitch as the engine turns over faster. As the accelerator pedal is released, the sound drops in pitch and becomes quieter. The exercise is carried out in a slow three beat rhythm, the *largo* rhythm, with the 'accents' or 'stresses' produced by small abdominal muscle contractions or 'kicks'. Initially the unaccentuated upbeat is followed by one accentuated or stressed beat and the accented beats are then increased to two and three. Although the abdominal muscles seem to be used most efficiently and easily when released a little between each kick, the general effect is that the abdominal wall continues to move inwards throughout phonation, albeit jerkily.

The early stages of the Accent Method are so relaxing they are almost hypnotic and patients usually respond to them quickly. They are carried out first with fricatives and breathy close vowels in strict alternation with the therapist who 'models' the required vocal quality and rhythmic structure. The close vowels are /i-u/, i.e. those with a high tongue position. The therapist and patient can model and monitor the abdominal accents or kicks by placing a hand on each other's abdominal wall to check the work is being done correctly. To prevent any misunderstanding of the touching that this type of monitoring requires, teachers of the method suggest that the back of the hand is used. A rhythmic rocking forwards and backwards in synchrony with the inspiration and expiration/phonation reinforces the breathing pattern and rhythmic structure.

The aim of the exercises is to condition the patient to produce well-controlled airflow coordinated with soft, breathy phonation in modal (chest) register and low pitch. 'Breathy' phonation in this context refers to minimal air escape and is totally unrelated to the air turbulance associated with constriction. Where the word 'breathy' appears in this chapter it will always apply in this context.

Traditionally the rhythms are accompanied by a drum beat. This is not essential, and although useful with patients who have a sense of rhythm, it can be disruptive where patients do not, as they become anxious about keeping in rhythm and lose touch with the purpose of the exercise. The exercises are usually introduced with the patient lying down, then sitting and finally standing, but there is room for flexibility, depending on the patient's skill and previous experience with breathing techniques.

Once the largo rhythm is well established the pace is increased to a four/four rhythm (*andante*). The principle remains the same, with the therapist modelling the voicing and rhythm while the patient repeats it. The number of stresses increase gradually in varying rhythmic cadences up to four or more contractions of the abdominal muscles. The breathy close vowels are gradually replaced by other vowels or consonant/vowel combinations, allowing the therapist to tailor the sounds used to develop the effect required, for example, improving oral/nasal resonance balance or altering tongue position. Prosody may be introduced so that the patient imitates the stress and intonation patterns modelled by the therapist, including variations in intensity (loud/soft contrasts). When the patient masters andante, the pace is increased by the therapist and the number of stresses also increases to five or more (*allegro* rhythm). For experienced professional voice-users, such as singers, the complexity of the accentuation/stresses may be increased to between 13 and 21 to further enhance abdominal muscle control.

The Accent Method is not a static technique, and as soon as the patient can carry out the exercises standing, arm movements similar to the gestures used naturally in speech are introduced to help bring further life to the prosody. The whole body can be rocked to the rhythm preventing the knees from locking and the body from tensing up. As the patient becomes experienced in babbling the sequences of sounds they can develop a rhythmic nonsense 'conversation' with the therapist, relying only on prosody, intonation, accentuation/stress and duration to convey meaning. It is a little like listening to a conversation through a wall where the words cannot be clearly heard but the listener is left in no doubt as to the type of communication going on or to the mood of the speakers.

As the patient progresses through the graded series of exercises, rhythmic coordination of breath and phonation is trained and the glottal resistance gradually increases to produce a clearer, less breathy tone. Rather like working with a knot in a shoe lace, it is infinitely easier to tighten a loose knot than unpick a tight one.

Acoustic analysis of phonation produced by patients pre- and post-Accent Method therapy demonstrates the following changes:

1. changes in fundamental frequency (lower for those with voices judged as perceptually high, and higher for those judged perceptually as too low);
2. reduction in jitter (cycle to cycle perturbation of the fundamental frequency);
3. improved pitch range for intonation;
4. increased intensity with reduced shimmer (cycle to cycle amplitude perturbation);
5. improved ability to stress the important words in speech or song;
6. enhancement of the vocal spectrum particularly in the formants F_2/F_3;
7. increased ability to vary vocal timbre (see section on speech spectrography in Part 13)

(Smith and Thyme, 1976; Frøkjær Jensen, 1983; Thyme and Frøkjær Jensen, 1983; Thyme and Frøkjær Jensen, 1987; Kotby et al., 1991).

Physiologically, the Accent Method aims to train the patient to use simultaneous vocal onset, where breath is released as the vocal folds close, to prevent the development of hard attack and glottic constriction.

Clinical experience suggests that the Accent Method is extremely successful in helping patients relax the cricothyroid muscles, develop modal voice and reduce constriction, both at the level of the glottis and generally in the vocal tract. The increase in subglottic pressure that underpins this method seems to have a number of effects in most patients. Observation of the larynx using a nasopharyngeal fibrescope shows that as patients produce fricatives in the early stages of the technique, the larynx seems to rise as the subglottal pressure increases. This tendency needs to be opposed by extrinsic muscle activity to stabilize the larynx (sternothyroid/sternohyoid) and an increase in vocal fold closure. The hyoid bone and base of tongue attachments appear to move forwards and upwards with each stressed/accentuated beat. This movement increases the antero-posterior pharyngeal space and gives the impression that the larynx has tilted forward, providing excellent visualization. These observations are based in clinical practice and need further verification. The secondary vocal tract constriction produced by the lips/tongue is believed to create back pressure, aiding vocal fold closure and duration of the closed phase (Laukkanen et al., 1996).

The fricatives and close vowels that are initially used to establish the basic vocal set for the Accent Method are produced at the front of the mouth, reducing the likelihood of tongue backing. Activity in the extrinsic laryngeal muscles that anchor the larynx may encourage the lower pharyngeal constrictors and suprahyoid musculature to release. A further strength of the Accent Method is that the technique involves long periods of '*practice babbling*' to establish the target set. As a result, patients are prevented from using their habitual voicing pattern for quite long periods as practice sessions may go on for 20 minutes or more. This makes carryover into spontaneous speech much easier and maintenance more reliable than many other techniques. A further advantage is that training tapes can be easily made during the session for additional home practice.

Estill's Compulsory Figures

Jo Estill was a singer by training who became interested in the physiology of the singing voice towards the end of her singing career. Her interest led her into the field of voice research and the development of her system of Compulsory Figures. Using such techniques as EMG, electroglottography and voice signal analysis, together with X-rays of the phonating larynx and laryngeal fibre endoscopy, Estill studied various voice qualities associated with different styles of singing. As a result of her research she was able to synthesize a series of vocal manoeuvres that allow singers to develop specific control over individual muscle groups within the vocal mechanism. When the control developed by these manoeuvres is applied to the singing voice, singers discover they have greater range and flexibility of style without fear of damage or strain to the larynx. Because the manoeuvres are based on careful observation of normal laryngeal function, they can be applied to **any** type of voice use. They have proved valuable not just in the teaching of singing, but also in the training of others wishing to develop their voice, whether professional or not. Perhaps even more importantly, the work allows singing/voice teachers, voice coaches, and speech and language therapists to identify and resolve specific vocal problems that have resulted in fatigue or damage to the vocal folds.

Estill describes the vocal manoeuvres as 'Compulsory Figures', rather as skaters have compulsory figures through which they work to acquire the skills they need to skate proficiently. Early on in her work the concept of the necessary effort that is involved in singing and speaking is introduced. This helps develop kinaesthetic feedback, enabling students to recognize and locate the degree of work involved in their own voice production. The 'effort' can then not only be identified, but quantified and controlled. Excessive effort that is involved in constriction is then possible to locate and special vocal manoeuvres can be applied to release it.

The compulsory figures are designed to achieve independent control of:

*   glottal and ventricular constriction;
*   the soft palate (velar port control);
*   three types of glottal onset;
*   vocal fold mass;
*   vocal fold plane;

- thyroid cartilage tilting;
- aryepiglottic constriction;
- control over the tongue and supraglottic vocal tract;
- anchoring of the head, neck and torso;
- vocal tract length and width

(Estill, 1996).

The increased control developed by the different figures allows the singer (or speaker) to manipulate the vocal tract specifically to produce a number of distinctive voice qualities. These include speech, falsetto, sob, twang, opera and belt qualities. Initially, each of these vocal qualities has a specific vocal tract prescription: for example, clear twang would require:

- a tilted thyroid cartilage (can be done without tilt but tilting is easier to begin with);
- thin vocal folds (twang with thick fold is possible but likely to be traumatic);
- a closed velar port;
- no anchoring of the head, neck or torso;
- a raised larynx;
- a raised, tense tongue;
- aryepiglottic narrowing.

'Twang' vocal quality is the gesture that best demonstrates the activity increasing medial compression of the vocal folds. (see Chapter 5).

It is not possible to explore all the manoeuvres and vocal qualities in this chapter as Estill in her manual describes six voice qualities with 27 different options. Many are already familiar to speech therapists as they have been adapted from traditional techniques but synthesized into an extremely creative system. A few that are particularly useful in voice therapy will be mentioned below, but it is recommended that speech and language therapists working regularly in the field of voice attend a recognized course on Estill's Compulsory Figures. The application of the system to dysphonic patients produces excellent results and the therapist will gain great confidence in their own voice use having mastered the manoeuvres and qualities themselves. As more therapists begin to work regularly with professional singers and actors, this work is likely to become more widely used, forming an excellent basis for voice therapy.

Humming/uh huh

This excellent technique has been around for as long as voice therapy itself. It is described in most of the major text books on therapy and also has a long history in the teaching of singing and voice (Green and Mathieson, 1989; Morrison et al., 1994). One of its major features is that it requires minimal involvement of the vocal tract beyond closing the lips. The tongue is in a neutral position, the soft palate lowered and the air released through the nose. There are many ways to teach the technique, but the easiest seems to be to begin with releasing breath through the nose audibly, as if the patient is exhausted. Then to allow voicing to come in on the breath, as if the patient were rather disdainful of something, producing a sort of nasal grunt. When viewed endoscopically, it can be seen that the position of the vocal folds resembles an extension of that seen in quiet breathing (Lawrence, 1987). The aryepiglottic folds and the arytenoid tips form a gothic arch appearance that is retained into phonation. Apart from the vocal fold closure, very little other muscular activity is seen. The closure is gentle and there is relatively little medial compression. However, the closed phase is adequate to produce good mucosal waves (see chapter 9). Because of its close relation to the position for quiet breathing, the larynx tends to be in a neutral position (neither raised nor lowered) with an open visor. Stiffening of the muscle body of the vocal fold may not occur initially, but soon develops as the technique progresses.

From the initial 'Mhuh' the length of the phonation is extended gradually into a hum. The kinaesthetic 'markers' of vibration on the lips and a slight sense of air pressure in the nose are noted, along with the ease of phonation and the low, rounded, resonant sound produced. Where an interarytenoid chink is present, the 'gothic arch' configuration of glottal closure described above appears to decreases abductor tension in the lateral cricoarytenoid (LCA) and posterior cricoarytenoid (PCA) muscles, allowing the interarytenoid chink to close. Chapter 5 describes the actions of PCA and LCA in persistent abduction, which is thought to be responsible for the interarytenoid chink.

The relatively neutral position of the vocal tract for humming appears to release excess supraglottic and extrinsic laryngeal muscle tension. Undifferentiated constriction of the supraglottic spaces prevents the formation of resonating cavities to enhance the glottal sound source. It should not be confused with the specific narrowing of the aryepiglottic folds, middle constrictor or raised tongue associated with the generation of specific formants (see Chapter 13).

The hum is gradually extended into M + vowel syllables (mmmmee, mmmah, mmmoh, etc.), followed by: M + vowel + nasal consonant syllables/words (e.g. moon, man, morn, etc.) and double syllables using nasal consonants (meaning, mining, morning, etc.).

These ideas can be dovetailed into the Accent Method structure if desired or simply extended through phrases and sentences into speech.

As with all techniques, there are certain patients who are unable to release the supraglottic tension and remain constricted in their production of the target sounds, despite having managed to close the interarytenoid chink. Ways of dealing with these difficulties will be discussed later.

Glottal fry/creak

Glottal fry is produced with short, bulky vocal folds that remain in their closed phase for much longer periods than usual. In its purest form the air is released in tiny puffs that can be heard as individual beats or clicks. To initiate creak the patient is asked to produce the lowest voice they can, making it like the opening of a creaky door in a horror film. Most patients are able to reproduce creak, especially when attention is drawn to places in their conversational voice where they produce it naturally.

It can often be heard in laid back 'NASA' American accents ('errrr Houston, we have a problem'). Once the raw sound is well established, patients will often comment on how easy it feels and most can count and say the days of the week using creaky speech quality. Boone and McFarlane (1988) recommend that patients allow themselves to run slowly out of air while producing a vowel as this often triggers creak.

It is often noticeable that there is some posterior movement of the whole larynx. This seems to be associated with short, thick folds, medial compression and increased tension in the pharyngeal constrictors. The cricothyroid visor is open and can be easily palpated. Patients are then asked to alternate creaky voice with clear voice in automatic speech, keeping the vocal set for creaky speech constant as they move to clear speech. Immediately most will notice a lower richer voice that feels easy to produce.

Yawn-sigh

This is another technique that is extremely well established in the literature on voice therapy. It takes a vegetative manoeuvre and builds on the muscular changes that take place in the larynx naturally during its production. The larynx drops downwards and the visor opens more widely than usual. The extrinsic straps muscles of the larynx tend to move it forward as well as down while the pharyngeal constrictors relax, the tongue backs and the jaw is opened widely and displaced forwards.

The voice quality produced during a yawn can be utilized to direct the patient's attention to the release of laryngeal and pharyngeal constriction and the change in quality to a breathy unconstricted tone. Care must be taken that the breathy phonation really is released as it is quite possible for constriction and false vocal fold activity to creep into breathy quality, even on yawn-sigh. As with most techniques, it is best to work first with single syllables, in this case vowels, and build the desired features gradually nearer to conversational voice through a graded sequence of words, phrases and sentences.

Viewed endoscopically, the drop of the larynx can be seen and the vocal folds are characteristically shorter and more lax. Closure is minimal and the sound breathy, gliding down in pitch. These features make it successful in opening the visor in Muscular Tension Dysphonia (MTD) (Morrison et al., 1983) patients and in closing the interarytenoid chink, but may also make it more difficult to develop through graded exercises keeping the benefits (full fold closure, open visor and relaxed vocal tract) without also involving some unwanted features, such as lowered larynx and backed tongue position. These problems are best dealt with early, by monitoring laryngeal position (with a finger on the thyroid cartilage or the thyrohyoid space) and careful attention to tongue and jaw position.

Froeschels' chewing

Chewing is a technique that is particularly helpful for patients with tight jaws and tongues, poor resonance and poor clarity. The technique was originally designed by Froeschels for stammerers. It is based on the idea that the muscles used for chewing and for speaking are the same and that speech originally develops from the movements of feeding and, in particular, chewing. The patient observes their lack of oral movement during speech in the mirror and then practises exaggerated chewing movements, with the mouth widely open so that the tongue can be seen moving within it. Gentle nasal voicing is then introduced with the chewing. The nasalization may be used to tune the formants (see Pahn's nasalization).

Boone suggests that the syllable 'yam' is used to ensure that the tongue continues to rise, fall and move forward during the exercise rather than become backed and frozen in the floor of the mouth. Gradually other speech sounds are introduced, beginning with strings of nonsense syllables and progressing to words and phrases, while the patient keeps a wider jaw opening and exaggerates tongue and articulatory movements.

This technique is useful for diverting attention away from the laryngeal area. It releases the tongue and jaw nicely and the type of phonation characteristically produced is very akin to that of humming, with strong nasal resonance in open-mouth chewing or nasally released in closed-mouth chewing (Froeschels, 1948, 1952).

The release of the jaw undoubtedly affects the extrinsic musculature of the larynx allowing it to drop down. As tight jaw and tongue muscles are closely correlated with habitual laryngeal raising, this effect of the technique needs to be drawn to the patient's attention and maintained using palpatory monitoring.

Sob (from Jo Estill's 'Compulsory Figures')

'Sob' quality is produced on a lowered larynx and thinned vocal folds. It is characterized by gentle vocal fold closure with the arytenoid tips together and braced slightly back. It is possible that this slight backward pull is accomplished by the posterior cricoarytenoid muscles, which, while paying out **a little**, remain active in stabilizing the arytenoids against the pull of vocalis and the interarytenoid.

It is easiest for the patient to produce sob quality in the mid to high vocal range initially, where the vocal folds are automatically stretched and thinned. Sometimes it is helpful to begin by asking the patient to produce a soft whimpering noise, like a small dog whining, in order to tilt the thyroid cartilage and initiate simultaneous onset in thin fold (position 1 in Figure 7.1). This seems to position the vocal folds nicely in preparation for the 'sob set' and can then be held while the patient glides down in pitch and lowers the larynx, opening the visor and reducing the tension on the vocal folds (position 2 in Figure 7.1). At lower pitches sob produces complete glottic closure and counteracts constriction effectively. The only drawbacks can be the reduced vocalis mass, which tends to restrict vocal intensity, and the lowered larynx, which can become tiring for sternothyroid and sternohyoid muscles. Patients may need to be encouraged gradually to return to the set for speech quality that requires a neutral larynx position and greater vocalis mass, while holding onto the gentle closure they have experienced while in the sob set.

Inspiration/expiration

This technique is particularly helpful for reducing excessive medial compression (also known as hypervalving) and false vocal fold phonation. It can be valuable

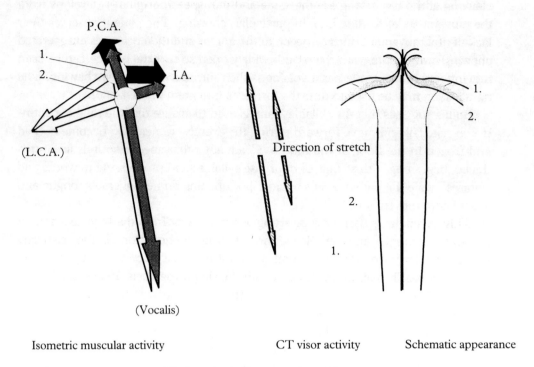

Isometric muscular activity   CT visor activity   Schematic appearance

Black arrows indicate muscle activity

Figure 7.1 Estill's Sob as an exercise. The slight change in arytenoid position between 1 and 2 occurs as the pitch is lowered.

when these features occur in combination with antero-posterior compression.

The patient is requested to produce voice on gentle inspiration. If they find this difficult to achieve it can often be elicited initially by asking them to produce a sharp, voiced inspiration of shock, for example, the reaction if you arrived at the airport and your partner asked you for the tickets, which you realized you have left at home. While this suggestion may produce a rather more forceful sound than is necessary, once the sensation is established, the effort involved can be reduced. When the patient can produce gentle voicing on inspiration reliably, he or she is asked to leave everything in the vocal tract feeling the same and to reverse the air through the same glottal aperture. The voicing produced is low and breathy, but gentle closure is usually maintained. The vocalis mass tends to be reduced and can be difficult to increase as the exercises progress towards speech quality. It does, however, provide good sensory feedback of true vocal fold control and is relatively easy to work into vowels and syllables. It is sometimes helpful to work through single vowels preceding each with /h/, before introducing other consonants and gradually reducing the characteristic breathiness.

Viewed endoscopically, inspiration/expiration shows the vocal folds to be held slightly apart. The aryepiglottic folds maintain their 'gothic arch' position and the entire length of the vocal folds is visible. There is no excessive effort observable in the supraglottic vocal tract.

This technique is very drying in the early stages and it is important to keep phonation very gentle and breathy to prevent friction and irritation to the vocal fold mucosa. Patients should be advised to sip water frequently during their early practice of the inspiration phase to 'milk' extra mucus squeezed from the laryngeal ventricles and through the closed glottis during swallowing. Gradual increase in closure and mass to progress to speech quality needs to be carefully monitored to avoid constriction.

Release of laryngeal constriction/hyperadduction

This is also known as 'retraction'/'deconstriction'. Estill has produced helpful exercises aimed at reducing glottal and ventricular constriction and her concepts are valuable to voice therapy as well as singing. During her research, Estill noticed that singers who hyperadduct the glottis tend to produce 'echoing' activity in the false vocal folds (ventricular bands). She looked for manoeuvres that release the hyperadduction and found that laughing accomplishes this naturally and has the added advantage that anyone can do it (Estill, 1991). If done silently, laughing produces an open laryngeal posture that can be 'held in place' during speech or singing, removing constriction and false vocal fold activity. Estill combines the 'silent laugh' manoeuvre with all her exercises on voice quality to prevent constriction becoming involved in voice production.

A similar effect can be achieved with the 'silent inhalation' of air advocated in the Coblenzer exercises. Patients are asked to breathe in through the mouth silently as if delighted or 'breathing in a wonderful perfume'. A sense of glottic widening can be felt and if this aperture is maintained as the air is released on phonation, the voice sounds and feels free of constriction (Coblenzer and Muhar 1976; Coblenzer 1980).

Patients can check that they have achieved the released laryngeal gesture successfully by holding the laminae of the thyroid cartilage lightly between the thumb and first finger as they silently laugh or inhale. A slight widening of the thyroid laminae can be felt and the larynx drops minimally down and forward (Bagnall, personal communication). The cricothyroid visor also opens.

Coblenzer Method

Professor Horst Coblenzer was a professional actor who devised a holistic method for developing efficient respiration, phonation and speech. His method is based on research into the role of the diaphragm in phonation, which he carried out with a lung physiologist, Professor Franz Muhar. It has also grown out of practical experience and application of Gerda Alexander's relaxation and exercise system 'Eutonia'. The main aim of the Coblenzer system is to develop speech that provides effective communication but is economic of effort. Although originally designed for work with singers and actors, it has many useful exercises and applications for working with dysphonic patients.

Coblenzer is now a Professor at the Max Reinhardt Seminar für Musik und Darstellende Kunst in Vienna. A contact address for further information on this method can be found at the end of this chapter.

Glottal onset/glottal attack

See the earlier section on coordinating breath and voice for a description of this technique.

Forcing exercises

The group of exercises described in the literature as 'forcing exercises' usually refer to isometric 'pushing exercises' that produce strong glottal closure of the type used to seal air into the lungs while lifting, straining and giving birth. Some therapists include all glottal closure exercises under this heading. It is, however, important to differentiate between the exercises designed to encourage control of the true vocal folds and phonation onset, and those that are designed to overcome **insufficiency** of glottal closure, as would be found in, say, vocal fold paralysis or bowing. In fact, it is possible to consider all of the traditional group of 'hypofunctional' voice disorders as candidates for forcing exercises. However, as we have previously suggested, many apparently hypofunctional states are likely to be the end states of hyperfunctional conditions, and as such, may not respond well to the increased effort required in forced glottal closure.

Let us first remind ourselves how forcing exercises are usually carried out. The patient is often asked to sit, placing his hands on the edges of his chair, and to try to lift his body weight as he holds his breath forcibly. He then releases the pressurized air in his lungs suddenly on a vowel. The vowel 'er' is perhaps the easiest sound to make but it can soon be varied. Another similar technique involves pressing the palms of the hands together firmly at chest level (as if exercising the pectoral muscles) and pushing as the air is sealed into the lungs with strong glottal closure. Vowels can gradually be prolonged in length and the force reduced as the patient gets the feeling of glottal closure and can repeat it reliably. Eventually the effort involved should become the same as that used in the gentler glottal onset group of exercises.

These exercises are often effective in the short term, but unless the aetiology of the condition is understood, and other features of the dysphonia addressed in therapy, their effectiveness may be short-lived. In some cases, forcing exercises can become contributory to further breakdown in muscle compensation so that, in the long run, glottal insufficiency increases.

How then can we decide when and how to use these exercises? Initially, the patient is examined using observation and palpation for signs of muscular effort that may suggest forcing exercises would be inappropriate. If muscular effort is observed as the patient speaks and is similar to that seen when forcing is carried out (e.g. the strap muscles stand out, the jaw clenches, etc.) then exercises that reduce **general** effort and encourage very specific work may be more appropriate. The Accent Method, humming and sob are all techniques that appear to encourage gentle fold closure and are probably better to try initially.

Where video techniques are available to film phonation in these patients, the therapist can look for signs of effort within the larynx, in particular the position of the arytenoid tips. It is easy to become fixated on the phonatory portion of the folds and to forget that closure is achieved by the approximation of the vocal processes.

Let us take the case of a patient with a unilateral vocal fold paresis, where the paralysed fold is poorly positioned. Forcing exercises will only be useful in this case where the innervated side shows signs of inadequate movement and is **not** bowing. Clinical experience tells us that this is rarely the case. The innervated side will most commonly be making enormous efforts to create some form of closure. These efforts can be seen in fullness and/or adduction of the false fold on the working side, with a constricted appearance of the pharyngeal space. In addition, the arytenoid on the paretic side may be tilted too far forward. When signs like these are present, it is probable that the patient is physically unable to close the phonatory gap, and surgery in the form of a thyroplasty will prove to be the best form of treatment. Thyroplasty is most effective when followed by voice therapy and manipulation of the tight muscles of the working side.

In cases of paresis where the working fold is bowing, it is worth trying to reduce the amount of effort and stretch involved in phonation, rebalancing the phonatory system with increased airflow before resorting to surgery. It is important to remember that many patients find falsetto produces the most stable voice in terms of quality, and this will involve closure of the cricothyroid visor and stretching of the vocal folds. The same rules apply in this case as with any case of bowing, i.e. the visor needs to be opened and the voice brought down to modal phonation. The bowing may disappear completely, allowing the innervated fold to compensate once more. These principles may be particularly valuable to remember for those patients who have a long-standing unilateral paresis, but who usually compensate successfully until infection or vocal overuse causes them to 'fall off their perch' and lose the delicate balance they normally maintain.

Forcing exercises are sometimes suggested for patients with bowing folds. As stated above, it is not logically the first choice of treatment, given an understanding of how we believe bowing develops. Video examination of patients with bowing vocal folds will show the effort involved in phonation. The arytenoid tips may be crammed together, tightly closing the posterior portion of the vocal folds. They may even override each other in their effort to produce closure in some patients. There is often evidence of false vocal fold activity, further demonstrating the enormous efforts being made to produce and sustain closure. Forcing is unlikely to help this group of patients, whose problem may be more related to an inability to bulk up vocalis because of prolonged stretching, rather than inability to produce vocal fold closure.

Forcing exercises may have a place in cases of psychogenic dysphonia where glottal closure is insufficient and little effort appears to be given to speaking. Where patients are depressed, their general muscle tone and levels of activity are low. It is, of course, important to ensure that the condition is not the result of a neurological or endocrinological problem and that more appropriate forms of treatment, such as psychiatric assessment, are being carried out. Where voice therapy is appropriate in these cases, forcing exercises would still be last on this clinician's list of 'things to try'. Techniques to produce gentle vocal fold closure would be first, followed by glottal onset exercises, always in conjunction with careful exploration of the psychological factors involved with a view to psychotherapy referral.

Where examination of the larynx shows any signs of inflammation or damage to the vocal fold mucosa forcing exercises are contraindicated.

Cough prolonged to a hum

This technique is closely related to glottal onset and forcing exercises. The patient is asked to produce a gentle cough to adduct the vocal folds and produce voice. Gradually the cough is moderated to a gentle throat clearing that can be prolonged into a hum. Therapy would then proceed as for humming. This technique can be useful, especially in cases of conversion aphonia, to achieve vocal fold closure. However, it also runs the obvious risk of being abusive and is best replaced by gentler techniques for adduction as soon as possible.

Plosive consonant closure (the hamster technique)

This technique is particularly useful to achieve vocal fold closure without forcing or strain. Patients are asked to fill the cheeks with air and to seal it into the oral cavity firmly with the lips and closure of the soft palate. They are then asked to push the air against the lips so that the cheeks fill out rather like those of a well-fed hamster. The air is released suddenly on the plosive /p/. Once they can sustain good oral pressure, patients produce /b/ in the same way, and full vocal fold closure is usually achieved without constriction. The technique progresses through /b/ with different vowels and into syllables. The syllables are most effective when initiated and closed with plosives that are strongly released. Double syllables (baby, bobby, etc.) and phrases (baby boy, bubble bath, etc.) can be practised until the feeling of good closure is conditioned. The patient should then be able to transfer these skills to other practised sounds and spontaneous speech fairly easily.

Vocal range - sirening

Sirening is an exercise designed to improve vocal range rather than voice quality, unlike the exercises described above. However, it is valuable to include as it can help patients learn to gain control of the cricothyroid visor, allowing smooth changes in vibrating vocal fold mass in order to shift from thick to thin folds. It also encourages flexibility of vertical laryngeal position.

The patient is asked to glide up and down through the vocal range on a quiet 'ng' sound, with the tongue high in the mouth as it would be for the sound at the end of the word 'singing'. Phonation is initiated with simultaneous onset. With rising pitch, the visor is closed and the vocal folds thinned. The patient is asked to start low down in his or her range and glide up and back through it, gradually getting higher like a siren on an emergency vehicle. The sound produced, however, is very quiet.

Vocal range exercises can also be produced on a higher airflow using /v/ or a rolled /r/. The rolled /r/ in particular seems to depend on a high airflow to maintain the 'rolling' or trilling quality of the /r/. If the airflow drops the trilling stops. When practising with patients it is useful to point out to them the enormous amount of work going on in the upper insertion of the rectus abdominis muscles, just under the rib cage. The higher in the range the patient goes, the harder these muscles can be felt to work. (This is in contrast with chest register, where increased muscular work in the abdominal obliques is apparent around the groin area.) The larynx can also be felt to rise significantly with rising pitch and to lower again as the pitch drops.

Twang (Estill)

This technique is very useful in resetting the higher vocal tract resonances (formants) (see Chapter 13) to produce a characteristically bright, rather piercing, quality that is perceived as being intensely loud. This quality is excellent at cutting through background noise and is therefore taught to both singers and actors to enable them to be heard clearly in large auditoria without vocal strain. It is also excellent for teaching patients to shout safely and is an important component in 'belt' singing quality (Estill 1988, 1996). (See also Chapter 8.)

The bright quality perceived in twang has been associated with aryepiglottic narrowing. Estill's "recipe" for twang involves learning to control the aryepiglottic sphincter which constricts to form a laryngeal tube within the existing tube of the vocal tract. She suggests that this laryngeal tube creates a separate resonator which is responsible for the extra brightness in phonation (Estill, 1995). The aryepiglottic sphincter and its effects on phonation are now being researched (Buscemi et al., 1995; Titze, 1995).

It is possible that there are other muscular adjustments that will also tune the vocal tract to produce the 2.5-3 KHz formant (the singer's formant) giving a bright ring to the voice (Miller and Schutte, 1990). Endoscopic observation repeatedly suggests that it may be associated with marked contraction and narrowing (waisting) of the lateral pharyngeal walls at the level of middle constrictor. This finding, however, has not, to our knowledge, been fully researched and remains an area of interesting speculation.

Aryepiglottic narrowing, seen at endoscopy, produces antero-posterior compression of the larynx but without excessive pharyngeal constriction or hyper-valving. The aryepiglottic folds move from their 'gothic arch' position seen in breathing and relaxed phonation (Lawrence, 1987) to an almost horizontal position, while the anterior commissure may be obscured by the base of the epiglottis. It is possible that the aryepiglottic narrowing observed is related to activation of the lateral cricoarytenoid muscles which provide strong medial compression but without false vocal fold activity. This type of medial compression would certainly provide the longer closed phase of the vibratory cycle that is reported by Estill (Estill, 1995).

To achieve this quality in its raw form, the tongue needs to be high in the mouth with its sides against the upper side teeth (Estill, 1996). It is easiest to begin with nasal sounds or heavily nasalized consonants. Estill provides a clear recipe for producing the quality. She suggests setting the vocal tract initially by imitating a cat yowling (meeyow), ducks quacking, children in the playground taunting each other ('You can't get me, na na-na na na') or a wicked witch's cackle. Some accents may have this quality as part of their characteristic production, for example, Australian, but for many patients it becomes a quality they can voluntarily call upon if they wish to increase volume and be heard through noise, or alternatively to express assertiveness and anger. It is excellent for giving an angry voice its 'edge' but is less appropriate for seducing your partner over a quiet dinner - unless you wish to give lessons to the entire restaurant!

There are courses available on learning how to carry out Estill's Compulsory Figures, including the figure for twang (see list of Useful Addresses).

Pahn's nasalization

Dr Johannes Pahn is a consultant phoniatrician working in Rostock, Germany. His 'nasalization method' is designed to release the oropharynx, nasopharynx and velum, and to free the laryngeal position to enable flexibility in the choice of reso-nance. The new 'phonation programme' is then conditioned in through a steady progression from the raw, nasally released sound, to heavily nasalized vowels, sylla-bles, phrases and sentences. Once the new pattern is established, the nasalization can be gradually phased out while the improved vocal efficiency is maintained. The system can be used to tune the 'singer's formant'. (For further information about training in this system see the list of Useful Addresses.)

Resonance work

For a definition of resonance see the glossary at the end of Chapter 9.

Resonance work relates to balancing the oral/nasal resonance in spoken or singing voices, releasing inappropriate vocal tract constriction and tuning the vocal tract to enhance specific resonances. Constriction within the vocal tract can either promote or inhibit resonance (see Chapter 13). It is the specific control and place-ment of constrictions in the supraglottic vocal tract that determines whether indi-vidual harmonics are damped or enhanced.

There are many good exercises designed to develop palatal control and balance the oral nasal resonance in speech and singing. The work mostly involves auditory and kinaesthetic training to enable the patient to differentiate between oral and nasal resonance, and to identify a target balance between the two in therapy. Estill describes useful exercises that can be used to gain voluntary control over the palate so that this balancing act can be more easily achieved.

Frequently voices are described as lacking in resonance when inappropriate constriction occurs in the vocal tract 'damping' or reducing its normal resonant features. Work described in the section on palpatory monitoring will help to release vocal tract constriction and restore resonance.

Tuning the vocal tract to produce specific resonances is also very valuable. Techniques that are useful here include humming, twang and Pahn's nasalization.

Tongue position

The position of the tongue during speech and singing is closely related to changes in resonance and voice quality (Laver, 1980). Patients who habitually pull the tongue back in the mouth have a characteristic 'covered' or 'plummy' sound to their voices. Boone and McFarlane (1988) describe it as 'hollow-sounding cul-de-sac resonance'. Those who carry the tongue too far forward tend to have a rather thin lispy quality to their speech that is often associated with immaturity. There is much argument about whether the tongue should be held high or low in the mouth, especially in singing (see Chapter 8). Raising the back of the tongue is essential for tuning the second and third formants, e.g. the /i/ vowel, and Estill includes exercises to raise the position of the tongue in the mouth for certain voice qualities. Clinical experience seems to support her findings of improvements in vocal quality and resonance when the body of the tongue is high, but to some extent it may depend on the sound patients or singers wish to achieve.

It is important to remember that the base of the tongue is anchored to the hyoid bone and therefore any activity of the back of the tongue will be met by an equal bracing of the suprahyoid musculature (geniohyoid, mylohyoid stylopharyngeus, styloglossus, stylohyoid, digastric and middle constrictor). This will inevitably affect laryngeal position for better or worse. Excessive tongue tension can be problematic as it is easily generalized into the pharynx and laryngeal suspensory system, restricting vocal range and damping resonance. Muscles that are habitually working outside their comfortable range of effort, tend to produce discomfort, shorten and lose their flexibility. External palpation of the muscles in the base of the tongue gives a good indication of how much work is going on during speech or singing and the habitual muscle tone. It can provide useful feedback, as the patient and therapist design exercises to reduce the amount of tension in this region (see Chapter 6 on palpation and manipulation).

Kinaesthetic and auditory skills

As with the breathing work discussed in the last section, voice therapy also relies on *looking*, *listening* and *feeling* to support work that is aimed at making changes in vocal technique.

Looking

Where a video recorder is available, patients can be recorded speaking spontaneously in the clinic. This is particularly useful for work in voice groups. If video is not available, patients can always observe their speech in a mirror and look for indications of tension in the throat, shoulders and face, and watch for any habitual laryngeal movement.

Listening

The different aspects of voice quality can be difficult to analyse at the best of times, but for patients with poor auditory skills or who are unaware of their vocal problems it can be a nightmare. Their concept of pitch may also be hazy, especially when applied to voices. It is therefore useful to introduce some simple ear training to help patients identify different vocal qualities and understand the terms used by the speech and language therapist.

Normal voices can be recorded and paired samples played to patients who are then asked to identify which voice was higher (or lower). The same can then be done for voice quality, for example, which voice was clear and which hoarse?, which was creaky and which breathy? Discussion of the voice samples quickly leads into the realms of attitude, as patients will like some voices better than others and will also attribute such things as age, physique and personality type to certain voice qualities. They will often begin to reveal their anxieties about how others see them and make assumptions based on their voices. Working through attitude change and helping dysphonic patients examine their voice quality more objectively can be extremely valuable in restoring confidence and providing strategies to cope with their disorder. Working in a voice group provides excellent scope for this type of work as patients can share their experiences, anxieties and solutions, as well as support each other in vocal exercises.

Feeling (palpatory monitoring)

Palpatory monitoring is a term that can be used to describe a simple way for patients to feel whether the movements they make are achieving the therapy aims. It has been touched on before by Aronson (1985), Boone and McFarlane (1988) and Case (1991) when they discuss digital manipulation, but the ideas suggested here have grown out of interdisciplinary work with our clinic osteopath, Jacob Lieberman. The most useful areas to monitor are:

- the base of the tongue
- the thyrohyoid muscles and ligaments
- the cricothyroid visor
- the larynx as a whole.

The base of tongue can be felt by placing the thumbs up under the hollow of the jaw, below and behind the chin. If pressure is exerted, the tongue can be felt lifting up against the roof of the mouth (depending on the amount of pressure used). In this way it is easy to monitor effort in the geniohyoid, mylohyoid and genioglossus muscles. These muscles will be particularly active when the larynx is pulled forward, or when the tongue pulls backwards and downwards (so called tongue backing). Palpation of these muscle groups during speech makes it easy to identify habitual patterns of use and monitor desired changes during therapy. Palpation using pressure or massage can also be used to interfere directly with habitual patterns in order to restrict or alter muscle behaviour (see Chapter 6).

The *thyrohyoid muscles and ligaments* are discussed in Chapter 6 and are extremely important in raising the larynx and controlling pitch during intonation in speech (Vilkman et al, 1996). They can usually be readily identified by patients with a little guidance, especially as they may be tender to the touch. It is best to start by helping patients to identify the top of the thyroid cartilage with an index finger. Using the thumb and index finger they then trace along the upper borders of the thyroid until their fingers lie either side of it. By sliding slightly upwards, the fingers should fall into the thyrohyoid space or gap. The thyrohyoid muscles overlie the thyrohyoid membranes and when they contract the space or gap closes. When finding the thyrohyoid muscles, it may help if the patient lifts the chin, hyperextending the neck and displacing the carotid sheath posteriorly. The head posture can then be returned to normal with the patient's fingers well away from potential hazards.

Monitoring the thyrohyoid gap with the thumb and index finger can help the patient learn to inhibit habitual laryngeal raising. They can also learn to release or lower the larynx. The latter can be particularly effective in releasing lower pharyngeal constriction and associated laryngeal backing, as in order to lower the larynx, the oblique fibres of the thyropharyngeus have to relax. It can also be used to ensure that the raising does not recur because the larynx position for phonation is returned to neutral, as it would be found in breathing.

To locate the *cricothyroid visor* patients should place an index finger on the top, anterior aspect of the thyroid cartilage (the thyroid notch), then slide down over the front until the finger falls into a small ditch (or space) between the lower border of the thyroid and the upper border of the cricoid cartilage. The space is known as the cricothyroid space or 'visor' and it opens and closes with changes in vocal pitch. This movement, or lack of it, can be felt as the patient glides up and down through their pitch range, closing as the larynx rises and the pitch increases, and opening as the larynx lowers and the pitch decreases. It is also noticeable that the cricoid cartilage tends to move forward, becoming more prominent, with laryngeal lowering, but appears to pull back at the top of the pitch range (see Chapter 5).

It is helpful to begin by training palpatory awareness first using the therapist's CT visor movement as a model, then helping patients find their own. To detect CT movement it is useful to contrast a yawn, when the visor opens widely, with a high-pitched squeak like the sound of a mouse. Patients may be confused at first by the raising and lowering of the larynx that accompanies these manoeuvres, especially as they may well be using excessive laryngeal movement to compensate for the lack of movement in the visor. However, once identified, patients can learn to monitor the rest position and smooth control of the CT visor during exercises, speech or singing (see Chapter 8).

Habitual movement of the larynx as a whole during speech can be monitored by placing three fingers over the front of the larynx, spanning the cricoid cartilage, thyroid cartilage and hyoid bone. In this way it should be possible to detect any tendency for the larynx to move, together with the direction. Laryngeal movement in any direction that is reliably initiated at the onset of phonation and released as it ceases can be considered to be a habitual 'setting' that is likely to involve hyperfunctional muscle use. Although laryngeal position during speech depends to some extent on vocal pitch and the chosen vocal quality (for example, twang would necessarily involve a high larynx), it does appear to have a rest or neutral position in the neck where it lies for breathing. Its position during speech needs to be flexible to allow for the necessary movements required by voluntary changes in pitch range and quality. Habitual settings away from the neutral position reduce flexibility and vocal quality options. Habitual shortening of the suspensory muscles that these settings may require can lead to fatigue, discomfort and excessively tight muscle tone. The most common clinical finding is an habitually raised larynx, but other settings also regularly identified include:

• habitual laryngeal lowering;
• anterior movement;
• posterior movement (backing).

Frequently the latter two settings are found in combination with laryngeal raising.

Having identified any habitual setting, exercises to reset to a less tiring neutral laryngeal position can be designed and monitored.

Classification of phonation patterns based on physical appearance: the application of appropriate therapy techniques

Let us now look at some of the most common vocal 'pictures' that videostroboscopy puts up on our screen in the voice clinic. There do seem to be recurring patterns that we recognize and which other clinics have reported (Koufman and Blalock, 1982; Belisle and Morrison, 1983; Koufman and Blalock, 1991; Morrison et al., 1994). We will describe the ones we see most frequently, relate them to those already described in the literature, and try to determine how they are produced. We will then try to apply our knowledge of how voice therapy techniques affect the larynx to select appropriate exercises for each pathological set.

Type 1: Morrison's muscular tension dysphonia: the large interarytenoid and posterior glottic chink (Morrison Type 1 Laryngeal Isometric Disorder)

This common pattern was first described by Morrison et al. and Belisle and Morrison in 1983 and later renamed Laryngeal Isometric Disorder (Morrison, Rammage et al., 1994). The anterior two thirds of the vibrating portion of the vocal folds are pressed tightly together while the posterior third, together with a wide interarytenoid chink, remains open (Figure 7.4). This vocal posture alone will produce marked dysphonia, characterized by a low, constricted, breathy/harsh quality with poor pitch control for upper registers. There may also be frequent pitch and voice breaks. If left uncorrected, trauma to the mucosa at the junction of the anterior two thirds with the posterior third frequently occurs, producing polypoid degeneration/soft nodules. Morrison et al. (1983) report that the posture is associated with an extremely tight suprahyoid musculature. In some cases the arytenoid cartilages are tilted forward, obscuring the interarytenoid chink, as the

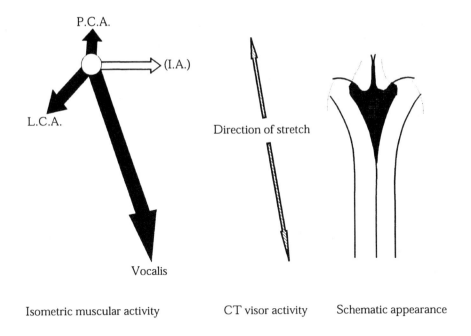

P.C.A.

(I.A.)

L.C.A.

Direction of stretch

Vocalis

Isometric muscular activity   CT visor activity   Schematic appearance

Figure 7.2 Muscular tension dysphonia

posterior cricoarytenoid (PCA) muscles fail to provide sufficient opposition to the anterior pull of vocalis, under tension from the cricothyroid mechanism.

Personality traits may well play a part in the development of this muscular pattern. It is frequently found among healthy young women who exercise heavily and are often trying to shout instructions while out of breath, for example, aerobics instructors or riding instructors. These people may also appear extrovert, being loud, noisy and the 'life and soul of the party'. The dysphonia is often considered socially acceptable because of the association with fun-loving, vocal, lively people. Under the facade, however, anxiety and insecurity may lurk.

Our clinical experience suggests that the problem arises in response to a persistent muscle set appropriate for forced respiratory movements. The vocal folds appear to be forcibly abducted by the combined action of the posterior cricoarytenoid (PCA) and lateral cricoarytenoid (LCA) muscles. Superimposed onto this muscular set is the additional activity necessary to produce phonation, i.e. increased vocalis activity, opposed by the already tensed PCA. These two muscles form a 'strap' (including the vocal ligament) further tensioned by closure of the cricothyroid visor (see the section on the cricothyroid visor in Chapter 5). Medial compression depends largely on the LCA, but this appears to be already active in its abductor capacity in tandem with PCA. It is, therefore, unavailable to perform its usual role working with the interarytenoid to produce medial compression. The LCA's companion in its sphincteric adductor/medial compression function, the interarytenoid, may either be inhibited by the high levels of PCA activity or simply overcome by the persistent (possibly locked) abduction. At present these comments remain supposition until further research has been carried out. However, the hypothesis does fit closely with the clinical features observed on stroboscopy.

How, then, could we expect to alter this muscular pattern, given that the patient will have no idea what they have done, or how they have altered their voice production. As far as they are concerned, this 'problem voice' just comes upon them and they have no control over it. Based on the observations discussed above, it would seem logical to aim our therapy towards synchronizing abduction and adduction so that they no longer overlap. To do this, the strain must first be removed from the system by opening the cricothyroid visor. It is then possible to work towards organized vocal fold closure, removing the tendency for an abducted set to persist.

In summary the therapy aims are to:

1.   open the cricothyroid visor;
2.   establish full vocal fold closure reducing/eliminating the interarytenoid chink;
3.   reduce suprahyoid and pharyngeal muscle tension;
4.   eliminate any habitual laryngeal raising during speech.

The therapy techniques are described more fully earlier in this chapter so only their usual effects on the vocal tract, as observed at laryngeal fibre endoscopy, will be listed here. Those most likely to be valuable with MTD are as follows.

The Accent Method

1.   It usually opens the cricothyroid visor successfully as it establishes modal voice.
2.   Full fold contact is a major feature of the technique, eliminating the interarytenoid chink.
3.   The extrinsic muscles that anchor the larynx inferiorly (sternothyroid and sternohyoid) are usually successfully activated, eliminating habitual laryngeal raising and releasing the excessive suprahyoid and pharyngeal muscle tension associated with MTD.
4.   The long periods of 'practice babble' condition the target muscular set, making carryover into spontaneous speech easier.

Sob

1.   Effective at producing full vocal fold closure.
2.   Releases supraglottic tension.
3.   Low larynx position counteracts laryngeal raising.

Humming/mhuh huh

1.   Excellent at closing the interarytenoid chink.
2.   Releases suprahyoid and pharyngeal tension very well.
3.   Effective in opening the CT visor as it usually establishes modal voice.

Froeschels' chewing

1. As with humming, it releases the jaw, suprahyoid and thyrohyoid muscula-ture.
2. It usually eliminates the interarytenoid chink effectively.
3. CT visor releases if modal voice is established.

Other methods that may also be helpful include:

- Pahn's nasalization – similiar effects to humming.
- Gentle glottal onset – especially for closing interarytenoid chink.
- Creak/glottal fry voice – especially opening the CT visor.
- Yawn-sigh – especially for releasing suprahyoid tension and gentle fold closure.

What to do when what you do doesn't work

Problems with the Accent Method

1. Some patients do not release the cricothyroid visor and continue to use excess medial compression. In these cases try *palpatory monitoring of the CT visor* during *yawn-sigh*, which opens the visor and neutralizes laryngeal raising. Then use CT monitoring with the Accent Method together with breath before voice onset to reduce excessive medial compression.
2. Some patients cannot close the interarytenoid chink. Check that the visor has released, then try the Accent Method with gentle *glottal onset* to help the closure.
3. Suprahyoid muscle tension remains a problem. Check that any habitual laryngeal raising has been eliminated. Ensure that this does not creep back by monitoring the thyrohyoid muscles and thyrohyoid gap. If the suprahyoid muscles are still tight, try massaging the base of the tongue during production of the Accent Method.
4. Check that the patient is not controlling the 'accents' at the glottis. Ensure the changes are occurring with airflow.
5. Try other methods mentioned above.

Problems with sob

1. The visor may not open and the thin fold setting may persist. Try *gentle glottal onset* to establish modal voice and palpatory monitoring to ensure that the visor has opened.
2. The laryngeal lowering may need to be released back to a neutral setting.

Problems with humming

1. The CT visor does not always release. Try *creak, yawn-sigh* and *Accent Method* in combination with *palpatory monitoring* of the CT visor.

2. Suprahyoid musculature does not always release. Try *chewing, palpatory monitoring* at the thyrohyoid level, massage of the base of tongue, or *yawn-sigh* to lower the larynx.

Problems with chewing

1. Nasalization may tend to persist. Use in combination with palatal work.
2. Pharyngeal muscles may not release. Check for habitual laryngeal raising and counteract it with *yawn-sigh* and *palpatory monitoring* at the thyrohyoid level.
3. CT visor may not release. Try *creak, glottal onset, palpatory monitoring.*

Type 2: Lateral contraction (glottic and/or supraglottic hyperadduction) (Morrison Type 2)

Looked at endoscopically, patients with this type of phonation habitually use their voices with stretched, thinned vocal folds, and the circumference of the laryngeal vestibule is distorted from its broadly rounded shape, becoming a narrower oval (i.e. from an apple to a pear shape).

There is often visual evidence of hyperactivity in the false vocal folds, reflecting the efforts of the underlying musculature to provide medial compression (see Figure 7.3). It seems likely that the problem here is one of vocalis muscle fatigue due to persistent inappropriate cricothyroid activity. Eventually, the muscle and ligament stretch, so that in the final stages of the syndrome they become bowed and are no longer able to achieve full closure or medial compression (Morrison

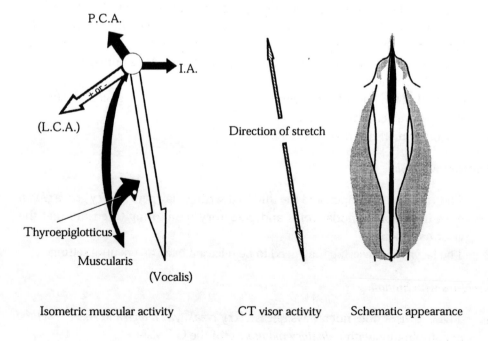

Isometric muscular activity   CT visor activity   Schematic appearance

Figure 7.3 Lateral compression of of the supraglottis

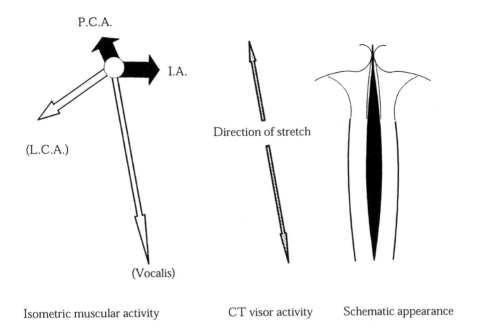

P.C.A.

I.A.

(L.C.A.)

Direction of stretch

(Vocalis)

Isometric muscular activity   CT visor activity   Schematic appearance

Figure 7.4 Bowing as an end stage of persistent cricothyroid visor tension

Type 5: psychogenic dysphonia with bowed folds). The remainder of the thyroarytenoid muscles, which lie in the aryepiglottic folds forming a sphincter (muscularis and thyroepiglotticus), appear to be recruited to try to counteract the vocalis stretch. A similar effect may be seen in a fatigued athlete (e.g. a marathon runner three quarters of the way through the race), where the 'proper' muscles involved in running are fatigued and no longer able to sustain the work required of them adequately. Other muscles, less suited to the task, are then recruited to try to shore up the flagging, fatigued muscles.

Vocal fold bowing that represents the end stage of this habitual phonation type is very familiar to clinicians (see Figure 7.4). In the early stages, prior to decompensation, the supraglottic vocal tract may show lateral compression. This may reflect activity in the middle and inferior constrictor muscles. Palpatory findings inevitably show a closed cricothyroid visor, together with tight thyrohyoid muscles. The larynx is usually raised for phonation and there is often evidence of hyperactivity in the geniohyoid group of muscles. The only good thing about the configuration is that the forward tilting of the larynx makes it much easier to examine.

The most important feature of this phonation type is the habitually closed cricothyroid visor and this therefore needs to be given priority in treatment. The main aims of treatment are to:

1. Open the CT visor and reduce vocal fold stretching.
2. Increase vocal fold mass to enhance successful medial compression.
3. Reduce the supraglottic lateral compression by releasing the pharyngeal musculature and eliminating any habitual laryngeal raising.

Useful techniques to achieve these aims are as follows.

Palpatory monitoring

This provides the patient with a means to monitor success in opening the visor. The introduction of palpatory monitoring should be judged by the therapist according to their assessment of the patient's needs and ability to cope with touch. There are times when the technique should be introduced first, followed by monitoring once the target voice quality is established, and times when monitoring can be safely introduced before the technique.

Yawn-sigh

1. Provides an excellent way to introduce laryngeal lowering. During a yawn the cricothyroid visor is widely open (see Chapter 6 and Vilkman et al., 1996), more so than it would be for modal speech.
2. The laryngeal lowering counteracts habitual laryngeal raising and can be used to eliminate it.
3. The laryngeal lowering may also release the pharyngeal musculature, reducing the lateral compression.

Creaky voice/glottal fry

1. Opens the CT visor.
2. Increases vocalis mass.
3. Counteracts lateral compression. In creaky voice the circumference of the laryngeal inlet is tightened antero-posteriorly.
4. The lateral thyroarytenoid muscles provide strong medial compression to produce the excessively long closed phase.

The Accent Method

1. Opens the visor.
2. Restores symmetry to the vocal tract shape.
3. Releases the suspensory muscles that habitually raise the larynx, allowing it to drop.
4. Encourages gentle modal voicing that can be gradually built into a speaking voice.

Useful additions to the recipe are palpatory monitoring of the cricothyroid visor and thyrohyoid monitoring to prevent laryngeal raising.

Humming

1. Usually opens the visor nicely, but not necessarily - beware!
2. Restores vocal tract symmetry and resolves supraglottic lateral compression and forward pull.
3. Produces nice vocal fold closure.

Twang

1. Increases medial compression and closed phase.
2. Counteracts lateral compression as aryepiglottic activity produces specific antero-posterior compression.

What to do when what you do does not work

Problems with yawn-sigh

Laryngeal lowering may make it difficult to adapt voicing exercises based on yawn-sigh into normal modal voice. The aim of treatment is, after all, to teach smooth control of the visor movement, not speech with a habitually lowered larynx. If this problem arises try one of the other techniques listed above.

Problems with creak

Patients with habitual lateral compression may have great difficulty in finding the 'vocal set' for creak. In an ideal world patients respond immediately to demonstration of the sound and being asked to do an imitation of a creaky door. However, if they experience difficulty try the following intermediate steps:

(a) employ yawn-sigh to lower the larynx and open the visor;
(b) use palpatory monitoring to make sure that the visor does not close;
(c) introduce gentle glottal onset to ensure thick folds and full closure;
(d) reduce airflow through the closure to minimal so that it is released in small bursts.

Boone and McFarlane (1988) suggest phonating (or speaking) until the air runs out, which will also usually trigger creak.

The other problem tends to be that patients produce excess constriction in the glottic and supraglottic structures in their attempts to produce the sound from imitation. The steps described above will be valuable in dealing with this, but in addition, it will be important to carry out some work on kinaesthetic awareness of constriction and its release.

Coblenzer's silent air intake is useful to release constriction and can be added into the steps given above (see section on deconstriction).

Problems with humming

The visor may not open and the vocal fold mass may remain thinned. Where this happens, try working on vocal onset and mass, e.g. creak and/or gentle glottal stops.

Problems with twang

Patients sometimes find this a difficult set to acquire and it can easily lead to constriction. It is also important to remember that twang requires a high larynx, closed visor and thinned vocal folds so it may not necessarily be appropriate to use with cases of lateral compression. However, where patients have problems producing twang, try combining the exercises with a higher, more forward tongue position and work to deconstrict the larynx (see section on deconstriction).

Type 3: Antero-posterior (A-P) supraglottic contraction (Koufman's 'Bogart-Bacall' Syndrome, Koufman and Blalock, 1991)

Visually, this phonation type shows compression of the laryngeal vestibule from back to front, so it appears wider than it is long. The anterior portion of the vocal folds is often obscured by the epiglottis and base of tongue activity, while the posterior portion may be obscured by the arytenoid tips, which appear to be pulled forward. There is often visual suggestion of increased medial compression with activity in the false vocal folds. These patients are the most difficult to view during phonation as the larynx disappears, seeming to tilt forward underneath the backed base of tongue.

This phonation type varies in degree. In its mildest form only the antero-posterior compression of the laryngeal inlet is seen. The vibrating portion of the vocal folds is still visible. As the problem becomes more severe, less and less is seen of the vocal folds and they may look quite thinned **despite** their shortness and the muscular work that appears to be going on around them. In the most severe form, false vocal fold phonation may be present. Clinical experience suggests that false vocal fold phonation tends to occur when:

(a)   the muscles of the true folds are failing and bowing is present;
(b)   the vocal folds are so stiff that extra effort is required to produce phonation;
(c)   total vocal effort occurs in the absence of true fold pathology, usually where emotion, abuse or excessive physical training (e.g. weight lifting) are primary factors.

Palpatory findings are always variable between patients and cannot be assumed in advance. This phonation set may occur with an habitually raised or lowered larynx. Where the larynx is raised, the thyrohyoid muscles are likely to be tight and there is often hyperactivity in the geniohyoid and mylohyoid muscle groups. Where the larynx is habitually lowered, the hyoglossus may be active because of the associated tongue backing.

In many patients with this vocal set the cricothyroid visor is frequently **closed**, a finding normally associated with thinning and lengthening the vocal folds. That the vocal folds still look short suggests that the PCA muscles may be working outside their normal range of contraction, and are unable to oppose the combined activity of LCA, interarytenoid and the cricothyroid visor. They therefore stretch, releasing the tension on the vocal folds despite the closed visor. In these cases there may be surprisingly little vocalis activity, giving the vocal folds a thinned or even slightly bowed appearance on laryngoscopy. A-P collapse, therefore, may have little relationship to the length of the closed phase of the vibratory cycle.

There is often visual evidence of brisk activity in the strap muscles and perceptually the voice may sound constricted and harsh with a hard glottal attack, pharyngeal constriction and poor resonance. It is possible that the breathy quality in the harshness comes from incomplete closure posteriorly, but this cannot be seen because of the arytenoid tips (see Figure 7.5).

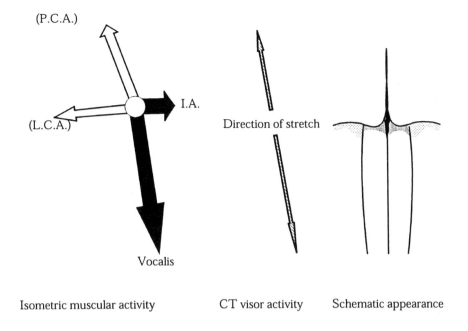

(P.C.A.)

I.A.

(L.C.A.)

Direction of stretch

Vocalis

Isometric muscular activity   CT visor activity   Schematic appearance

Figure 7.5 Antero-posterior collapse (*syn:* 'Antero–posterior compression')

Therapy techniques

The aims of therapy are to:

(a) Open the CT visor where this is closed to eliminate stretching of the vocal folds, thus reducing the strain on PCA.
(b) Activate PCA to oppose vocalis and stabilize the posterior end of the vocal folds.
(c) Reduce the forward tilting of the larynx and tongue backing.
(d) Stabilize the flexibility of the laryngeal movement to restore range.

The Accent Method

1. Opens the visor.
2. Reduces glottal constriction.
3. Helps resolve habitual laryngeal raising or lowering.
4. Can be adapted to resolve tongue backing by working on babbling sequences to condition forward placement.

Sob

1. Activates PCA to oppose vocalis.
2. Decreases glottal hyperadduction and medial compression.
3. Laryngeal lowering tends to release pharyngeal constriction.
4. Counteracts any tendency to tongue backing.

Yawn-sigh

1.   Lowers the larynx for patients with habitual laryngeal raising.
2.   Opens the CT visor where this is closed.
3.   Releases glottal hyperadduction.
4.   Releases pharyngeal constriction.

The following techniques can be helpful in conjunction with the above techniques.

Breath before tone and simultaneous onset

1.   Reduces glottal hyperadduction.
2.   Reduces likelihood of false vocal fold involvement.

Humming

1.   Releases glottal constriction.
2.   Releases vocal tract constriction.
3.   May help to open the CT visor and increase vocal fold mass.

Sirening

1.   Releases constraints on the vertical movement of the larynx.
2.   Encourages smooth change of the vibrating mass of the vocal folds. This is particularly important where the visor is open and the larynx tightly constricted.

Release of laryngeal constriction

1.   Reduces hyperadduction and restores laryngeal symmetry.
2.   Releases false fold adduction.
3.   Secondary release of pharyngeal constriction because of the slight lowering of the larynx.

What to do when what you do doesn't work

Problems with the Accent Method

This may not necessarily release glottal or pharyngeal constriction in some patients. Where this happens try combining with *palpatory monitoring* of the thyro-hyoid muscles and *yawn-sigh* to release the larynx down. Techniques that release laryngeal constriction will also help, as will *breath before* tone onset.

Problems with sob

Sob is produced with thinned folds on a lowered larynx. It will only be effective in opening the CT visor where it is moved down into the lower pitch range. There may be difficulties adapting a gradual increase of vocal mass and removing laryngeal lowering. *Glottal onset* can be used to stiffen the vocal fold mass and *palpatory monitoring* of the CT visor ensures that it remains open.

Problems with yawn-sigh

This may be difficult to adapt the vocal quality into spontaneous speech once the laryngeal lowering has been released.

Problems with breath before tone/simultaneous onset

These exercises may not release pharyngeal constriction or open the CT visor on their own. They are probably best combined with *palpatory monitoring* of CT visor and thyrohyoid muscles. Care must be taken to make sure that constriction does not persist.

Problems with humming

Humming may not open the CT visor or necessarily release hyperadduction. Try in conjunction with *onset work*, *deconstriction* and *palpatory monitoring*.

Problems with sirening

Some patients have trouble in gliding through their vocal range, especially from the lower range upwards. Try *sob* initially to produce thin folds and glide down from high to low notes. Then try sirening again. Vary the sound used, trying a rolled /r/ and /v/ as well as the 'ing' sound.

Problems with deconstriction

Some patients may have difficulty in grasping the concept and carrying over the manoeuvre into spontaneous phonation. Best used with other methods, e.g. *humming*, *Accent Method*, etc.

Type 4: Conversion aphonia/dysphonia (Morrison Type 4 Conversion Aphonia/Dysphonia)

A diagnosis of psychogenic aphonia (or dysphonia) is usually made where patients appear unable to produce phonation voluntarily, despite vocal folds that look normal, are fully mobile and achieve closure and phonation for vegetative functions such as coughing, gagging, laughing, etc. When patients are asked to phonate during clinical examination, the vocal folds either come briskly to the midline and then fail to maintain their contact, or stop slightly apart and fail to contact each other. They may also be held in the position for whispering as described by Morrison et al. (1993).

Traditionally, patients with this presentation were considered to be 'hysterical personalities' with implications of secondary gain and bland affect (see Chapter 9). Clinical experience, however, suggests they may have more in common with the psychosomatic group of patients, where the symptoms are a response to distress and conflict. Many are anxious and depressed about the voice loss and respond very quickly to voice therapy once the underlying conflict has been uncovered. True hysterical conversions do occur, but these are quite rare. The patients seem untroubled by their symptoms in any deep sense and while they may describe them as 'a nuisance' they smile and appear to quite enjoy soldiering on. A little investigation into the history surrounding the onset of the problem may well illustrate the famous secondary gain. These patients are notoriously difficult to treat and may require psychotherapy. They are often very resistant to the idea that their symptoms have a psychological base and need very careful and tactful management.

Therapy for this client group depends very much on the views and experience of the therapist involved. Many therapists feel strongly that any counselling work crosses our professional boundaries and should not be carried out in voice therapy. Others, many of whom have counselling training, see it as an integral part of their work and combine it very successfully with traditional voice work. There can be no hard and fast rules, but it is unusual for these patients to resolve with voice work alone. Usually they need to develop some insight into the nature of their symptoms and acknowledge their emotional difficulties. Once this has taken place, they may respond extremely well to voice therapy, as their need for a voice problem has been reduced. Frequently this process of insight develops over six sessions of voice therapy and needs to be very skilfully guided. It is wise for therapists to seek supervision from their psychotherapy or psychology colleagues where possible in these cases.

The aims of therapy in cases of psychogenic dysphonia are to:

1.   Help the patient achieve insight into the nature of their symptoms and seek appropriate counselling/psychotherapy.
2.   Develop kinaesthetic awareness of general body tension and specific laryngeal control.
3.   Work through exercises that produce vocal fold closure and phonation towards maintaining normal speech.

Therapy techniques

1.   Glottal onset, plosive consonants, forcing exercises and cough/throat clearing into a hum, gargling. All of these usually produce reliable vocal fold closure and good kinaesthetic awareness of vocal fold movement. It is fairly easy for patients to achieve phonation from an initial closure into words, phrases and speech, but they may well need combining with other systems and exercises to complete the carryover into spontaneous speech.
2.   Accent Method, humming and creaky voice. These techniques may be used alone initially to see if they work, or used later to assist transfer of phonation into spontaneous speech.
3.   General relaxation exercises and visualization techniques/self-hypnosis techniques. These may increase body awareness and improve anxiety states. They can be combined with general work on breathing.

Vocal fold paresis

Voice therapy for vocal fold paresis depends very much on the assessment findings at laryngoscopy. In most cases, patients put enormous amounts of muscular work into trying to achieve vocal fold closure and normal phonation. The effort can be observed in the false vocal folds, arytenoid tips and pyriform fossae (see section on forcing exercises). Where these signs are observed, the therapy aims will be to reduce the muscular tension to an appropriate level and increase the air support. Where palpation reveals a closed CT visor, exercises designed to open it and restore modal voice should be carried out. Regular reassessment is vital, as many of these cases cannot compensate and will require surgical intervention in the form of a medialization procedure (see Chapter 11).

In such cases it may be helpful to try the lateral manual compression test which has been shown to be extremely useful in determining whether medialization will be beneficial (Isshiki, 1989, Blaugrund et al. 1991). The thyroid alae are squeezed between the thumb and middle three fingers using different degrees of pressure as the patient phonates. Where there is audible improvement in phonation the medialization procedure is likely to be successful. The converse, however, is not necessarily true, as the test may have been done using the wrong site or inadequate pressure, or the thyroid cartilage may have become calcified and too stiff to be compressed. With guidance from an experienced surgeon, speech therapists can learn how to use this test. Patients, too, may find compression helpful in improving phonation, or alternatively they may prefer to displace the larynx gently towards the normally innervated side, which also often produces a stronger voice.

In the rare cases where patients are not putting enough muscular effort into phonation, exercises such as *glottal onset, twang, plosive consonants, gentle cough into hum* and, if all else fails, *forcing exercises* are required. All these exercises will work best when introduced in tandem with work to increase the airflow, and further support from airflow techniques such as the Accent Method should be provided once compensation has begun to take place.

Spasmodic dysphonia

Voice therapy for adductor and abductor spasmodic dysphonia can be effective in providing symptom relief for some patients, although it is well recognized that these problems can be intractable.

Adductor spasmodic dysphonias respond fairly well to techniques that reduce medial compression and encourage very gentle vocal fold closure. The Accent Method, sob, humming, yawn-sigh, and Froeschels' chewing may be good techniques to try in conjunction with laryngeal manipulation and laryngeal monitoring.

Abductor spasmodic dysphonia prevents the patient from being able to maintain vocal fold closure reliably, resulting in sudden brief breaks in phonation leaving only audible air escape. These breaks may occur anywhere during speech, breaking up the flow and impairing communication. The listener often attributes the symptoms to nervousness on the part of the speaker, which, by the time they have suffered from the disorder for a while, may well be true. Techniques that improve medial compression, such as twang and Pahn's nasalization may be beneficial here, as may creak. Airflow techniques, such as the Accent Method may also be useful as they tend to increase the smooth flow of one word into the next and, when coupled with prolonged speech such as would be used in stammering, they can be remarkably effective.

The emotional ramifications of both types of spasmodic dysphonia are reminiscent of stammering, in that avoidance of certain difficult sounds and words is common, together with marked anxiety about speaking situations. Work on attitude change and self-perception can be very valuable with these patients, particularly when the symptoms are severe. Ultimately, however, they may respond best to botulinum toxin (see Chapter 10).

Puberphonia (Morrison Type 6: Adolescent psychogenic dysphonia with bowed folds)

Occasionally postpubescent males with normal endocrinology retain the higher pitch of their prepubescent years, using habitual falsetto quality in speech. There has been much speculation as to why this should happen and it is generally thought to relate to emotional difficulties (Aronson, 1985) combined with voice production habits that develop to maintain pitch stability across the period while the voice is breaking (Colton and Casper, 1990).

On examination these patients are found to have lengthened and thinned vocal folds, which may also be bowing, depending on the length of time the voice has been used in this way and the amount of strain placed upon it. To produce this picture, the CT visor is closed and the larynx habitually raised during speech. The natural, low (modal) voice can usually be heard in spontaneous coughing, laughing or other vegetative gestures. It is very important to eliminate any vocal fold pathology as many patients with vocal fold sulci present with high pitched, weak voices that may sound perceptually similar. These patients, however, rarely use pure falsetto quality.

There is enormous variation among puberphonic patients. Some are unaware of how high pitched their voice sounds and have only sought help because they have been teased, or others have worried about them. These patients are usually not 'in touch' with their modal voice and cannot produce it at will. Other patients are aware that they have two voices, one high and one low, but lack the control and courage to switch to modal voice. As a result, puberphonics have the reputation of being either extremely easy or extremely hard to resolve. Usually, the greater the psychological component, the harder it is to treat these patients, as unconscious resistance may hamper therapy success. In these cases it is wise for the therapist to seek supervision and try to redirect the patient towards counselling.

Therapy aims with puberphonics are to:

1. Open the cricothyroid visor, restoring modal voice.
2. Resolve habitual laryngeal raising.
3. Transfer the use of a modal voice into everyday speech.

Laryngeal manipulation by an expert is invaluable with these patients if available. However, other techniques that are useful include:

1. Laryngeal monitoring: the patient needs to learn to open the cricothyroid visor, lower the larynx and then use thyrohyoid or CT visor monitoring to maintain the modal voice produced.
2. Voice exercises that open the CT visor and bulk up the vocal folds: glottal onset, cough into hum, glottal fry/creak, plosive consonants and forcing exercises (used sparingly) are all appropriate.
3. Once modal voice is established, conditioning systems are useful to train modal voice into speech (e.g. the Accent Method, humming, etc.).
4. Speech assignments (as would be used for stammerers) are useful to generalize modal voice into social situations. Patients often find it hard using the 'new voice' with family and friends and need support over this period.

What to do with problems

Traditionally, therapy for puberphonics has concentrated on putting pressure on the upper borders of the thyroid cartilage (in the thyrohyoid gap) to pull the larynx down, counteracting habitual laryngeal raising (Aronson, 1985). Where puberphonics fail to respond to this approach, or to palpatory monitoring, they may lower the voice if gentle pressure is put on either side of the thyroid cartilage, pushing it slightly up and back. This inhibits the forward thyroid tilt that closes the visor and the raised, forward pull of the whole larynx in speech (Kotby, personal communication, 1986).

As already stated, patients who are particularly resistant to speech therapy may respond better if referred on for counselling/psychotherapy or laryngeal manipulation.

Appendix 7.1

Relaxation exercises - notes for patients

Posture
Line up the ear with the shoulder, the shoulder with the hip and the hip with the ball/middle of the foot. Make sure the crown of the head faces the ceiling and the chin is down.

When sitting, choose a chair good low back support. Make sure the shoulders (and chest) are down, and your hands are resting in your lap. Your feet should be ready to take your weight, with the ball of your foot under or slightly back from the knee joint.

Check in the mirror that your shoulder are down and symmetrical and that your head is not tilted.

Try standing against a wall with the back of your head, shoulders and lower back all touching the wall. You will probably need to move your feet away form the wall, often quite a distance to begin with. You can reduce the distance as you improve your posture.

Lie down on the floor with your feet flat and your knees bent. Feel the lower back touch the floor. Push the back of your head against the floor, then relax. Repeat 5 times

Shoulders
1. Raise your shoulders up towards your ears, (allow them to be a little rounded) hold the position **but breathe** then let go. Repeat 5 times

2. Drop your head down to your chest, then pull your shoulders down towards the floor, hold the position **but breathe** then let go. Repeat 5 times
3. Rotate shoulders in a circle 10 times each way.

Neck
NEVER FORCE OR STRAIN
1. Correct the head posture(see above) then slowly and gently turn your head from side to side as far as is comfortable. Repeat 4 times to each side.
2. Drop your head down on to your chest and then allow the upper back to curve forwards. Uncurl the upper back feeling the head come almost up the midline. Correct head posture again. Lift the chin to look at the ceiling (do not go right back) then drop the chin down and in and correct the head posture again (see above).
3. Tilt the head from shoulder to shoulder (keep facing straight ahead or turn your head slightly towards the shoulder you are tilting away from). Use the weight of your head to stretch the muscles in the side of your neck.

Jaw
Put your jaw through its normal; range of movements a few times quite quickly.
1   Forwards (so that the lower teeth come in front of the upper ones),
2   side to side
3   in a chewing circle (both ways) -

Chew for one minute. Try the chewing with and without voice.

Gently open and close the jaw feeling the muscles. If you feel the muscles bulging out allow the jaw to open, dropping it down and back, and the bulging should disappear (unless you open overly wide). Try to maintain this type of opening when practising vocal exercises.

Tongue
Imagine that you have a caramel stuck in your top left back tooth. Try to massage it free for 20 seconds. Then move your imaginary caramel to the bottom right back tooth (also 20 seconds) the bottom left back tooth, (20 seconds) the top right back tooth (also 20 seconds) up under the top lip and down under the lower lip (20 secs each).

Keeping the tongue tip against the lower front teeth see how far along the top side teeth you can slide the back of your tongue.

Massage - First find the pulse in your neck. Always work in front of this

Base of tongue/suprahyoid muscles
Using your thumbs, press up firmly in the horse-shoe shaped hollow under your chin and pummel the muscles at the base of your tongue. Use this technique to monitor tongue tension in your vocal exercises, speaking (and singing) trying to prevent the tongue pushing your thumbs down.

Firmly stroke up and backwards from under the lower jaw to the first bone of your voice box (the hyoid bone). (Remember to let the jaw drop down).

Thyrohyoid muscles
Find the top of the thyroid cartilage (Adam's apple) with your index finger. With your thumb and index finger feel out along the edges for the thyroid cartilage then slide them up into the small space between the thyroid cartilage and the hyoid bone above it. **Remember to let the jaw drop**. Notice whether this area is tender. Massage gently but firmly until the discomfort begins to ease.

Placing the thumb and index finger on the top edges of the thyroid cartilage pull gently down (making sure you have dropped the jaw down). Notice how tender areas release their tension and become more comfortable to touch.

Cricothyroid muscles
Slide your index finger gently down over the front of the thyroid cartilage until it falls into a small space. Massage gently either side of the space where the thyroid and cricoid cartilages border one another.
Gently move larynx from side to side a few times. Again make sure the jaw is relaxed down.

**These exercises have been gathered from many places and from many colleagues with thanks.
The massage has been largely developed with Jacob Lieberman**

Appendix 7.2

Assessment Checklist

Voice Clinic, Queen Mary's Hospital, Sidcup, Kent

Affix patient label
here please

General posture:

Posterior neck muscles and
shoulder muscles:
C/D shelf
Hyperextension
Anterior/Posterior Weightbearing
Other

Anterior cervical muscles
Tension Checklist:

Jaw (including suprahyoid,
jaw and base of tongue tension)

Extrinsic strap muscle tension:

Laryngeal movement
Sternocleidomastoid
symmetry
Tension during speech
Laryngeal rotation:
Laryngeal movement during
speech:

Extrinsic laryngeal muscle tension:

Thyrohyoid membranes:
Cricothyroid visor:
- at rest
- range of movement while
sirening

Articulatory Set:

Malocclusion:
Tongue position:
Lip spreading/rounding
Articulatory movement during
speech:
Pharyngeal tension:
Hypernasality:

Breathing:

Pattern at rest:
In speech:
When asked to breathe in:
Lower throat filling:

Voice assessment

Pitch:
Volume:
Quality:
Comfort:
Stamina:

s/z ratio

/a/
/i/
/m/
counting

Tape recording:
Rating Scales:

Please ring other studies completed:
EGG (Laryngograph) / Pitch
Analysis / Spectrography / Airflow
Studies (Aerophone II) /
Phonetogram

Signed:..

Date:................/.................../.................

References

Andrews ML (1991) Voice therapy for children. San Diego, CA: Singular Publishing Group Inc.

Aronson AE (1985) Psychological puberphonia. In Clinical voice disorders: an interdisciplinary approach, 2nd edn. New York: Georg Thieme Verlag, p 148.

Barlow W (1973) The Alexander Technique. New York: Warner Books.

Belisle G, Morrison MD (1983) Anatomic correlation for muscle tension dysphonia. Journal of Otolaryngology 12: 319-321.

Bielamowicz S, Kreiman J, Gerratt BR, Dauer MS, Berke GS (1996) Comparison of voice analysis systems for perturbation measurement. Journal of Speech and Hearing Research 39: 126-134.

Blaugrund SM, Taira T, Isshiki N (1991) Laryngeal Manual Compression in the Evaluation of patients for Laryngeal Framework Surgery. In: Vocal Fold Physiology, (Eds) Gauffin J, Hammarberg B. Singular Publishing Group Inc. San Diego. pp 207-212.Boliek CA, Hixon T, Watson PJ, Morgan WJ (1996) Vocalization and breathing during the first year of life. Journal of Voice 10: 1-22.

Boone D (1980) The Boone voice program for children. Oregon: CC Publications.

Boone DR, McFarlane SC (1988) The voice and voice therapy. Englewood Cliffs, NJ: Prentice-Hall Inc.

Bunker M, Stew J, Epstein R (1996) Teaching about voice. Bulletin of the Royal College of Speech and Language Therapists 526: 10-11.

Buscemi S, Yanagisawa E, Citardi M, Estill J (1995) The role of the aryepiglottic sphincter in the performance of the *messa-di-voce*. Paper presented to the 1st World Voice Congress, Oporto, Portugal.

Case JL (1991) Clinical management of voice disorders, 2nd edn. Austin, TX: Pro-Ed, p 206.

Coblenzer H, Muhar F (1976) Atem und Stimme. Wien: Österreichischer Bundesverlag.

Coblenzer H (1980) Therapie der Sprach, Sprech und Stimmstorungen 3. Stuttgart & New York: Gustav Fischer Verlag.

Colton RH, Casper JK (1990) Puberphonia-stabilisation. In Understanding voice problems. Baltimore: Williams and Wilkins, p 78.

Dickson DR, Maue-Dickson W (1982) Anatomical and physiological bases of speech. Boston: Little, Brown and Co.

Donnelly P, Kellow BM (1989) An experience in setting up a joint voice clinic: four years on. Newsletter of the Voice Research Society 3: 199.

Enderby P, Emerson J (1995) Does Speech and Language Therapy Work?: a review of the literature. London: Whurr Publishers, Chapter 9. pp 151-165.

Estill J (1988) Belting and classic voice quality: some physiological differences. Medical problems of performing artists. Philadelphia, PA: Hanley & Belfus, Inc.

Estill J (1991) Laryngeal constriction and retraction. Symposium of the British Voice Association.

Estill J (1995) Voicecraft: a user's guide to voice quality. Vol 2, some basic voice qualities. Santa Rosa, CA: Estill Voice Training Systems.

Estill J (1996) Primer of Compulsory Figures (Level One). Santa Rosa, CA: Estill Voice Training Systems.

Everson SA, Goldburg DE, Kaplan GA, Cohen RD, Pukkala E, Tuomilento J, Salonen J (1996) Hopelessness and risk of mortality and incidence of myocardial infarction and cancer. Journal of Psychosomatic Research 58: 2.

Fawcus M (Ed.) (1986) Voice Disorders and their Management. London: Croom Helm Ltd.

Fawcus M (Ed.) (1990) Voice Disorders and their Management, 2nd edn. London: Croom Helm Ltd.

Feldenkrais M (1949) Body and mature behaviour. New York: International University.

Froeschels E (1948) Twentieth century correction. New York: Philosophical Library.

Froeschels E (1952) Chewing method as therapy. Archives of Otolaryngology 56: 427-434.

Frøkjær Jensen B (1983) Acoustic-statistic long time analysis of the voice. Proceedings of the XVIIIth IALP Congress, Washington DC, USA.

Fry DB (1979) The physics of speech. Cambridge University Press.

Gelfer MP, Andrews ML, Schmidt CP (1991) Effects of prolonged loud reading on selected measures of vocal function in trained and untrained singers. Journal of Voice 5: 158-167.

Greene M, Mathieson L (1989) The Voice and its Disorders, 5th edn. London: Whurr Publishers.

Harris S, Harris D, Neemuchwala P (1995) Group voice therapy. Bulletin of the Royal College of Speech and Language Therapists 513: 11-12.

Harris T, Lieberman J (1993) The cricothyroid mechanism, its relation to vocal fatigue and vocal dysfunction. Voice forum. Journal of Voice 2: 89-96.

Harris TM, Collins S, Clarke DD (1986) An interdisciplinary voice clinic. In Fawcus M (Ed.) Voice disorders and their management. London: Croom Helm, pp 283-292.

Hillman RE, Holmberg EB, Perkell JS, Walsh M, Vaughan C (1989) Objective assessment of vocal hyperfunction: an experimental framework and initial results. Journal of Speech and Hearing Research 32: 373-392.

Hodkinson E (1990) Therapy and management of the dysphonic child. In Fawcus M (Ed.) Voice disorders and their management, 2nd edn. London: Croom Helm, pp 83-95.

Hoit JD, Hixon T (1991) Body type and speech breathing. In Hixon T (Ed.) Respiratory function in speech and song. San Diego, CA: Singular Publishing Group Inc.

Isshiki N (1966) Classification of hoarseness. Japanese Journal of Logopedics and Phoniatfics 7: 15-21.

Isshiki N (1989) Phonosurgery: theory and practice. Springer-Verlag, Tokto, Berlin, Heidelberg, New York. pp 83-84.

Jacobsen E (1938) Progressive relaxation, 2nd edn. University of Chicago Press.

Kotby MN (1995) The Accent Method of voice therapy. San Diego, CA: Singular Publishing Group Inc.

Kotby MN, El-Sady SR, Basiouny SE, Abou-Rass YA, Hegazi MA (1991) Efficacy of the Accent Method of voice therapy. Journal of Voice 5: 316-320.

Koufman JA, Blalock PD (1982) Classification and approach to patients with functional voice disorders. Annals of Otology, Rhinology and Laryngology 91: 372-377.

Koufman JA, Blalock PD (1991) Functional voice disorders. Otolaryngologic Clinics of North America 24: 1059-1073.

Laukkanen A-M, Lindholm P, Vilkman E, Haataja K, Alku P (1996) A physiological and acoustic study on the voiced bilabial fricative /ß:/ as a vocal exercise. Journal of Voice 10: 67–77.

Lauri E-R, Alku P, Vilkman E, Sala E, Sihvo, M (1997) Effects of prolonged oral reading on time-based glottal flow waveform parameters with special reference to gender differences. Folia Phoniatrica et Logopedica, in press.

Laver J (1980) Phonetic description of voice quality. Cambridge University Press.

Lawrence VL (1987) Suggested criteria for fibreoptic diagnosis of laryngeal hyperfunction. Video presentation. Proceedings of the Voice Research Society, London. UK. (Video available from The British Voice Association, London.)

Levy SM, Heiden LA (1990) Personality and social factors in cancer outcome. In Friedman HS (Ed) Personality and disease. New York: John Wiley and Sons.

McAllister A, Sederholm E, Sundberg J, Gramming P (1994) Relations between voice range profiles and physiological and perceptual voice characteristics in ten year old children. Journal of Voice 8: 230-239.

Mathieson L (1993) Vocal tract discomfort in hyperfunctional dysphonia. Voice 2: 40-48.

Miller DG and Schutte HK (1990) Feedback from spectral analysis applied to the singing voice. Journal of Voice 2:4 pp 329–334.

Morris C (1992) Shared problems - shared success. Bulletin of the Royal College of Speech and Language Therapists 485: 4-5.

Morrison M, Rammage L, Nichol H, Pullan B, May P, Salkeld L (1994) The management of voice disorders. San Diego, CA: Singular Publishing Group Inc., pp 54-63.

Morrison MD, Rammage LA, Gilles M, Belisle DM, Pullan CB, Nichol H (1983) Muscular tension dysphonia. Journal of Otolaryngology 12: 302-306.

Pahn J (1964) Der therapeutische Wert nasalierter Vokalklange in der Behandlung funktioneller Stimmerkrankungen. Folia Phoniatrica 16: 249-263.

Proctor DF (1980) Breathing speech and song. Wien: Springer-Verlag.

Roy N, Leeper HA (1993) Effects of the manual laryngeal musculoskeletal tension reduction technique as a treatment for functional voice disorders: perceptual and acoustic measures. Journal of Voice 7: 242-249.

Rubin JS, Sataloff RT, Korovin GS, Gould WJ (1995) Diagnosis and treatment of voice disorders. New York: Igaku-Shoin.

Sataloff RT (1984) 'How I do it' head and neck and plastic surgery. A targeted problem and its solution: efficient history taking in professional singers. Laryngoscope 94: 1111-1114.

Sederholm E, McAllister A, Dalkvist J, Sundberg J (1995) Aetiologic factors associated with hoarseness in ten-year-old children. Folia Phoniatrica et Logopaedica 47: 262-278.

Smith S, Thyme K (1976) Statistic research on changes in speech due to pedagogic treatment (the Accent Method). Folia Phoniatrica 28: 98-103.

Smith S, Thyme K (1981) Die Akzentmethode. Vedbæk, Denmark: Danish Voice Institute.

Stemple JC, Stanley J, Lee L (1995) Objective measures of voice production in normal subjects following prolonged voice use. Journal of Voice 9: 127-133.

Sundberg J (1987) The science of the singing voice. De Kalb, IL: Northern Illinois University Press.

Thyme K, Frøkjær Jensen B (1983) Results of one week's intensive voice training. Proceedings of the XVIIIth IALP Congress, Washington, USA, pp 984-989.

Thyme K, Frøkjær Jensen B (1987) Analyses of voice changes during a 10 month period of voice training at the education of logopeds in Copenhagen. Proceedings of the 1st International Voice Symposium, Edinburgh, UK.

Titze IR (1994) Principles of voice production. Englewood Cliffs, NJ: Prentice-Hall.

Titze IR (1995) Source-vocal tract interactions in the singer's formant. 1st Pan European Voice Conference, London, UK.

Vilkman E, Sonninen A, Hurme P, Körkkö, P (1996) External laryngeal frame function in voice production revisited: a review. Journal of Voice 10: 78-92.

Wilson DK (1987) Voice problems of children, 3rd edn. Baltimore: Williams and Wilkins.

Some useful addresses

For further information about some of the therapy techniques mentioned in this chapter.

Accent Method
Kirsten Thyme-Frøkjær, Danish Voice Institute, Ellebuen 21, DK-2950, Vedbæk, Denmark

Alexander Technique
The Society of Teachers of the Alexander Technique, 20 London House, 266 Fulham Road, London SW10 9EL, UK

Coblenzer Technique and Pahn's Nasalization
Åse Ørsted, Institute for Speech Disorders, Rygards Alle 45, Hellerup, 2900 Denmark

Estill's Compulsory Figures for Voice
Jo Estill, 67 Airport Blvd East, Santa Rosa, California 95403, USA

Feldenkrais
The Feldenkrais Centre, 10 Fernside Court, London NW4 1JT

Pilates
The Alan Herdman Studios, 17 Homer Row, London W1H 1HU, UK

Abigail Ben-Ari, The Belsize Studio, 74a Belsize Lane, London NW3 5BJ, UK

Singing and therapy

DINAH HARRIS

This chapter is divided into two sections. The first covers general considerations for the singing teacher working in a voice clinic, the second examines clinical practice and includes practical exercises and ideas for remedial treatment. A glossary of common singing terms, descriptions of voice types and a list of useful references is included at the end.

General considerations

> *It is the best of all trades, to make songs,*
> *and the second best to sing them.*
>
> Hilaire Belloc

This chapter is aimed at different groups working with singing voices, including those singing teachers who are permanent members of voice clinic teams and wish to discover what techniques others are using, and those teachers working with singers in a more traditional teaching environment who would like some information about how we manage singers and their problems in our voice clinic.

We also hope the chapter will be of use to speech therapists working with singers where there is no singing advisor attached to the voice clinic, and to laryngologists working with professional singers.

It should be remembered that there is no available training for remedial singing teaching in Britain, and the teachers involved in this area have borrowed, adapted and invented from many different sources, including speech therapy techniques, voice teaching, body work and the other members of the clinical team.

Caveat. There are no right or wrong ways to do things; this is what one singing teacher does in one voice clinic. It offers practical ideas but in no way pretends to be the definitive way of working with singers.

This clinical practice has been evolved by the dictates of time, space, equipment and NHS contracts: i.e. six sessions, grossly limited space, no piano and a pitch pipe provided by the teacher. Ideally, in the future, funding would allow for many more sessions, a studio with a suitable acoustic, a piano, a music library and excellent audiovisual equipment. Speech therapists would provide joint sessions with video transnasal fibreoptic laryngopharyngoscopy, airflow measures, spectrography and more – in other words, a performance medicine clinic. In our dreams!

The role of the singing teacher in the voice clinic

It is most important that the singing teacher actually attends the voice clinic rather than simply receiving referrals, as nothing in singing pedagogy constitutes a suitable preparation for clinical practice. Teachers are likely to receive their training from the other team members, adding their own experience and skills. It is extremely advantageous to work closely with the speech therapist and, whenever possible, to attend therapy sessions. The singing teacher and speech therapist will find that frequently the singing and speaking voice mirror the same problems - a high level of anxiety, insufficient airflow, hypervalving, reduced range, voice breaks, discomfort and lack of stamina. Therefore it is important to address these issues together. The singing teacher should be able to work with the singers' speaking voices as well as their singing voices, as NHS contracts do not allow for long courses of therapy.

It is not the singing teacher's remit to give formal singing lessons on the NHS. Indeed, this would be fairly difficult within an NHS context because funding a piano or an electronic Midi keyboard will be low on the list of hospital priorities. More often than not you will find yourself in an acoustically tiled treatment room (the dimensions of a fairly generous cupboard), with a pitch pipe in your hand. The aim should be to return the singer to their preproblem level of performance. Anything more than this is a bonus.

Shared aims and differences between the singing teacher and the speech therapist

Speech and singing therapy in general share the same aim: in so far as it is possible, to restore the patient's voice to a comfortable, reliable instrument.

This is often easier for the singing teacher to achieve as his or her patients are much less likely to have permanent vocal damage, serious neurological damage or other disease. Singers are on average a younger group in a voice clinic's patient intake, and have a much higher level of body awareness. Apart from the usual run of singer's pathologies (bleeds, nodules, polyps, scars, etc.), their problems tend to be associated with technical imbalances and malfunctions, muscular tension and, above all, with stress and anxiety.

The difference between working in a voice clinic and a private voice studio

There are many differences between working in a studio and a voice clinic. As a teacher in a traditional studio setting it is normal to have an ongoing pedagogical relationship with the student over a number of months or years. The teacher has many aims, including establishing a technique that will allow the singer to respond to many and varied vocal tasks with a flexible and reliable instrument that will enable them to fulfil their vocal and artistic potential. It is important to encourage the student to have the courage to expose their response to the musical, literary and emotional text, which can make reticent British characters feel rather vulnerable. The teacher will aim to introduce the student to the wealth of (suitable) repertoire available to them and work with them interpretatively.

In a voice clinic setting little of this applies. Both time and the nature of the singer's needs will dictate quick and basic 'plumbing'. Whether the singer is having postoperative therapy or therapy to reduce a nodule or hyperfunction, the main concerns will be the same: to release hypertonic muscles; to balance appropriate subglottic pressure to appropriate valving; to find the best and widest possible vocal range; to re-establish stamina, comfort and quality; to halt abusive vocal habits; and to offer emotional support.

By now, any speech therapist readers will be saying, 'I can do that!', and how right they are. One of the main differences between a studio and a voice clinic is that the latter will provide a great deal of advice and help from the other team members that is not available to most singing teachers. This is very reassuring. At best, teaching singing is dark and lonely work, but someone has to do it.

What the speech therapist and singing teacher can learn from each other

The work of the speech therapist and remedial singing teacher would appear to be fundamentally similar. In our voice clinic we have happily stolen ideas and techniques from each other without apology. Learning to sing is very much to do with learning to coordinate and finely control the balance between many different muscles, and speech therapy techniques have a great deal to offer in precisely identifying and working these different groups in an organized way. It is easy to extend these techniques into the singing voice. From the speech therapist's point of view it is to be hoped that the inventiveness and the grasp of imagery and metaphor of the singing teacher will add a certain flexibility in dealing with voices. They will also add to the therapist's understanding giving him or her a knowledge of the performer's anxieties, the unpublished realities of daily professional life, repertoire, voice types and the practical details of how the wide spectrum of the music business works.

The singing teacher can gain from the therapist the kind of vocal education that is simply not available to teachers in this country. He or she can acquire an overall view of the voice as both a speaking and a singing instrument, a much clearer and more precise picture of what can go wrong with voices, and an exact understanding of the anatomy and function of the vocal instrument.

Who are we treating?

The groups of professional performers that one is likely to come across roughly divide into five:

- Western classical tradition trained singers;
- music theatre singers (who are usually also highly trained);
- occasional clients from other traditions (e.g. Indian classical singing);
- leading actors who are prepared to 'have a go at singing' (often without any singing training or 2 months' worth of lessons 10 years ago);
- pop, rock and band singers (who will have had little or no voice training).

Classically trained singers

This group of singers have much shorter contracts than the others, and within a few weeks their diaries may range from an oratorio performance, to a run of six opera performances, to a radio broadcast of baroque music, to a concert of contemporary or 'squeaky gate' music. So they are rarely bored, but frequently worried about how they are going to find time to learn their new repertoire for the next few months. Vocally of course, they take life seriously. They will try to get enough sleep, not get hung over too often and pay attention to the state of their voice, of which they are perpetually and acutely aware. They are no more neurotic than the general population of patients, but know instantly when their voice is not responding in the way that they are used to. They work hard, taking lessons throughout their performing lives, even when they are established. They frequently regard their voice as an almost separate entity from themselves, which is how it often feels. They are at risk from pushy or unsympathetic agents, fourth-rate conductors or opera company managements; and those who work in professional choruses or choirs have to cope with perpetual sight-reading, which means that they are never vocally prepared for what is coming next, as nothing is ever 'sung in'. Their own insecurities or ambitions may make them accept too much work. They live in fear of 'doing themselves permanent (and unspecified) damage', and for most classical singers it would be more acceptable to be diagnosed as a typhus carrier than the owner of a nodule.

Music theatre singers

These singers are sometimes well trained. The vocal demands on them are very different to those on the classically trained singer. For the classical singer (regardless of the style of the music) the vocal set will remain largely the same. The music theatre singer will often be required to produce many different qualities of voice, from a ballad quality for pre-1960s shows, to belt and rock. They therefore require a much more flexible and bolder use of the voice. They will be expected to give eight shows a week and, in some cases, be available to stand by as understudies for other roles (often 'covering' several other performers). This is testing, particularly in the winter months when most of the cast will be laid low at one time or another, and often several members of the cast at once. You cannot produce good vocal support when gastroenteritis has rendered your fundament untrustworthy!

Singers from other classical traditions

The Indian classical singer requires (among other things) to be able to sing sitting down with crossed legs while producing long passages of 'pressed' phonation with greatly enhanced higher formants. We have little experience of the tradition but can help with posture and breath control.

High profile actors

This group comprises high profile actors who have little experience in singing, but have been seduced by a management or director into thinking that anyone who acts can sing. This is tantamount to saying that anyone who can run for a bus can sprint like a 100-metre Olympic gold medallist. They may well have had a few singing lessons some years previously, but will not necessarily have kept up with their voice work. As the rehearsal period intensifies, so does their terror. They may feel both vulnerable and incompetent as they begin to realize how different singing and speaking may feel, and often become seriously panicked. They need an enormous amount of emotional support and as much work on relaxation, low abdominal breathing and support as it is possible to provide. They usually end up giving a wonderful performance and walk away with every available theatre award.

Rock, pop and band singers

This group will usually have had no voice training and are deeply suspicious of singing teachers, particularly those of a classical bent, and often with good reason. A rock singer is unlikely to benefit from the finer points of bel canto. There are several megastars who would be considerably less famous without vocal pathology. Their problems begin only when the vocal pathology renders them incapable of performance. They are deeply serious about their work, and these days usually lead a (mostly) exemplary life. The days of unlimited sex and drugs with your rock and roll appear to be over.

The band singer will perform mostly at functions (ladies' nights, weddings and 21st birthday parties). He or she may be semi-professional, working at another job during the week to keep the wolf from the door, and looking forward greatly to the weekend 'gigs' where his or her heart really lies. In six sessions it is not possible to provide a full singing technique. Therefore we would suggest that one follows the basic speech therapy rules and ensures that the voice is produced with a good subglottic pressure rather than indiscriminate muscle tension and hypervalving, which may lead to vocal abuse. The singer may need to be made aware of vocal hygiene. It is also important to check that the body posture is viable and that the microphone is at a good enough angle for the head position not to be hyperextended. It does have to be acknowledged that there are many singers in this category who have had long and trouble-free careers, and who have clearly found a vocal production that may sound abusive but manages to fool us all. It would be fascinating to film Phil Collins's or Tina Turner's vocal tract with a fibre nasendoscope while in performance to find out just how they do it and escape scot-free.

What is a singer?

I do but sing because I must,
And pipe but as the linnets sing.

Alfred, Lord Tennyson

It is almost easier for a singer to bear the fact that they have a pathology, than to discover that muscular tension and emotional stress have caused voice loss. When an amateur singer develops voice problems it is a disappointment and sadness. For a professional singer it is tantamount to a bereavement. A professional singer will describe voice loss like losing a limb. They have an ambivalent relationship with their voice (note how singers sometimes refer to 'the' voice, rather than 'my' voice.) When they have a voice problem it is as if their familiar instrument takes on a sinister life of its own, rather like a vocal 'alien'. It is not only their livelihood that is at risk, but also their sense of identity: 'If I cannot sing, who am I?' Everybody tends to define themselves by what they do, rather than who they are. The very special nature of the singer's relationship with his or her voice makes this an almost unbearable responsibility.

There is an appalling anxiety in having to perform with an instrument that is unreliable. Agents, managements and conductors are not always sympathetic or understanding. Colleagues may be supportive, but it is often difficult to discuss problems as the singer is fearful that the 'powers that be' may find out and fire them. Thus a sense of secrecy and shame is engendered. Singers are well used to living with fear, but the dread and terror of having to perform with a malfunctioning voice is difficult to describe.

Their knowledge of anatomy is usually negligible but their biofeedback/kinaesthetic awareness is good. Many teachers will take the attitude that to inform the pupil of the functional anatomy and science of singing will in some way impede the artistic flow and imagination. We have in no way found this to be true. Singers are always anxious to learn about the working of their instrument and are delighted to find out what is going on. Any other instrumentalist can see, touch and feel what they are doing to their instrument from the word go. A singer does not have this luxury. Our sensations when we sing are not necessarily an accurate picture of what is physiologically occurring. Singers are obsessional, diligent and desperate to 'sort things out'. If you ask for ten per cent, they will give you one hundred and ten.

When you play the 'Phantom of the Opera' or 'Sweeney Todd', the vocal demands are obvious - not least that twice a week there are days when two performances take place. The length of a show contract in a long-running success is often a year with a week's holiday, and artists will sometimes want a change of scene and spend their holiday singing something else somewhere else, rather than falling silently in a heap on a beach. This does not leave much time for the recharging of batteries.

For classical singers the demands are different. Unless you are a superstar you are unlikely to be expected to sing so often. Wise and established operatic stars are likely to limit the number of performances they give per year. Other lowlier artists do not have that choice, and the complaint is that they suffer from a feast or famine of booking. In a full-time company, singers will often rehearse one opera in the morning and perform another at night. If they are freelance singers they may be learning repertory for a concert or a broadcast in the afternoon.

Operatic roles also make very different demands on singers. Wagner specialists sing for hours on end. Siegfried (in 'Siegfried') probably sings in total for about 2 hours, and Violetta in 'La Traviata' for about an hour and a quarter. However, the Queen of the Night in 'The Magic Flute' sings two arias and a short ensemble, and all the public hears (or cares about) is whether she can sing a series of extremely high notes - twice. Not for nothing do opera singers sometimes feel that they are taking part in a boxing match or a high-wire act, rather than a creative act. There is a truly gladiatorial element to audiences, not to mention critics.

General problems

Of course, we've all dreamed of reviving the castrati; but it's needed Hilda to take the first practical steps towards making them a reality ... She's drawn up a list of well known singers who she thinks would benefit from ... treatment ... It's only a question of getting them to agree.

Henry Reed

Fatigue

General exhaustion is disastrous for performers. As their energy levels drop, the 'support' or supply of air pressure under the vocal folds becomes inconsistent. This is when vocal damage is likely to occur. By the time music theatre performers reach the second show on a Saturday night they are seriously tired. They don't always notice vocal deterioration with the speed of a classical singer, as they are not working in an acoustic environment and the overall feeling of exhaustion may mask it. There is this strange belief in the theatre world in a mythical being called 'Dr Theatre' (not to be confused with the theatre doctor), who will mysteriously help the actor get through a show no matter how disastrous the mental or physical state he may be in (e.g. should he have broken his ankle, be running a temperature of 102°F, be throwing up every half hour or lost the spouse that morning). We subscribe rather more readily to Nöel Coward's song, '*Why* must the show go on?'

Pay and illness

West End show singers are usually paid for rehearsals and by the week, whether they appear or not. Most classical singers are freelance and are paid by the performance and if forced to cancel will lose their fee. It is not unusual for a rehearsal period that can last for up to 4 or more weeks to be unpaid. Consequently, a run of ill health lasting for a few weeks can be a financial disaster to a young classical singer. Singers on full-time contracts in an opera house are in a much happier position, as they are salaried

Understudies/covers

Show singers are contracted for a run of the show, but are sometimes inadequately understudied. A new understudy may not be ready to go on, and while there may be a second understudy, it is not uncommon for most of a cast to be suffering from the same virus and for both understudies to be unable to go on as well as the principal. The resilience of singers will usually mean that another member of the cast will offer to learn the role and play it that evening. The production company may have cut costs by booking cheap, inexperienced covers, who they are reluctant to put on stage. The actor playing the role is sometimes leant upon to appear by the company manager when ill, as the understudy is 'not really up to it'.

A 'swing' has the unenviable task of understudying several different roles in the same show. They must know each role back to front, as in the height of winter they may find themselves singing several different roles in one week. A swing also has to know the separate vocal lines in the ensembles for each role as they may have to sing the alto line at the matinee and the soprano line at the evening performance.

It is not unusual for the management to have omitted to book any understudies at all, relying on the unremitting good health of the cast. You can well imagine the anxiety this produces for the performer, and the moral blackmail that may well ensue. Unfortunately in the present financial climate all companies are fighting for survival and the performers' needs are, alas, among the last things to be considered.

It is possible when faced with a voiceless singer and no understudy, to suggest that the singer 'walks' the show and someone else sings the role from the orchestra pit with the musical score. No one will thank you for it but it is better than having to cancel the performance altogether. Opera managements are much more realistic and understand that there are times when a singer must simply shut up in order to complete the run of shows over the next few weeks. In the big companies they are well covered, or may, as Covent Garden does, fly someone in who will sing the opera with virtually no rehearsal, often meeting his or her fellow artists for the first time on stage.

In music theatre the understudy is expected to remain in the theatre until the artist he is covering has made his final entrance on stage. In opera companies the understudy is supposed to remain at the end of a telephone where he may be reached, until the early afternoon. This can lead to problems should the artist performing that night suddenly find his health deteriorating after 2 pm, but makes the process of understudying less tiresome.

Foldback and 'sound design'

This is an essential part of music theatre and pop and rock concerts. There is a substantial amount of sound amplification on stage, and pop and rock bands will have monitor speakers in front of them to 'fold back' their own voices to them, as the sound level on stage is punitive.

In music theatre the band is often to be found in another part of the theatre rather than the orchestra pit. For this reason it is totally impossible for a singer to monitor his or her voice as there is no natural acoustic. The singers will usually wear tiny radio microphones in their wigs or on their costumes, which will enable them to sing from any position on the set and be heard as clearly as if they were hugging the proscenium arch.

Foldback monitor speakers in the wings give a general mix of the sound that is occurring on stage and from the band, but there is no individual monitoring facility as is the norm in a recording studio. If these are not well adjusted and the sound level is too high, everyone on stage will sing louder to try to get some aural feed-back on their own voice. (The Lombard Effect makes a singer or speaker automat-ically attempt to voice about 20 dB louder than the ambient noise level. This can have catastrophic vocal results if the performer can't hear himself think, let alone sing.) Accordingly, the sound level will mount and the singers become increasingly vocally exhausted as they negotiate their way through eight shows a week. The same is true of the alternative. The foldback level may be too low and the singers 'push' themselves vocally in order to try and hear themselves in the artifically 'dead' acoustic.

A sound technician sits in front of a large console and balances (or doesn't) the mix that results from the various microphones. This means that the performers are entirely in the hands and ears of the engineer rather than being able to judge the balance for themselves. A classical singer will always, if possible, give themselves the opportunity to test their voices in the acoustic of the concert hall or theatre before the performance, although the feedback will change once the space is filled with an audience.

Nerves - or lack of them

There is undoubtedly a certain amount of nervous tension about performing. There are a few lucky people who sail through the whole business nerve-free, but they are rare. It should be remembered that many famous artists suffer from appalling nerves, to the extent (it is rumoured) that one generously proportioned diva had to be pushed on stage at the beginning of her career.

Apart from the 'normal' terror of stage fright, which goes with the territory, nerves may be caused by other factors, such as an inadequate technique or the growing realization that the singer has taken on a role whose demands are too heavy or vocally taxing.

Mirella Freni, who has sustained a huge international operatic career for longer than most other singers around, is quoted as saying that the most important word in a singer's vocabulary is 'No'.

'Loss of nerve' is a very different business. This terrifying distress never goes away with 'a nice holiday' or a period of voice rest. It is psychogenic in nature and is often greatly helped by psychotherapy or counselling.

Stress

Stress is rarely due to a single factor. Problems always seem to come in droves. They may be professionally engendered by such things as vocal deterioration or a singing technique that has always seemed secure no longer appearing to work.

There can be a feeling of emotional paralysis due to too much pressure from too many engagements, and a panic about lack of time for learning the new reper-toire required. This can be just as distressing as too little work. Singers may realize that the role or concert is beyond their present capabilities. They may be fearful of displeasing the agent/company manager/conductor/director/opera intendant or singing teacher, or of being 'found out'. They may be physically exhausted owing

to too many train or car journeys or flights, swiftly followed by too many performances. All this is generally accompanied by a marked lack of self-esteem.

Financial anxieties abound. Performing is at best an unreliable source of
income. When it becomes open knowledge that a performer has had a run of bad
shows or has been in an overwrought state the work tends to dry up, regardless of
how well the performer is doing at present.

Domestic factors can also play a part. Relationships are often difficult to maintain for a performer. Children, spouses and partners often suffer, as much of a
performer's life is spent away from home. They may well resent the fact that they
are constantly left to keep the home fires burning. There are problems with
collapsed relationships, divorce and infidelity (always a risk on tour, as travelling
around the globe can be exciting, but often very lonely).

Problems with the singing voice may be indicative of emotional stress elsewhere. Psychodynamic counselling or therapy may be helpful to ensure that the
problems are dealt with in an appropriate place rather than spilling over haphaz-
ardly into the singer's professional life. (Useful addresses are included at the end of
Chapter 9.)

Singers' voice problems are not necessarily due to a single factor, but can have a
whole bouquet of causes, although the singer will often wish to attribute the problem to a single cause.

Clinical practice

Far from the madding crowd's ignoble strife,
Their sober wishes never learned to stray;
Along the cool sequestered vale of life
They kept the noiseless tenor of their way.

Gray's Elegy

General assessment

Joint voice clinic diagnostic visit

We are lucky enough to be able to hold a joint voice clinic at Queen Mary's Hospital Trust, Sidcup, which involves all four members of the team being present at
the initial voice clinic appointment. This has great advantages from everyone's
point of view (although patients may find it a little intimidating for the first few
minutes). For this singing advisor it is an absolute necessity. It is possible to meet
the patient in an informal but clinical situation, be present when the medical diagnosis is made, and observe and assess for oneself while also enjoying the feedback
from the other team members. It is important to see the larynx in action rather
than reading about it in a letter of referral, and to take part in deciding the
management plan.

The medical case history

A case history for the medical notes is taken during the initial voice clinic visit. There are certain items in the usual medical and social history that are particularly relevant to singers:

Gastro-oesophageal acid reflux ('heartburn')

This can alter a singer's use of voice. If you feel acid rise up your oesophagus to the back of your pharynx, you are likely to tighten every available muscle in your vocal tract in order to protect your airway (Jones et al., 1990). Good abdominal support is likely to exacerbate this problem. If you push your stomach contents up through your diaphragm you can feel the tidal wave of acidified lunch. It is advisable to avoid late night meals and alcohol, spicy foods and to seek medical treatment.

Menstrual problems

A fairly recent hysterectomy or severe menstrual cramps will impede easy and energetic abdominal support. In the premenstrual period and during the first few days of menstruation the vocal folds may become oedematous and the mucosal veins may dilate, causing the voice to sound 'off colour'. The blood vessels in the vocal folds become more prone to damage with an increased risk of microbleeds. In German opera houses it is still sometimes an agreed part of the contract that female artists are not required to sing during the first few days of menstruation (Abitbol et al., 1989). Singers should sing warily at this point in their cycle.

Hormones

The contraceptive pill can affect the extreme top of a voice, and it is always worth checking if a singer has been on any hormonal/steroid treatment, as various treatments in the past have resulted in a masculinization of the voice. It is not unknown for a light soprano to drop to mezzo range (Damste, 1967; Sataloff, 1990). On the other hand, pregnancy may result in fluid retention causing minimal vocal fold oedema that may affect the vocal range and clarity of tone. The increased blood supply necessary to support pregnancy may result in vocal fold haemorrhages. The increase in body weight may alter posture and 9 months' tenancy will affect abdominal breath support.

Neck and shoulder problems

Whiplash injury or chronic pain in the shoulders, neck or back will greatly effect posture, and therefore the singing voice. (See Chapter 6 for details on management.)

Hydration

Every singer alive complains of catarrh. Check the water intake, and tell them to carry bottles of designer water with their music and to remember to drink it. Tell them to inhale steam nightly over at least 3 weeks and avoid cold cures, which have a drying effect. Hydration is the name of the game. (Singers are always impressed, but also somewhat revolted, by the fact that humans appear to swallow a litre or so of 'goo' per day.)

Asthma

There are a considerable number of singers who are asthmatic. It is important to know what they are inhaling, and if it is a steroid, whether it is delivered via a spacer. This will provide a cloud of steroid spray, a higher proportion of which will reach the bronchi rather than settling on the vocal folds. Deposits of steroid in the mouth and pharynx may be flushed away with a drink of water after inhalation. Swallowing pumps mucus (with the steroid lying on it) out of the larynx. Beware of fungal infections ('thrush'). If the asthmatic is not very proficient at using the spray, enough steroid may remain in the vocal tract (rather than the lungs) to precipitate a fungal infection. This produces quantities of thick white sticky mucus and irritation, and will need medical attention. The same problem can arise after long or repeated courses of antibiotics (see Chapter 10).

Tonsillitis

Singers can lose work through frequent bouts of tonsillitis. However, if the tonsils are removed, the vocal set feels quite different and it takes a while to get accustomed to it. The surgeon should suggest that 2 months of singing retraining will be required.

Smoke, dust and chemicals

Theatres and rehearsal rooms are often very old and have layers of dust accrued over many years, and they are not cleaned with the same frequency or care as hospitals or railway stations. Many dressing rooms are underground or do not have windows that open, and are air-conditioned. Colleagues may smoke in rehearsal or dressing rooms and may not always be cooperative about no-smoking zones. The production's special effects may involve smoke machines or dry ice machines, and stage management and directors are inclined to get rather overenthusiastic with them, leaving the singer blinded and choking on a cloud of fumes .

Social life

Beware the sociable singer and the busy, noisy pub after the show. It is better to leave the first night party early if there is to be a second night performance. Indeed, it is preferable to forego the first night party altogether, but a therapist does need to be realistic!

Voice rest

The singer may have put himself or herself on a stretch of voice rest for weeks or even months in an attempt to cure what feels like vocal fatigue. By the end of this period the result will usually be an even tighter vocal set as they will be in a state of immense anxiety and muscular tension. Once the laryngologist has seen them and given the 'all clear' it is advisable to begin rebalancing the vocal gesture as soon as possible. Within our voice clinic, periods of voice rest in excess of 10 days are never recommended. Even complex surgery of the vocal folds (or a bleed into a fold) physically heals within 10 days. There is therefore no physical reason for suggesting a longer period of voice rest. However, if a singer is physically and psychologically exhausted, voice rest may be used as the only possible excuse for a break. This should not be confused with healing of laryngeal damage. An athlete expects to go back into rehabilitative training immediately after damage has been healed. The same should apply to singers.

Drugs

There are many singing myths and as many remedies: gargling with various arcane mixtures to reduce laryngitis, special lozenges and magic sprays. These may help the confidence but are unlikely to improve the voice. Local anaesthetic sprays are more dangerous. They work by reducing sensation in the larynx, and while the singer may feel more comfortable, they are much more likely to oversing and thus inflict real damage on their vocal folds.

Some years ago performers were prescribed beta blockers to help them through a fear of auditions or 'rough patches'. While these **are** an improvement on the use of alcohol, cocaine or cannabis (which is even more damaging than tobacco) to allay nerves, they have the effect of not only damping down the effects of adrenalin, which causes the terror, but also reducing the noradrenalin, which gives the dramatic edge to the performance. The singer finds that he or she feels tired, lacking the requisite energy to perform, unable to give of their best and miserable, albeit with a stable heart rate (Dehorn, 1991). We would suggest that it is most important to identify the underlying cause of the nerves and set about rectifying this, rather than dealing with the symptom.

Anaesthetics and intubation

Sometimes it is possible to have a general anaesthetic without the need for a tube to be passed through the vocal folds (Harris et al., 1990) Singers should be reminded to advise their anaesthetist of their profession **before** being put under a general anaesthetic. Anaesthetists may not always listen.

Hobbies

A singer who is working out in the gym, using heavy body building equipment or lifting weights may turn into the body beautiful, but it may also give him the straps tight and the grunted hard attack.

An advice session for the patient without a therapy contract

In this age of extracontractual referrals it is no longer possible, because of financial constraints, to treat all patients who do not live locally. Therefore, whenever possible, having made a diagnosis in the voice clinic, an advice session for an 'out of contract' patient can be both helpful and reassuring. It is also worth suggesting to the patient that their singing teacher is welcome to telephone the singing advisor (should they wish) for any clarification or elaboration of the diagnosis and for a bit of moral support. Teachers tend to feel a certain degree of responsibility for their students.

First therapy session

> *The siren waits thee, singing song for song.*
>
> Walter Savage Landor

Additional information: singing history and social details.

Apart from having the patient's personal details together with the speech therapy observations and medical diagnosis, the singing advisor needs to be aware of other additional 'singing' information:

- Age is important. Are the patient's goals realistic, given his or her maturity or lack of it?
- Where has the patient studied, with whom and for how long? Are they with a teacher at the moment? In some cases, have they ever had a teacher?
- Voice type. Have they ever changed voice type, especially recently (i.e. moved from soprano to mezzo, or baritone to tenor)?
- Warm ups. Does the patient warm up before singing? Does it take longer to get the voice running than it used to? As singing is an athletic pursuit, it is most important that muscles are gently warmed up before embarking on any heavy duty vocal activity.
- Repertoire. Are they singing suitable repertoire for their age, standard and development?
- Present and future professional engagements. What work are they contracted to do in the next few weeks or months?
- Emotional state. Is anyone leaning on them? Agents, conductors, opera company chiefs, company managers, singing teachers? (Ask tactfully!)
- Family. Are they trying to support a family with an instrument that they feel is no longer reliable or employable?
- Are they working in other employment in order to pay the rent? If so, the singer may be exhausted from teaching classes or individual pupils 8 hours per day. Other unsuitable activities may be waiting tables, serving in shops and bars, or answering telephones. Whichever of these provides their main income, they will find they have very little energy left to sing with by the end of the day.

What does the **client** want to change?

> *She was a singer who had to take any note above A with her eyebrows*
>
> Montague Glass

How does the patient perceive the problem? Singers usually have a very clear picture of the symptoms of their problem.

- Loss of quality. They may complain that their singing and/or speaking voice has become husky, breathy, 'unfocused', lacking clarity, harsh or pressed.
- Loss of stamina, singing or speaking. How long are they singing for per day? How do they warm up and for how long? Are young singers attempting to sing

for 3 hours on end, or do they find at the end of 20 minutes that they are sung out? Do they know how to 'mark' in rehearsal? Do they warm down?

- Discomfort. Where precisely? This gives a good clue as to which muscles may be hyperfunctioning. Many singers have a very good grasp of which muscles are causing them discomfort, i.e. tongue tension (geniohyoid, mylohyoid, genioglossus), tight jaw (masseter, pterygoid muscles, temporalis), thyrohyoid membrane, cricothyroid, sternocleidomastoid, the posterior muscles of the neck and shoulders. They just do not always know the anatomical names.
- Reduction in range. Does the singer complain that the 'top' appears to have gone, that they cannot sing through the passaggios smoothly, or that they are unable to access the lower range of their voice?
- Reduction in dynamic range, i.e. inability to sing out fully or sing softly. They may complain of breaks in the flow of tone when singing quietly, rather like a loose connection.
- Voice onset problems. Are they having problems with simultaneous or easy voice onset and only able to produce hard glottal attack?
- Vibrato. Are they reporting changes or problems with vibrato? A wide, slow, uneven vibrato, a fast narrow 'flutter' or even total absence of vibrato? (Beware the early music singer - 'straight' singing, although aesthetically loved and admired by many, is often the result of low airflow, hypervalving and little breath support. Whereas many singers use this with enormous success, other voices may find it both inhibiting and tiring.)

It can be helpful to ask the patient what they have been told by their singing teachers, speech therapist or doctor. This information may easily have been misinterpreted or misunderstood.

Physical assessment (see Appendix 7.2)

> Swans sing before they die - 'twere no bad thing
> Did certain persons die before they sing
>
> ST Coleridge

The following areas should be included in the assessment of any singer/professional voice user.

Breathing pattern

What type of breathing pattern does the patient use habitually? (clavicular, abdominal, chest; noisy or quiet? see Chapter 7). Any examination of the breathing pattern should include the abdominal muscles.

Many singers mistake rigid inflexible abdominal muscles for 'support', without being absolutely certain of the meaning of the concept. It is important to understand that 'support' refers to the ability to sustain subglottic pressure and airflow, rather than a vague muscular contraction of the abdominal wall unconnected to this.

Posture (at rest and in singing position)

These should be, but are not necessarily, the same.

General body posture Anterior or posterior weight-bearing and asymmetrical body use (see Chapter 6). Weight-bearing and body symmetry will influence postural alignment. Anterior weight-bearing gives the typical gymnast's stance, with an overly hollow back, high chest and hyperextension of the head and neck.

Posterior weight-bearing gives the 'pregnant woman stance'. The weight is on the heels so that the hips are thrust forward, the shoulders move back and the head and neck are hyperextended. Frequently the lower back takes most of the strain and can lead to problems later.

Asymmetry of the spine may be reflected in asymmetrical muscle use through-out the body, including the vocal mechanism. Where the spine is properly adjusted there is no temptation to raise the chest by contracting the abdominal muscles or the strap muscles. It is interesting to note that a rotated body or head, or an asymmetrical positioning of the shoulders, will often result in a rotated larynx (see Chapter 6).

Head position As the head weighs approximately 14 lb it must be correctly balanced. Anterior translation of the head position affects the length of the strap muscles and the tension in the paravertebral muscles, and markedly changes the quality of the voice. Try it. Sustain a note and change the head position while doing it.

A head tilt may rotate the larynx, as will singing out of one side of the mouth. Where the chin is perpetually held high the larynx automatically raises.

Tight strap muscles (see Chapter 6) The following may lead to tight strap muscles: asymmetry, 'held' shoulders, head tilt, chest held too high.

Habitual voicing mode for speech

Singers who have problems with their singing voices will usually try to protect their speaking voices. Unfortunately this is not always done in the most efficient or effective way of dealing with the problem. They may resort to a technical falsetto (lengthened and thinned vocal folds with little or no closed phase to the vibratory cycle) in order to take the weight out of their speaking voice. If the speech runs on an inadequate airflow with hard onsets it is likely to be mirrored in singing. Frequently singers imagine that a creaky voice is in someway 'saving' their singing voice. It is important to disabuse them of this. For speech, 'Chest is best' (Titze, 1994).

Thick/thin fold, vocal fold tension (i.e. open/closed cricothyroid visor; see Chapter 5) If the singer habitually speaks in falsetto with a closed visor and thinned folds they are likely to have an inadequate chest register (modal voice). Some sopranos are still being told not to use 'chest' when speaking, as it 'will inhibit their high notes'. In speech it is important to be able to open the cricothyroid visor (CT visor) to produce chest (modal) voice and to close it now and again for brief excursions into head voice (falsetto with a short closed phase), but this usage is not nearly sophisticated enough for singing. Difficulty in closing the CT visor can result in restriction of the mid and upper pitch range in singing. As the cricothyroid mechanism is the primary pitch control mechanism, especially in the singing voice, it is most important that singers should be able to use the full, free range of the joint with the greatest flexibility and coordination.

Resonance balance and focus (i.e. oral/nasal resonance balance, pharyngeal/oral resonance balance) Resonance is the enhancement of the sound signal (produced by the vibration of the vocal folds) by the vocal tract, and is essential in shaping the different vowel sounds. In singing, the size and shape of the vocal tract is deliberately altered in order to achieve the specific changes in resonance that create an aesthetically pleasing sound.

Changes in resonance to create specific vowel sounds and voice qualities depend on the ability to vary the shape of the vocal tract to tune specific formants (see Chapter 13). Formant tuning is the result of the combined action of laryngeal position, tongue position, soft palate position and the pharyngeal constrictor muscles (Sundberg, 1987; Titze, 1994).

The habitual resonance balance used by the patient in speech may affect both the tongue and palate position for singing. If they have difficulty with the control of the velopharyngeal valve during speech it is likely that the same problem will be present in their singing technique. Equally, the position adopted by the tongue and pharyngeal musculature during speech will affect the pharyngeal/oral resonance balance (see section on backed tongue).

Hard glottal attack Where there is a preponderance of these in speech, there is a strong possibility that the patient will have difficulty producing simultaneous onsets when singing 'staccato' or a note beginning with a vowel.

Breathy voice It is well understood in the world of speech therapy that a breathy voice may not necessarily be due to hypovalving, but may be the result of a hyperfunctional voicing pattern and the presence of a posterior glottal chink (see Chapter 7). This possibility is not always appreciated by singing teachers, and the pupil is sometimes encouraged to 'bring the vocal folds together more strongly' to 'focus the voice'. This sometimes results in the singer dropping the airflow and, even more unfortunately, tightening all the laryngeal musculature still further indiscriminately, thickening the anterior folds, which are already in contact, while failing to approximate the posterior third of the folds.

Backed or depressed tongue/tongue grooving or scooping Should the speaking voice be produced with a backed or depressed tongue, there is a strong possibility that the same pattern will occur in the singing voice. Singers often depress the larynx in order to make a 'richer' or 'darker' tone, and this may well affect their ease in accessing the top range. This darkened tone is much loved in the UK, so beware! Western classical tradition requires a lower larynx posture than most other styles, but unfortunately there is a general lack of definition as to what is low and what is depressed. The difference can be checked by gentle external palpation of the tongue base together with the sternothyroid and sternohyoid muscles in the sternal notch (see Chapter 1).

Over-extension of jaw/tension in jaw How does the jaw drop – forwards and out or down and in? It needs to be acknowledged that there is no absolute agreement in singing teaching about this. In our clinical practice we would prefer that the jaw should release inwards and down without a muscular bulge around the jaw joints as this should produce freer use of the jaw.

Rigid abdominal muscles Many singers mistake rigid inflexible abdominal muscles for support, and are not absolutely certain what the purpose of support is. It is important that the concept of support is understood as the sustaining of an even subglottic pressure and airflow, rather than as a vague abdominal muscular contraction of the abdominal wall unconnected to this.

Assessment of the singing voice may, in fact, be done much later than the above assessment, after certain other prerequisites have been tackled. The reason for not even listening to the singing voice early on, often not until three or four sessions have taken place, is that until certain basic mechanical functions have been corrected, good singing is going to be limited.

Treatment and vocal exercises

There is a delight in singing, 'tho none hear
Beside the singer

Walter Savage Landor

As mentioned earlier in this chapter, because of the financial constraints on the NHS, it is not always possible to employ both a speech therapist and singing advisor to treat a singer in the six sessions that are normally allotted to a patient. It is therefore vital that the speech therapist and singing teacher are both able to practise techniques with regard to the singer's speaking and singing voices.

We feel very strongly that our job is to set the essentials of good voice use in place. It is important to remember that any patient can produce any exercise wrongly. It is the skill of the teacher or therapist to spot the errors and use their talents and experience to rectify them. It is vital for both patient and therapist to understand what the exercise aims to achieve.

There are no new 'singing' muscles. All the muscles employed in singing are also used for vegetative activities such as swallowing, vomiting, coughing, sneezing and yawning. Some of these are helpful for singing and some not.

We would hope to:

(a) reduce inappropriate muscular tension and discomfort in the larynx, neck and shoulders;
(b) introduce a fully functional abdominal breath support system with flexible and responsive abdominal muscles, well coordinated with phonation;

(c)   establish good postural habits;

(d)   encourage the optimum resonance balance, i.e. oral/nasal/pharyngeal compo-
      nents;

(e)   establish the full range of the voice and resolve problems with the *passaggios*
      by working on cricothyroid visor flexibility;

(f)   provide education in functional vocal anatomy and hygiene;

(g)   provide emotional support.

Many of the following treatment techniques and exercises will have been
covered in other chapters. However, we would suggest that all these things are even
more essential for singers than for most other professional or amateur voice-users,
as singing is fundamentally an athletic pursuit. The technique of singing is a
supremely complex balancing act, requiring fine-tuning of a considerable number
of muscles. It is therefore important that the basics are properly laid down.

Any speech therapy exercise can be usefully adapted for the singing voice. First
principles remain the same, whether sung or spoken. The general rule seems to be
'If it feels good, the chances are that the singer is doing it right'.

Basic equipment

Ideally:

- a couch or floor mat for relaxation exercises
- a pitch pipe
- a mirror for patients' self-monitoring (a video camera would of course be an
  excellent acquisition)
- a tape recorder
- an anatomical model of the larynx or illustrations and diagrams
- a video of larynges in action.

Exercises

Posture

In their anxiety to communicate with the audience, or because of the concentration
required, singers often develop unusual postural habits. One would hardly expect a
violinist to play with the violin upside down as it would increase the technical difficulties of playing. Equally, no singer can be expected to give of their best when the
instrument is being held incorrectly. Unlike dancers, it is rare (and offputting) for
singers to watch themselves in a mirror. However, a great deal can be brought to
their attention in this way, much as they may dislike it.

Exercises for postural alignment (see Chapters 6 and 7)

Find the imaginary plumb line from the crown of the head, through the ear, shoulder and hip, so that the body weight is distributed behind the ball of the foot. The
crown of the head should be pointing towards the ceiling.

Singers/patients needing manipulation to rectify long-standing postural problems (scoliosis, low back problems, cervicodorsal shelves, etc.) are best referred on to osteopaths or physiotherapists.

The Alexander (Barlow, 1973), Feldenkrais and Pilates techniques are all useful in helping singers correct their posture (see Useful Addresses section at the end of Chapter 7).

Relaxation (see Appendix 7.1)

The following exercises should be performed sitting in a chair that supports the lower back. It is important to remind patients to correct their head posture between exercises and never to force movements further than they feel is comfortable. Many people hold their breath when concentrating and may need gentle reminders to keep breathing.

Shoulder exercises

These help to release shoulder tension. Singers carry a great deal of anxiety in their shoulders (and anywhere else you care to mention).

(a) Rolls - rotate the shoulders 10 times forwards, 10 times backwards.
(b) Lift ups - raise shoulders to ears; hold the position and release five times.
(c) Pull downs - pull shoulders down towards the floor; hold and release five times.

Neck exercises

Use gravity and the weight of the head to stretch the strap muscles.

(a) Head tilts - starting with the crown of the head towards the ceiling, tilt the ear towards one shoulder, stretching the strap muscles unilaterally. Then lift the chin upwards, to stretch the upper insertion of the sternocleidomastoid muscle. Try this five times each side.
(b) Looking over alternate shoulders - turn the head gently from side to side (keeping the crown of the head towards ceiling), as if you were looking over one shoulder. Repeat five times to each side.
(c) Drop the head forward and down, curling the top of the spine forward. Gradually uncurl the upper spine, straightening it until the head comes back to the midline. Lift the chin to look at the ceiling, then, using the ear as an axis, lower the chin down and in, while at the same time raising the crown of the head back up to face the ceiling again. The chin is tucked in, giving a sensation of a long back to the neck and a short front.

Massage

(See also Chapter 6, Feeling [Palpatory monitoring])

Singers as a breed tend to be quite tactile, and are not apprehensive of touching or being touched, as traditionally this has always been part of singing teaching.

It is often reassuring for singers to discover that they can not only touch their larynx and move it gently from side to side, but can also massage the muscles that cause them discomfort, i.e. the suprahyoid, thyrohyoid, cricothyroid, omohyoid, and/or sternocleidomastoid and trapezius muscles. They are profoundly relieved to discover that something at least is within their control. Massage is an atraumatic comforting method for getting in touch with the relevant anatomy. In fact, this is perhaps the moment to introduce the concept of basic functional anatomy, so that singers can learn to assess and monitor their own laryngeal position and cricothyroid muscle activity in various tasks.

Jaw exercises

Check the jaw joint opening and closure for bulging. Where there is evidence of jaw tension and rigidity, Froeschels' chewing exercises are very useful (see Chapter 7). It is possible to chew on humming (or 'nyum') while singing a small three or five note scale up and down.

Singers often try to overextend the jaw opening, which can lead to tightness and a forward-locked jaw joint. A more relaxed jaw opening can be achieved by suggesting that the singer imagines that he or she is opening the upper jaw upwards (no, this is **not** physically possible, but it does prevent hyperextension). This manoeuvre does not always provide enough opening for the top register, and some singers will still want a forward and downward movement of the jaw for notes above the upper passaggio.

Tongue exercises

External massage of the tongue base under the chin when speaking or singing will often release an habitually backed tongue. Any exercise that will move the tongue forward and up helps to stretch hypertonic muscles at the base of the tongue.

The 'tooth sweep' (demonstrated by Bonnie Raphael in her British Voice Association course for Instructions in vocal communication, London, July 1993)

The tongue tip is run slowly from the back left molar over the outer surface of the teeth to the other side and back again on the upper jaw. Repeat for the inside surface of the upper teeth. Then run the tongue tip from the back left molar of the lower teeth, over the inner surface and back; repeat for the outer surface. Swallow.

The 'great caramel search' (demonstrated by Kirsten Thyme-Frøkjær in her Accent Method Course run by the British Voice Association, London, November 1993)

Imagine a caramel stuck in the top left back molar. Try to dislodge it from the tooth with the tongue tip for 10-20 seconds. Repeat the process for the lower right rear molar, the lower left and the upper right molar. The caramel then magically reappears up under the upper lip, then down under the lower lip. Chase it out again and swallow.

Abdominal breathing, support and phonation

One of the most important factors in a singer's technique is the precise management of airflow and subglottic pressure. Clinical practice suggests that singing patients with voice problems often appear to have mislaid this ability and to have a very ambivalent attitude to air. They forget to breathe and are fearful of running out of air during or at the end of a long phrase. They become anxious lest they produce a 'breathy' or 'unfocused' sound. They therefore 'hoard' air, trying to take in 102 per cent of their vital capacity, using minimal airflow on phonation and regular use of residual air during speech. This can result in hyperadduction of the vocal folds, unreliable subglottic pressure and pressed voice.

It should be noted that in speech, loudness and pitch are typically interdependent, an increase in subglottal air pressure being generally reflected by a rise in pitch and loudness (Gramming et al., 1988). Singing, however, demands increasing skill in the manangement of airflow and subglottal pressure, as loudness and pitch have to be independently controlled, and also matched to the requirements for articulation and marking of significant tones (Gramming, 1991).

In singing pedagogy, as in speech therapy, it is a matter of some controversy whether it is necessary to train patterns of breathing or not. We, however, are of the opinion that the basis of all efficient voice use is the fine and changing balance between subglottic pressure, airflow, glottic resistance and the resonating vocal tract. It would seem impossible to achieve this without directly addressing the process of breathing and support. While it is true that breathing is scarcely an acquired ability, singing undoubtedly is.

Research has shown that classical singers use abdominal breathing, chest breathing or a mixture of the two (Hixon, 1991; Pullan and May, 1994). Show, pop or rock singers may use any of the above, but may also use clavicular breathing patterns. While it is possible to use clavicular breathing for belting (the style of singing with the longest closed phase, highest air pressure and greatest glottic resistance; Estill, 1994), we would advocate low abdominal breathing and support as being the simplest, most flexible and direct pattern to teach·for speech and singing. It is also the pattern of breathing most commonly taught by speech therapists, and it would therefore seem economical of effort to use the same pattern for singing and speech.

Hixon (1991) writes:

> The diaphragm is the most powerful of inspiratory muscles. Using it as the sole inspiratory driver leaves the rib cage free of inspiratory assignment and therefore able to engage instantly in continued expiratory activity for singing once diaphragmatic activity is terminated ... The diaphragm can be continuously mechanically tuned by the abdomen for inspiratory action regardless of the lung volume.

This is one of the major reasons why we favour abdominal breathing and support. Although we fully acknowledge that singers use different breathing patterns (chest, abdominal or a mixture of the two) with great success, by the time they are patients in the clinic their breathing and support systems have usually failed and need retraining. It is also possible that these have never been precisely coordinated in their singing training.

Singing patients are fairly obsessed by the malfunction of their larynx and vocal tract. Concentration on the activity of the abdominal wall is a wonderful diversionary tactic. It is a very long way from the internal and external lateral obliques to a throat, and the very activity of moving a patient's concern due south has many advantages. It is far quicker and simpler to contract the diaphragm onto the soft tissue of the gut than to lift the heavy bone of the rib cage. It means that singers can access a high lung volume in a very short space of time with minimal effort.

Lying down on a couch or mat in order to get in touch with tidal abdominal breathing is also hugely relaxing. To be given permission to concentrate on simply breathing in and out may prove especially comforting for patients who have been fighting a rearguard action with their voices for many months. One of the problems for singers with voice breakdown is that they are unable to stop analysing and listening, and to start feeling. Vocal life for them has become extremely complex, and the elementary act of learning to do nothing is most beneficial. To quote Ling (1976): 'Breathing first, then phonation, then articulation.' It is difficult to improve phonation unless the breathing and support pattern producing the sound source is functioning freely and flexibly. However, should someone invent a group of exercises that coordinate phonation, breathing and support, begin simply and gradually increase in complexity for rib or chest breathing, we should be very interested to hear from them.

One of the problems for singers is that the reason for 'support' is not always made clear to them in their training, and they are not always certain what the contraction of the abdominal muscles is actually doing. There may be vague allusions to 'use more support', but not how and with what and at which moment. Titze (1994) gives a concise description of the cycle of breathing and support: 'Assume that the task is to keep the airflow and lung pressure constant during phonation. This results in a constant decrease in lung volume during expiration, followed by a quicker increase during inspiration.'

The respiratory cycle may be divided into four separate phases, which require different patterns of muscular activity. We prefer to look at breathing out as an act that follows intake of air. Following inspiration, there are three distinct expiratory phases necessary to maintain an even exhalation of air at constant pressure from the chest:

(i) Inspiration

The primary motivators are the contraction of the diaphragm and the external intercostals. The internal intercostals and the abdominal wall are released, the rib cage expands and the diaphragm contracts downwards onto the gut, pushing it down and outwards, out of the bottom of the chest. This increases the chest volume.

(ii) First expiratory phase

At maximum inspiration there is a tendency for the rib cage and lungs to collapse down. This is called 'elastic recoil'. In this phase, elastic recoil alone will provide adequate air pressure for voicing. The recoil may produce a higher pressure than is required. This overpressure can be controlled by continuing (briefly) to keep the diaphragm contracted. This persistent contraction rapidly becomes unnecessary as the overpressure diminishes, and the diaphragm can then begin to release passively (Leanderson et al., 1984).

(iii) Second expiratory phase

There is now much less tendency for the lungs to deflate by recoil alone. The internal intercostal muscles begin to squeeze the lungs by contracting the rib cage until the elastic recoil is complete.

(iv) Third expiratory phase

The abdominal muscles and (often) back muscles (Hixon, 1991) are then brought into play incrementally to counteract the (by now) negative elastic recoil in the lungs, which would now naturally reinflate in tidal breathing. The moment at which the abdominal muscles join in is dictated by the intensity of the sound. While a long soft phrase will follow the above three distinct phases of support, singers seem to engage the abdominal musculature much earlier where increased intensity is required. Titze's research suggests that the vocal folds work most efficiently when lightly approximated rather than pressed together, when singing or speaking (Titze, 1995).

The Accent Method (see Chapter 7)

This is an excellent way to begin warming up a voice before singing exercises and to warm down after sustained periods of practice or performance. If the singer's speech pattern is part of their voice problem it is advisable to take the exercises into text. One of the technique's great virtues for singers is they do not have to sing for a few weeks and their only responsibility is to make noises for a while. Sometimes the patient will become aware quite early in the course of the exercises of changes in his or her speaking voice and is able to carry these through into everyday speech. In our experience it is the most effective system of exercises that addresses the balance between airflow, support, glottal resistance and phonation. It introduces simultaneous onset (see Chapter 13) and reduces glottal hypervalving and constriction in the vocal tract. The rhythmic structure is very attractive to singers, and because the sounds are often fairly ridiculous it creates a lighthearted atmosphere. The fricative sounds can then be introduced into the singing voice. These produce supraglottic back pressure, helping vocal fold closure and increasing the length of the closed phase, without dropping the air pressure. This is of great benefit both to breathy singers and to those using low air flow.

Other exercises to help get in touch with the abdominal muscles (see also Chapter 7)

(a) Blowing up lilos (or squeezing from the bottom of the toothpaste tube). This introduces the idea of maintaining the sensation of a constant subglottic pressure throughout a sung note or phrase.
   (i) Blow the lilo up slowly. Note increasing abdominal support.
   (ii) Sustain a sung note on a fricative consonant (e.g. zzzzzz,) as you blow up

the lilo.

(iii) Open into a sustained vowel.

(iv) Try short ascending and descending scales over a fifth on a vowel.

(v) Sing a nursery rhyme.

(vi) Work the new sensation into phrases that the singer knows and hates!

(b) Cumulative counting exercises. These exercises can be used either for speech or singing and facilitate fast diaphragmatic contraction with quick release of the abdominal wall and quiet breath intake. For example, '123 (breathe), 1234 (breathe), 12345 (breathe), 123456 (breathe)', etc.

(i) Do this slowly, with gaps for quiet inhalation.

(ii) Speed up so there are shorter gaps for quiet inhalation.

(iii) Increase the speed until the exercise becomes almost a breath/phonation continuum. After this Bach arias should prove much easier to negotiate!

(c) Rolled 'r's or 'lip bubbles' (for those who have tongue ties or short tongues). Make a 'temperature chart' or a 'silhouette of a mountain range' gliding the rolled 'r' or 'lip bubble' (like a horse sneezing or someone expressing that they are cold), up and down through the singing range (like a small boy making Harley Davidson motor bike noises). The external and internal oblique and transversus abdominal muscles will contract as the pitch and intensity rises, and release somewhat as the pitch descends. The exercise is useful for monitoring airflow; immediately the airflow drops the tongue trill will grind to a halt. This is not the pattern for the breath support of sung phrases, which tend to use the 'slow burn' or 'lilo' method of incremental abdominal muscular contraction, but does give flexibility to the use of the abdominal wall and associates the sensation of increasing subglottic pressure with increasing pitch. It is also possible to use fricatives (i.e. jjj, zzz, vvv, whoo) in the same way, as concentration on the sensation at the lips, teeth and tongue tip will bring the sound forward and release the tongue base.

Freeing the vocal tract

One of the most important aspects of working with singers is the process of persuading them to stop listening to themselves and to begin to concentrate on monitoring different sensations. They are their own sternest vocal critics, and are often unaware that when they hear their own voice conducted to them through bone, soft tissue and airwaves, they hear a distortion of the genuine sound. To quote Diane Forlano: 'If you are listening and I am listening, who is doing the singing?' Abandoning the internal critic is a major step in the direction of learning to drop old patterns and maintaining new ones.

Useful exercises

(a) Silent intake of breath through the mouth usually drops the larynx downwards. This releases the pharyngeal constrictors and produces very wide abduction (parting) of both the false and true vocal folds (see section on Deconstriction, retraction and release of hyperadduction in Chapter 7).

(b) Feel what happens at the onset of yawn: the palate lifts, the jaw releases and the tongue drops backwards releasing the pharyngeal constrictors and moving the larynx down (McKinney, 1994).

(c) The 'silent laugh' (Estill). This manoeuvre releases glottal and ventricular constriction (see Chapter 7).

(d) 'Sob' (Estill) (see Chapter 7). The 'sob' figure releases glottal hyperadduction and medial compression, lowers the larynx and releases pharyngeal constriction.

(e) Humming usually releases a backed tongue, glottal hyperadduction and supraglottic constriction. It introduces gentle adduction of the vocal folds along their full length. Exercises may be begun on a hum and, once good vocal fold closure is established, opened into a vowel.

Oral/pharyngeal balance of resonance or 'the diamond on the velvet'

'The diamond on the velvet' may sound typically 'pink fluffy cloud school of singing teaching'. However, like much singing imagery, although unscientific in nature, it describes for many listeners the ideal of a singer's oral/pharyngeal resonance balance.

Tongue positioning would seem to play a major part in helping to establish this. If it is retracted or the larynx depressed, the resultant tonal quality will be too dark and 'plummy'. If the tone is produced with pharyngeal constriction, a high laryngeal position and overemphasis on 'keeping the tone bright and forward', the tone will be too bright and 'hard' or 'metallic'. Generally, if the pharyngeal muscles and false folds are released, the jaw is loose, the tongue tip is lying gently behind the front teeth and the tongue blade feels spongy (when palpated externally), the necessary balance is easily achieved. A splendid Italian phrase describes this - *lingua morta* or 'dead tongue'.

Careful tuning of the frequency of specific resonances or 'formants' in the vocal tract is responsible for the 'bright' quality that penetrates through an orchestral accompaniment, also known as the 'singer's formant' (see Chapter 13).

A forward tongue position will also give greater clarity to diction, as it is difficult to manipulate the tongue tip at speed if the blade is retracted.

Oral/nasal resonance balance

A word about hypo- or hypernasality. It would appear to be rare for singers to suffer from hyponasality unless suffering from an upper respiratory tract infection or polyps. However, it is not unusual for the reverse to be true. To check for nasal air escape try holding a mirror under the nose during the release of vowels; if the mirror clouds over there is insufficient velopharyngeal valve closure.

Estill (1996) has excellent exercises for learning palatal control. These consist of learning to monitor the three different palatal positions that open, partially close and completely close the velopharyngeal port. Control is developed by gliding between one position and the next (i.e. 'ng' → (a nasalized 'ah') to the orally released vowel → 'ah'; phonetically /ŋ/ → /ã/ → /a/).

The role of the soft palate in resonance and vocal range

There is no general agreement in Western classical tradition singing pedagogy as to whether the soft palate should be given an increase in lift, in addition to the amount required to maintain appropriate closure of the velopharyngeal valve. Some teachers maintain that it should be lifted prior to the passaggio into head voice and others that it is positively detrimental to do so. It would seem to help the process of 'covering' the sound in the upper range, in conjunction with vowel migration (i.e. the process of adapting the vowel to a slightly 'darker' version of the true vowel) and a greater opening at the back of the jaw. However, to quote Meribeth Bunch (1995), 'When the intrinsic muscles of the tongue are contracted, the resultant action is most likely palatal depression'. If the tongue is either retracted or depressed it will tend to pull down on the palate, making the increase in lift extremely difficult. It would appear that it is largely a question of aesthetic taste (see Chapter 1 for a discussion of the palatal musculature). In belt quality the palate is liable to be held lower.

Simultaneous onset (or coordinated attack)

Singers are frequently anxious about the 'vocal attack' of a note. They will often use a hard glottal attack or an aspirate attack, when the ideal is a simultaneous onset of glottal closure with expiratory airflow. Usually the process of being able to increase air support and decrease hyperadduction (Accent Method) will teach simultaneous onset. However, if this fails there are other techniques to try that may help.

(a) Staccato, starting with a snort of voiced air down the nose co-ordinated with abdominal support, e.g. 'Hmm' (release) 'Hmm' (release) 'Hmm' (release) (breath before tone). 'Ah' (release) 'Ah' (release) 'Ah' (release) (remove breath before tone). These can then be developed into small staccato exercises.

(b) Onset exercises (Estill) (see Chapter 7). In these, much as in the palate exercises, the patient learns to distinguish and produce the three different types of onset.

Range, passaggios and the cricothyroid visor

It would appear from our clinical practice that problems with the *passaggios* can be greatly improved by an easier and more efficient use of the cricothyroid mechanism. As with most joints, a full range of movement is required for flexible function. It would seem that many lower passaggio problems for women are to do with the singer's inability to control the opening and closing of the joint in a smooth way, and to judge the amount of muscular tensioning in the CT muscles required at different pitches around this break point. It would also appear to be an important factor for male voices shifting from modal into 'head' voice.

A female classical singer has the choice around the lower passaggio to sing in full modal voice. This is thrilling and dramatic as an effect, but if used as a constant, aesthetically less pleasing. Our observation of singers without pathology or technical problems shows that they may close the visor a little in order to sing in a low mixed voice. This is more efficient, mechanically sound, but much harder for the singer to judge. They may also keep it closed and sing in low 'head' voice that is pure but lacking in excitement.

We find that show or rock singers, when belting, are more likely to use a relatively open visor and thick folds to a higher point in their range. They will none the less deliberately raise their larynx to shorten the vocal resonator and tilt the thyroid cartilage forward slightly. Many singers experience problems when they try to take modal voice with a lowered larynx into a higher range. We would suggest that this is using a high 'chest' quality. Belting, however, is a precise balance between:

- an open CT visor;
- thick folds;
- high laryngeal position;
- high tongue position;
- low (closed) palate;
- high subglottic pressure;
- low air flow;
- efficient use of breath support;
- aryepiglottic sphincter constriction (see Chapter 1).

It produces the longest closed phase of all the styles of singing. Whereas it is anathema to many classically trained teachers, it is a fact of vocal life, and performed correctly, it requires as fine vocal balance as a Verdi aria. However, when dealing with malfunctioning voices it is important to address the basic requirements before tackling 'belt' voice. (Estill (1996) gives a clear 'recipe' for belt voice and also the vocal tract 'options' that can be used to vary it in her Compulsory Figures.)

Cricothyroid visor versus laryngeal height

It is enshrined in much Western classical singing pedagogy that the larynx must remain low at all times. However, there appear to be a wide range of vertical laryngeal positions among classically trained singers. Unfortunately singers will often substitute extremes of vertical laryngeal movement for a freely functioning cricothyroid visor mechanism. We frequently find that they will 'back' their tongue position in order to depress the larynx and lengthen the vocal tract, rather than rely upon release of the cricothyroid muscles. This shortens and thickens the vocal folds in order to drop into 'chest' voice. Conversely, they may raise the larynx to assist an otherwise inadequate closure of the visor for 'head' register. Vilkman et al. (1996) have reviewed the work on laryngeal position, the cricothyroid visor and the effect on F_0. The required vocal fold adjustments for register shift are also made in a similar manner.)

Fibreoptic endoscopic observation of volunteers – healthy, professional singers without vocal problems – suggests that the middle constrictor muscle often plays a part in accessing 'head voice', and the phrase in singing pedagogy 'slim the tone as you go into head voice' may well be describing this muscular contraction. It may also assist to shape the vocal tract to produce the characteristic 'ring'.

Exercises for vocal range

(a) First make sure that the visor is open and the patient in modal voice. To do this, try asking the patient to produce very gentle 'creaky' voice without false fold intervention. This will usually open the visor and bring the patient into modal voice (see Chapter 7). The 'creak' can then be released into a modal 'hum' as the hyperadduction is released.

(b) It is then appropriate to use exercises to find free and flexible use of the CT joint to access the middle and 'head' registers. Try slow *glissandi* up and down to open and close the CT visor easily and smoothly. These can be performed on rolled 'r's and 'lip bubbles' (see section on abdominal breathing and support), fricatives and, when confidence is established, vowels. Palpatory monitoring of the cricothyroid visor is most useful (see Chapter 7).

(c) Sirening (Estill; see Chapter 7). We have noted in clinical practice that as pitch rises in soft singing or soft 'ng' sirening, there is a concomitant increase in rectus abdominis activity just below the area of the upper insertion (see Chapter 4). It is possible to find this by making small, high-pitched hums of delight. Our clinical experience seems to suggest that this is a method of controlling a very gentle subglottic pressure against a low glottic resistance, and has implications for 'floating' (see Glossary) the voice. The airflow through the larynx is not simply controlled by the closed vocal folds, but is in addition limited by using increased diaphragmatic and rectus tone, which is then firmly contracted to control exhalation. This produces the additional fine control of the diaphragmatic piston required to manage low pressure airflow.

(d) Octave leaps on a rolled 'rr', which then open into a vowel and glissando down

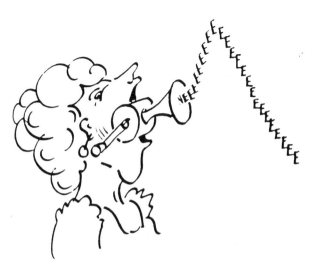

'Sirening'

to the original note, are also useful to extend vocal range.

Belt/twang (Estill's compulsory figures for voice)

See Chapter 7 for a fuller description. It is inadvisable to attempt 'belt' style
singing and 'twang' quality until a pattern of good abdominal breathing and
support has been established in conjunction with a free vocal tract and the ability
to produce simultaneous onsets.

Warm downs

It is unusual in the UK for singers to warm their voices down at the end of a performance. Bearing in mind the immense amount of time and energy spent during a
singer's career on warming up the voice, it is well worth considering the virtues of the
warm down. What is it in aid of? Muscles that have been heavily employed for some
hours need releasing into a looser, less athletic resting tone. Female singers frequently
report that after a performance requiring a lot of sustained high notes or a role with a
high tessitura, their speaking voice has markedly risen in pitch. This is unsurprising
as they spend much of their singing time in 'middle' or 'head' voice, with rarer excursions into modal/chest voice. It is therefore a wise move to release the cricothyroid
visor fully in order to return the speaking voice to modal. This can be accomplished
by some breathy glissandi downwards on fricatives such as 'jj', 'zz', 'vv' and 'whoo',
easing the voice down. The Accent Method is also useful for this.

We would recommend that any singing teacher wishing to work in a voice clinic
attends a course on both Accent Method and Estill's Compulsory Figures as both
techniques provide many useful tools, particularly when time and sessions are
limited (see Chapter 7 for further information).

Operations and singers

> In over a year and a half,
> I've only sung it once,
> And I don't suppose I shall sing it again
> For months and months and months.
>
> Joseph Tabrar

It is alarming enough for any patient to be required to undergo phonosurgery.
However, for a singer it is much more complex. A nodule will announce to the
world at large that the singer has insufficient technical expertise or nasty vocal
habits. Teachers may feel some sense of guilt, and the patient undoubtedly will. For
generations, nodules were the death knell of a career, and the prospect of developing them still makes a singer's blood run cold. The good news is, of course, that the
postoperative recovery period is short following a meticulous local excision. Bad
vocal usage can be speedily improved, and the singer returned to employment
fairly quickly, as the vocal fold cover is returned to its full function within a period

of a couple of weeks. It is always wise to follow any operation with a course of speech therapy in order to ensure healthy vocal habits and technique.

Pity the poor owners of sulci and cysts (see Chapter 2). The pathology may be congenital, and the singer blameless. Because the mucosa and deeper layers of the vocal fold have been seriously compromised, rehabilitation takes much longer and is more complex. It may take many months for the mucosal wave to establish itself where there was none before. It requires nerves of steel on behalf of the singer and the teacher. Many tricks will have been acquired by the singer to try to bypass a vocal fold that has lost or never had the ability to vibrate freely.

The owners of sulci may have used their singing and speaking voice in falsetto to avoid pitch breaks. They may well have sung with low airflow and low subglottic air pressure to reduce the risk of the tone 'breaking up'. They may have been to ENT departments where they have been viewed with a laryngeal mirror, and diagnosed as being the owner of spotless vocal folds.

Postoperatively, the therapist will need to employ techniques to shake the mucosa loose, with priority given to high airflow in chest register. It may be necessary to open the CT visor in order to find modal voice, and thus run the risk of engendering the very pitch breaks that the singer has always feared. The singer should refrain from employment for 2–4 months, as much adjusting of the singing technique needs to be done. The mucosa may not shake free for many months and is unlikely to normalize completely in less than 18 months.

Glossary of commonly encountered terms

Everyone suddenly burst out singing.

Siegfried Sassoon

This glossary has been compiled at the request of voice therapists to try and explain some of the terms commonly used in singing pedagogy. Unfortunately, there is not always general agreement, but we have done our best.

ABDOMINAL BREATHING – Respiration principally dependent on diaphragmatic activity for inhalation. The whole abdominal wall is released to allow the contraction of the diaphragm to move the abdominal contents downwards and outwards.

ARPEGGIO – The notes of a chord played or sung in succession either up or down.

ARTICULATION – (a) The various ways in which a performer may produce the notes in a phrase, observing staccato and legato notes, accents and slurs, which together shape the phrase. (b) In the teaching of singing it refers to both the clarity of the production of consonants (giving clear diction without interfering with the ease of the tone production) and the definition of the separate notes of a run.

ATTACK – The onset of voicing achieved by bringing the vocal folds together in coordination with airflow. A *hard glottal attack* (closure before onset of phonation) should be avoided whenever possible in singing as in speech. *Aspirate attack* (breath before voice) can be useful when teaching *simultaneous attack* or onset, where the release of air and vocal fold closure is coordinated, safer and more efficient in singing.

BEAT – A slow vibrato with too much variation in the range of intensity.

BEL CANTO – (Italian: literally 'beautiful singing') Style of singing and teaching belonging to the 18th and early 19th centuries particularly. Employs a smooth lyrical legato, and complex florid runs. It is found in the operas of Rossini, Bellini and Donizetti. It is also used in very vague terms to describe the 'mystique' of 'good singing'. As such it should be ignored.

BELTING – A style of music theatre singing associated with Ethel Merman and Broadway shows. Not to be confused with chest or modal voice. It requires a high laryngeal position, low air flow, high subglottic pressure, thick vocal folds and a relatively open cricothyroid visor. It has the longest closed phase of any vocal style.

BLEAT – A fast vibrato with too much variation of intensity, rather than a variation of pitch. Caused by excessive muscular tension.

BREAK – A sudden change in register (as in yodelling, or a 'crack' in the voice).

BREATHY – The opposite of a *focused tone*. The subglottic pressure and glottal resistance are not appropriately matched. This may be caused by *hypovalving*, poor medial compression, inefficient activity of the interarytenoids causing a posterior glottal chink, or vocal fold pathology.

CHEST OR INTERCOSTAL BREATHING – The lower abdominal wall is contracted and the external intercostal muscles swing the rib cage outwards and up.

CHEST REGISTER OR VOICE – The lower notes of a vocal range. Modal voice produced by short thick folds and a fully open cricothyroid visor.

CLAVICULAR BREATHING – The diaphragm and abdominal wall are held almost immobile, while respiration takes place by raising the shoulders and upper ribs in order to increase lung volume. This produces a shallow breathing pattern.

COMPASS – The full range of a singing voice or piece of music.

COVERING – A method of changing register towards head voice that balances the increasing brightness of colour by darkening the vowel (reducing the higher formants). Associated with reduced laryngeal raising, thus maintaining an evenness of colour and preventing a 'whitening' of the tone.

CRESCENDO – (Italian: getting louder)

DECRESCENDO/DIMINUENDO – (Italian: getting softer)

DRIVEN SINGING – The singing equivalent of pressed phonation. Hyperadduction with resultant insufficient airflow.

DYNAMICS – Varying degrees of loudness and softness of intensity or volume of sound. These are denoted by musical symbols.

FACH – (German: literally 'speciality' or 'pigeon-hole') Voice classification applied to the group of roles sung by a particular weight and timbre of voice.

FALSETTO – (Italian: diminutive of 'falso', meaning false or bogus) The lightest and highest vocal register, produced by a closed cricothyroid visor, with extremely thin vocal folds, which either do not touch at all or do so with a very short closed phase to the vibratory cycle. It is used interchangeably with *head voice* by some voice professionals. To quote Johan Sundberg, 'some types of phonation in the falsetto register use a complete closure in the glottal vibratory cycle and some do not, and the type of falsetto singing used by countertenors is probably different from other types of falsetto. The fundamental frequency control may very well differ between such different types of phonation in falsetto register' (Sundberg, 1987).

FLOATING – Very soft, high singing, in *head voice* (usually associated with sopranos). Perhaps the female equivalent of falsetto, but produced with complete but very light adduction of the vocal folds.

FLUTTER – A tone where the rate of vibrato is too fast.

FOCUS – The opposite of *breathy*. Clear, ringing and defined sound, well coordinated by the balance between subglottic pressure and glottal resistance, efficient laryngeal control and good *placement*.

FULL VOICE – To '*sing out*', i.e. to sing with full breath support at a relatively high sound intensity.

GLISSANDO – (French: glisser - to slide) To slide through an infinite number of microtones between two different pitches.

HEAD REGISTER OR VOICE – The upper part of the singer's range, produced with a closed cricothyroid visor, thinned, long vocal folds and a short but complete closed phase to the vibratory cycle. Sometimes used interchangeably with *falsetto* in male voices.

LEGATO – (Italian: bound together, tied, connected) The notes of a phrase sung smoothly, evenly and without breaks between them.

MANUFACTURED SOUND –Tone that sounds unnatural, untruthful. Usually the singer is copying someone else.

MARKING – A rehearsal technique employed to save the voice. A godsend if the singer is clever at using it. The techniques used are singing gently (i.e. *mezza voce*) at the correct pitch, transposing the high or low passages down or up an octave, or speaking the text in rhythm.

MASK – Rather like wearing a venetian carnival mask. The concept of feeling sensations in the face, particularly in the cheek bones, around the nose and the eyes, in order to *place* the voice.

MESSA DI VOCE – (Italian: placing of the voice) One of the most important exercises in the historical *bel canto* school of singing. The singer performs a slow *crescendo* and *decrescendo* on one long note, beginning and ending on a fine pianissimo.

MEZZA VOCE – (Italian: half voice) As opposed to *full voice*.

MIXED REGISTER OR VOICE – (French: voix mixte). *Middle voice.* The middle of the singing range. The intermediate or bridging area between heavy (chest) and light (head or falsetto) registers. Changing from light to heavy (or vice versa) without using this transitional register usually results in obvious pitch breaks.

OPEN THROAT – Ideally, the sensation of a vocal tract that is appropriately released (back of tongue, pharynx and without false fold activity). Unfortunately, it is not always understood by singers that the pharyngeal muscles are constrictors. Therefore when these muscles release the larynx forwards, the singer feels very little biofeedback. A lot of effort may be expended in trying to 'make space' by distorting the pharynx, backing the tongue and depressing the larynx, when all that is required is to 'let go'. To quote Diane Forlano, 'An open throat is a throat that is not closed.'

PASSAGGIO – (Italian: literally 'passage', 'transit') The area in a voice where it is necessary to effect a change in register, e.g. from a heavier to a lighter register (chest to middle voice or middle voice to head voice).

PLACEMENT – The idea of using the imagination to feel resonance variously on the hard or soft palate, the *mask*, or other areas in the head, before the tone begins.

PING or RING – The quality of voice produced by an abundance of high partials, giving brilliance to the tone, and the ability to be heard through a symphony orchestra.

PORTAMENTO – (Italian: literally 'carriage', 'bearing') Gliding from one note to another through intermediate pitches.

PRESSED PHONATION, TONE or VOICE – Hypervalving of the glottis with high subglottic air pressure and inadequate airflow.

PROJECTION – The ability of a voice to travel through large spaces and be heard over an instrumental accompaniment without compromising the beauty of tone or the clarity of the text.

REGISTER – A group of notes produced with the same vocal set and vocal fold length and mass that are alike in quality. The naming of voice registers in singing pedagogy is by no means universally consistent. Some teachers believe that there are three registers, some two, and some none at all. From an acoustic point of view there are two principal registers, modal and falsetto. Among singers the general consensus would appear to be that there are three main registers: chest, middle or mixed register (sometimes subdivided into lower and upper middle registers in the female voice), and head register. Falsetto is usually understood by singers to indicate the male voice when imitating the female voice or singing counter tenor.

RESONANCE – In *singing* terms, the description of a voice meaning its 'colour', 'quality' or 'timbre'. In acoustic terms it is what happens to the sound signal (which consists of a fundamental frequency and its partials, generated by the oscillation of the vocal folds in the airstream) when it is enhanced by the shape and size of the vocal tract cavity. The individual colour of a singer's voice is dictated by this.

SITTING ON THE BREATH – The sensation of well supported singing, where subglottic pressure is evenly balanced with appropriate glottal resistance.

SPIN - A free tone that projects and seems effortlessly produced. Usually the result of *sitting on the breath.*

SPREAD TONE - Tone that is unfocused, with poorly tuned formants (see Chapter 13).

STACCATO - (Italian: literally 'detached' or 'separated') The opposite of *legato.* Notes with a rest between them. In effect, a series of voice onsets.

STRAIGHT TONE - A tone without vibrato. It is sometimes used as a constant vocal quality for early music, rather than as a transitory vocal effect. Large and Iwata (1971) found that it was produced by lower airflow and greater glottal resistance than tone with vibrato. In order to supress spontaneous, involuntary vibrato, there may be a constriction of the supraglottis resulting in pinched or strained tone, or a widening of the supraglottis resulting in a flat, shallow or open tone (Dejonckere et al., 1995). It is an aesthetic much beloved by many baroque specialists, but not by all singing teachers.

SUPPORT - (Italian: appoggiare - to lean, to rest upon) The proper coordination of abdominal, intercostal and back muscles with the diaphragm in order to control and sustain appropriate subglottic air pressure. Much the same as squeezing the bagpipes.

SWALLOWED TONE - Tone that is produced by a depressed, backed tongue, and pharyngeal constriction. Unfortunately it can sound rather impressive and 'operatic' to the singer producing it.

TESSITURA - (Italian: texture) Where the majority of the vocal range required for a particular role or piece of music lies.

THICK FOLD - A term used to describe a vocal fold in which the body, the vocalis muscle, is very active. The fold is firm in texture and, as a result, a higher proportion of the muscle mass is actually involved in the vibration of the fold. From an acoustic standpoint, it is as if the 'virtual' oscillating mass has been increased and the fold is effectively 'heavier' (see Chapter 1).

THIN FOLD - A vocal fold in which the vocalis muscle is relatively inactive. The 'virtual' oscillating mass of the fold is effectively reduced and a lighter tone results. Thin fold is often associated with *falsetto* register when tightening of the vocal ligament has made the edge of the fold hard and thin, but it may also be produced when the ligament is lax, resulting in a light often slightly breathy voice.

TIMBRE - The individual colour of a voice given by its characteristic overtones.

TRILL - (Italian: trillare - to warble like a bird) A rapid alternation between the main note and the semitone or tone above it.

VIBRATO - (Italian: to shake or vibrate) To quote Seashore (1938): 'a good vibrato is a pulsation of pitch, usually accompanied with synchronous pulsation of loudness and timbre, of such extent and rate as to give a pleasing flexibility, tenderness and richness to the tone.' The rate of vibrato is reported to be between 4 and 7 cycles per second (Hz) in most literature, the average among singers being about 6 cycles per second. The cricothyroid muscles play a major role in the production and maintenence of vibrato, as the cricothyroid visor is the main pitching mechanism of voice and provides the variations (perturbation) in fundamental frequency. However, as the visor mechanism slightly abducts the vocal folds, the lateral cricoarytenoids and vocalis also increase in activity in order to maintain proper adduction during singing. Oscillation may also occur synchronously in other parts of the vocal tract, including the velum, tongue base, epiglottis and lateral pharyngeal wall near the larynx. The respiratory muscles should not oscillate during vibrato. Singers may try to develop a vibrato using the muscles of respiration. The effect is most unpleasant. (after Dejonckere et al., 1995.)

VOCALIZE – A vocal exercise consisting of a melody sung on a vowel without text.

WHISTLE REGISTER – A very high register in some female voices. It occurs beyond the high Fs sung by the 'Queen of the Night'.

WHITE TONE – Much the same as *straight* tone, with the addition that the tone is generally in head or falsetto register.

WOBBLE – A vibrato with an unpleasantly slow rate and wide variation of pitch, 'a friendly voice - it waves at you'.

(See also: Benninger et al., 1994).

Appendix 8.1

Singers' voice types

These voice types refer to the Western classical tradition of opera singing.

Soprano

Highest female voice

*   Light, high soprano or soubrette: Usually plays maids, flirts or children.
    Adele (Die Fledermaus), Despina (Cosi fan tutte), Gretel (Hansel und Gretel)

*   Coloratura: (Italian: literally 'colouring') Meaning a light, lyric or dramatic soprano who sings brilliant showy runs involving a lot of high notes. Vocal firework display artist.
    Queen of the Night (Die Zauberflöte), Olympia (Les contes d'Hoffmann)

*   Lyric soprano: Warmer and somewhat larger in voice. Gentle, warm-hearted, somewhat passive characters.
    Mimi (La Bohème), the Countess (the Marriage of Figaro)

*   Spinto: (Italian: literally 'pushed', 'daring', 'high', 'excessive') Can be any of these. Heavier in voice, bigger emotional range. They tend to come to a bad end.
    Madame Butterfly, Desdemona (Otello), Senta (Der fliegender Holländer)

*   Dramatic: Grand passions, big noise. Many of Verdi's ladies.
    Leonora (Fidelio), Tosca, Aida, Lady Macbeth

- Heavy dramatic: Rare like hens' teeth. Seriously powerful voice, tremendous stamina, capable of sustaining long Wagnerian roles. Mythical creatures.
  Brünnhilde (the Ring), Elektra, Turandot

Mezzo soprano

Lower female voice

- Lyric: Warm, flexible voice, able to sing coloratura. Young with good legs for the many trouser roles.
  Cherubino (the Marriage of Figaro), Rosina (the Barber of Seville)

- Dramatic: Darker and stronger. Glamorous, strong characters.
  Carmen, Dalila (Samson et Dalila)

Contralto

Lowest female voice

- Mature, heavy, very strong low range. Plays nurses, fortune tellers, gipsies and older female relatives.
  Ulrica (Un ballo in maschera), the Countess (The Queen of Spades), Erda (The Ring), Lucretia (The Rape of)

Counter tenor/male alto

Frequently are baritones singing mostly in falsetto with rare excursions into modal voice. Much the same range as the female contralto, but with less ease at the top of the voice. Baroque roles, originally for castrati.
Oberon (A Midsummer Night's Dream)

Tenor

The highest male voice

- Buffo: A highly skilled character actor (never the lead), but allied to skilful singing technique.
  Basilio (the Marriage of Figaro), Pedrillo (Die Entführung aus dem Serail)

- Lyric: Light, youthful, Mozart/Rossini type tenor.
  Tamino (Die Zauberflöte), Nemorino (L'Elisir d'amore)

- Italian: Romantic, heavier and louder. Pavarotti-esque.
  Faust, Rudolfo (La Bohème)

- Youthful heroic or tenore robusto: A great top to the voice, stamina. Born to command.
  Calaf (Turandot), Don Jose (Carmen), Radames (Aida)
- Heldentenor: Seriously loud, dark. Marathon man. Heroes and demi-gods. More hens' teeth.
  Otello, Siegfried (the Ring), Florestan (Fidelio)

Baritone

The average male voice

- Lyric: Young, smooth, charming. Frequently comic characters.
  Papageno (Die Zauberflöte), Figaro (the Barber of Seville)

- Cavalier: A term used infrequently in the UK. Dashing, romantic and heavier than a lyric. They tend to get the girl, but not always for long.
  Don Giovanni, Valentine (Faust), Eugene Onegin

- Character: Big strong personality, dark powerful voice, with an exciting high register. They do not always get the girl.
  Rigoletto , Escamillo (Carmen), Tonio (I Pagliacci)

- Heroic: Powerful, cruel and able to sing heavy Verdi. They have no great interest in the girl.
  Macbeth, Pizarro (Fidelio), Wotan (the Ring)

Bass

The lowest male voice

- Buffo: Excellent actor, varied roles that are often comic, duped or angry old men. Called upon to sing patter songs at unbelievably fast speeds. Can be a baritone or a bass-baritone.
  Leporello (Don Giovanni), Don Pasquale

- Bass-baritone: Darker and more dramatic than a buffo.
  Figaro (the Marriage of Figaro), Méphistophélès (Faust)

- Basso-profundo: Both in depth of voice and profundity of character. Imposing in personality and rich in voice. Verdi bass roles. Gods, kings, ageing soldiers and men of conscience.
  Sarastro (Die Zauberflöte), King Phillip (Don Carlos)

Remember, many singers think they have heavier voices than they do, and will yearn to sing heavier roles than their actual capabilities will allow (see Legge, 1990).

References

Abitbol J, De Brux J, Millot G (1989) Does a hormonal vocal cord cycle exist in women? Study of vocal premenstrual syndrome in voice performances by videostroboscopy-glottography and cytology on 38 women. Journal of Voice 3: 157-162.

Barlow W (1973) The Alexander Technique. New York: Warner Books.

Benninger MS, Jacobson BH, Johnson AF (1994) Vocal arts medicine: the care and prevention of professional voice disorders. New York: Thieme.

Bunch M (1995) Dynamics of the singing voice, 3rd edn. Wien: Springer-Verlag.

Damste PH (1967) Voice changes in adult women caused by virilization agents. Journal of Speech and Hearing Disorders 32: 126-132.

Dehorn AB (1991) Performance anxiety. In Benninger M et al. (Eds) Vocal arts medicine: the care and prevention of professional voice disorder. New York: Thieme.

Dejonckere PH, Hirano M, Sundberg J (1995) Vibrato. San Diego: Singular Publishing Group Inc.

Estill J (1994) Belting and chest voice compared. Paper presented to the 7th Pacific Voice Conference, San Francisco CA, USA.

Estill J (1996) Primer of Compulsory Figures (Level One): A user's guide to voice quality. Santa Rosa CA: Estill Voice Training Systems.

Gramming P (1991) Vocal loudness and frequency capabilities of the voice. Journal of Voice. 5: 144-157.

Gramming P, Sundberg J, Ternström S, Leanderson R, Perkins WH (1988) Relationship between changes in voice pitch and loudness. Journal of Voice. 2: 118-126.

Harris TM, Johnston DF, Collins SRC, Heath ML (1990) General anaesthetic technique for use in singers: the brain laryngeal mask airway versus endotracheal intubation. Journal of Voice: 4: 81-85.

Hixon TJ (1973) Respiratory function in speech. In Minifie F, Hixon T, Williams F (Eds.) Normal Aspects of Speech, Hearing and Language. New Jersey: Prentice Hall.

Hixon TJ (1991) Respiratory function in speech and song. San Diego CA: Singular Publishing Group.

Jones NS, Lannigan FJ, McMullagh M, Anggiansah A, Owen W, Harris TM (1990) Acid reflux and hoarseness. Journal of Voice 4: 355-358.

Large J, Iwata S (1971) Aerodynamic study of vibrato and voluntary 'straight tone' pairs in singing. Folia Phoniatrica 23: 50-65.

Leanderson R, Sundberg J, Von Euler C (1984) Effects of diaphragm activity on phonation during singing. Thirteenth Symposium: Care of the Professional Voice. New York: The Voice Foundation.

Legge A (1990) The art of auditioning. London: Rhinegold Publishing Ltd.

Ling D (1976) Speech and the hearing impaired child: theory and practice. Washington, D.C.: The Alexander Graham Bell Association for the Deaf, Inc.

McKinney JC (1994) The diagnosis and correction of vocal faults. Nashville: Genevox Music Group.

Pullan B, May P (1994) Basics of singing pedagogy.In Morrison MD, Rammage L (Eds) The management of voice disorders, vol. 11. San Diego: Singular Publishing Group Inc., pp 201-228.

Sataloff RT (1990) Endocrine dysfunction. In Sataloff RT (Ed.) Professional voice: the science and art of clinical care. New York: Raven Press.

Seashore CE (1938) Psychology of music. New York: McGraw-Hill.

Sundberg J (1987) The science of the singing voice. De kalb: Northern Illinois University Press.

Titze IR (1994) Principles of voice production. New Jersey: Prentice Hall.

Titze IR (1995) Pan European Voice Conference, London. Workshop.

Vilkman E, Sonninen A, Hurme P, Körkkö P (1996) External laryngeal frame function in voice production revisited: a review. Journal of Voice 10: 78-92.

CHAPTER 9

Psychogenic factors in dysphonia

PHIROZE NEEMUCHWALA

The people's voice is odd...

Alexander Pope

In this chapter I intend to accomplish two things. First, to explain a theory of how psychogenic dysphonia is created through the interaction of three distinct variables and second, to outline a structure in which patients whose dysphonia has been diagnosed as psychogenic can be treated in a group context.

Readers may be surprised to see the author of this chapter using the first person singular throughout. In a book of this nature one tends to find either impersonal expressions, e.g. 'It was noticed that...', 'One tends to find...', or the first person plural, e.g. 'We believe that...' I have elected to express myself in the first person singular for two reasons, first because the mistakes and omissions are mine and mine alone and second, because I wish to model the kind of self-expression that I exhort my patients to use in the groupwork for dysphonics that is the subject of the second part of this chapter.

The theoretical approach to group therapy techniques for treating psychogenic dysphonia and its practical application for a particular voice clinic

As a psychotherapist in private practice I had repeatedly come across patients who somatized their emotions in the normal areas of skin, sleep, musculature, digestion and back pain, but I had never encountered dysphonia as a symptom of emotional mismanagement until I was invited to start observing the voice clinic at Queen Mary's Hospital. I soon realized that a significant proportion of patients presenting with dysphonia were either causing or exacerbating their symptoms by muscle misuse and poor respiration caused by high levels of anxiety, anger or depression.

In discussion with colleagues at the clinic I learnt that we see similar personality types in patients but from differing ends of the telescope. They pitch up in the voice clinic saying 'I keep losing my voice', and members of the team notice their demeanour and wonder if they have a problem with the management of their emotions. They pitch up in my psychotherapy consulting room saying 'I'm always worrying, I can't sleep. No one is interested in what I have to say, and there's something wrong with my voice as well', and I start wondering if their strangulated-sounding and often fading voice has something to do with their statement 'No one is interested in what I have to say'. Could there be a psychomuscular mechanism by which this belief leads to a suppression of the volume and timbre of the voice? If there is, what is the pathway and what can be done about it?

Freud's earliest cases were mainly women who had become partly paralysed because of unsayable ideas that had somatized or dived down into the body. Freud coined the word 'innervation' for this phenomenon and treated it by talking to them rather than by prescribing more body-centred treatments (Freud and Breuer, 1895). The rest, as they say, is history. It appeared from our discussions that some of the most intransigent patients presenting in the clinic had problems with 'unsayable ideas' either revolving around chronic anxiety, long-term depression or with the expression of anger.

Clinical vignette 1

Ruth (not her real name), 62, presented with a husky whisper. She also presented with a fixed smile that was hiding her anxiety at being in the clinic. Her terror was palpable and her rictus incongruous. She had been unable to produce a normal voice for several months. I established that there had been a death in her family a while ago. I asked her to repeat the phrase 'I like sponge cake'. It came out as a husky whisper. I asked her to frown sadly and to say it again. She was able, to the surprise of all in the clinic, to produce her usual voice. The anxiety had met an inner rule, 'I must put a brave face on my pain: I must not let it be seen that I am suffering'. This chronic smile, forced and therefore doubly demanding on the relevant musculature, had distorted the normal muscle tone of her vocal apparatus. When she dropped the smile, her voice was immediately able to function almost normally.

In my clinical experience the problem is more often to do with anger and this is borne out by the fact that it affects more women than men (House and Andrews, 1987; Bridger and Epstein, 1993). Women are more socially discouraged when it comes to the spontaneous expression of anger. No personality type has been found to be particularly susceptible to dysphonia, but most of my patients have made significant improvements through a simple exploration of how they generate anger for themselves and how they ventilate or fail to ventilate their anger. I can only partially concur with Gerritsma (1991) regarding the finding of introversion in dysphonics. Teachers and actors, who are often seen in voice clinics, certainly do not fall into this category. It has also been asserted that there is a link between alexithymia (emotional woodenness) and psychosomatic illness (Kinzl et al., 1988). I do not dispute this, but I would stress that the dysphonics I have treated have been some of the most emotionally vibrant and alive patients I have ever worked with. I clearly remember the tears and rage of some of the patients referred from the voice clinic, many of whom appear as clinical vignettes below. In fact, these patients had such a vibrant emotional world that they had to evolve extraordinary release techniques in order to relieve the dysphonic symptoms. In time, they were able to celebrate the fact that the dysphonia had been the symptom that had encouraged them to seek psychotherapy and thereby ameliorate the quality of their relationship with themselves and with others via an improved understanding of how they generated their feelings, and then either succeed or fail in discharging them adequately.

Several psychological conditions have been associated with functional dysphonia, including major depression, dysthymic disorders, adjustment disorders and anxiety or depression, generalized anxiety disorder, conversion and phobic disorders, post-traumatic stress disorder as well as personality trait difficulties (Morrison and Rammage, 1994). What has not been remarked upon thus far is that the patient's ability to communicate and ventilate emotional thoughts and emotions is the crucial variable. Those emotions that do not leave the body will remain in the body and will damage the body, either through immunosuppression, via the endocrine system or though chronic muscular hypertonicity.

Somatic expressions for emotional responses that are felt in the body are seen in all cultures and range from above the pharynx to below the perineum, for example:

- 'That leaves a bitter taste in my mouth.'
- 'She bit off more than she could chew.'
- 'I find that story hard to swallow.'
- 'That really sticks in my throat.'
- 'I can't stomach him.'
- 'You make me sick.'
- 'He's a pain in the neck.'
- 'She's a pain in the arse.'
- 'It made my toes curl.'
- 'It made the hairs on the back of my neck stand up.'

The throat is the pathway for verbal communication, food and drink, crying, rage and the infant's cry for help and is therefore a nexus vulnerable to emotional conversion symptoms in the way that a latissimus dorsi or a gastrocnemius is unlikely to be.

As we discussed the range of auxiliary symptoms that our patients pitch up with, it became clear to us that a great deal of consultant time was being wasted treating symptoms that would either recur or find an alternative mode of expression. Some patients somatize their emotional problem in a variety of ways until one of the physical manifestations gets them the kind of psychotherapeutic attention that the emotion originally craved.

These symptoms speak of overactivity of the autonomic and voluntary nervous systems leading inevitably to generalized muscle hypertonicity arising from (largely unconscious) muscle misuse. In dysphonia it will be the intrinsic and extrinsic muscles of the larynx that are being ill-treated. In my view, all these symptoms, when caused by mismanaged emotions, can be grouped under the umbrella name displaced affect syndrome (DAS), and will respond poorly to medication. As long as the basic problem in the patient's life situation and the subsequent emotion, be it anxiety, depression or anger, is being inadequately dealt with, it will surface in one guise or another.

Clinical vignette 2

Barbara (not her real name), 40, suffered with colitis for many years until her dysphonia started. At this point, all gastroenteritic symptomatology ceased. Her dysphoria had found an alternative mode of expression, an even more 'visible' one. The voice clinic heard/saw/sensed/understood the communication that her unconscious was trying to make and referred her for counselling. A serious deficit in anger management skills was found and could then be addressed.

Six basic psychosomatic symptoms as seen by a psychotherapist

1. Headaches, migraines.
2. Musculoskeletal pain, usually neck, shoulder and back pains, sometimes manifesting as rheumatoid arthritis.
3. Dyspepsia, food intolerances, constipation, diarrhoea, eating disorders.
4. Sexual dysfunction, erection problems, anorgasmia, dysmenorrhea, vaginismus.
5. Disturbances of sleep, insomnia, early waking, leading to fatigue and apathy, depression or irritability.
6. Dermatological problems. Eczema, psoriasis, blushing, rashes, flushes.

Vocal dysfunction is not one of the big six, but it is one of the classic hysterical paralyses as discussed by Breuer and Freud a century ago.

I was asked to observe the clinic on Friday mornings. I did this for a month and I was then asked to design a provisional schedule for a pilot weekend workshop that would have as its goal the raising into consciousness of the way in which the mismanagement of emotions might be causing or exacerbating the symptoms, if only by mismanaged anxiety interrupting the normal quantum of breath available for voice production.

Information sheets about the weekend were offered to patients who were interested and in January 1993, the weekend was run. The group size was nine, this being constituted of four voice clinic referrals and five patients from my private practice in psychotherapy to bump up the numbers. Of the four dysphonics, all of whom, in my opinion, were psychosomatic to some extent, the two women refused to acknowledge any emotional role in the aetiology of their symptoms and the two men assimilated the weekend well – both entered psychotherapy and were relieved of all symptoms within 3 months. It should be stressed that the goal of the weekend was not to cure but to show where the cure might lie. Admittedly, a sample of four is statistically inadequate; however, 90 per cent of the patients referred for psychotherapy have obtained significant relief through improved self-awareness and improved emotional management. I currently receive a referral from the clinic every 2 months or so and all these patients have improved by at least 80 per cent. This body of work in once-weekly individual psychodynamic psychotherapy usually takes between 6 and 9 months and is accompanied by the reading of four self-help books.

In my observation of dysphonics, the cognitive–behavioural pathway by which emotions enter the body seems to be something like this (I have underlined the two most crucial variables and will attempt definitions below):

1.   Activating event + patient's interpretive matrix = quantum of affect.
2.   Affect + inadequate cathartic technique = strangulated affect.
3.   Strangulated affect somatizes and manifests as dysphonia with probably one or more of the six conversion symptoms as listed above.

Once the dysphonia is well established it becomes an anxiety-provoking threat all of its own, the patient fearing his or her dysphonia as much as he fears the more external activating events, which leads to breathlessness and a rerunning and exacerbation of the whole loop.

I shall illustrate this with an extended clinical vignette.

Clinical vignette 3

Alison (not her real name), 33, a secondary school teacher.

1.   Activating event. A recalcitrant pupil in her class continues to talk after being asked to quieten down.

     Patient's interpretive matrix. This describes how the patient interprets and processes the event. Alison's mind says 'They don't respect me. I don't deserve respect. I'm a rubbish teacher, this is terrible, I want to shout at them but I must never shout at anyone because then I would be just like my aggressive and violent father and that would be catastrophic so I had better just bite my lip.'

     Quanta of affect. Because of this processing, first anger was created, then sadness, then the desire to shout and then the self-given interdiction 'Thou shalt not shout'. This leaves Alison seething with frustration and confused. Most importantly, most of this process takes place below the threshold of consciousness. Alison's conscious mind merely notices the recalcitrant pupil and then feels ill at ease, tight and tense. She may never consciously acknowledge that her voice loss, dyspepsia and sleeplessness are connected to a self-esteem and anger management problem that ultimately has to do with her ambivalent feelings of anger, fear and sadness around her father.

2.   Inadequate cathartic techniques. Now comes the second crucial variable, the efficacity of the patient's cathartic techniques. Once the anger has been created by the interpretation of the activating event, what determines the

impact on the body is the extent to which the patient successfully discharges the affect from his/her body. What Alison's instinct (id) tells her to do is shout at the pupil, then her conditioning (superego) orders her to repress the shout. This I would describe as a highly inadequate cathartic technique. She is left with 'angry energy' running through her system. This has to go somewhere. Anger tends to manifest in a strangulation of some muscles. Our word anger, after all, comes from the Latin *angere*: to strangle. In Alison's case her mind successfully strangles the shouting she instinctively wants to do and goes even further … it leaves her with a tight throat for several hours.

3.   Later that day Alison notices that her throat is tight and that she can hardly speak. She loses her appetite but forces some food down and experiences severe indigestion. That night thoughts such as 'He will be in that class again tomorrow' haunt her and she has difficulty sleeping. She may, in time, consult the school nurse about the dyspepsia and later, her general practitioner for relief of the insomnia, and these symptoms will probably be treated as unrelated symptoms. She may well be prescribed different medications and even be sent to clinics for laryngoscopy and gastroscopy. These clinical procedures are valuable in that they rule out major organic pathology. However, none of these measures is going to provide long-term relief. The one sure way to help Alison is to take a whole body history, establish the recurring emotional inhibition, i.e. her difficulty with ventilating anger and the recalcitrant pupil, and then to refer her to someone trained in psychotherapy and anger management, so that her interpretive matrix and cathartic techniques can be worked on.

What group work can do is to alert the patient to awareness of psychosomatics and motivate her to accept how her mind is responsible for part of her problems. Alison will have to confront her father issues and her self-esteem issues. The need for one-to-one psychotherapy may be obviated if extended specialized group work is available. For a case such as this, about 6 months in once-weekly group work would be indicated. (Group work is contraindicated when the patient's anxiety level is such that a withdrawal from the group is likely. This would be damaging to the patient's already low self-esteem. With these patients, individual therapy should be undertaken with a view to preparing for group work.)

Let us explore in detail what we mean by the concepts of:

1.   the patient's interpretive matrix;
2.   the patient's cathartic techniques.

The patient's interpretive matrix (PIM)

This refers to the 'software' that the patient has in the hardware of his or her brain. Good, loving, secure parenting and schooling will build in effective, realistic and enjoyable programmes into the system. Poor, ambivalent, insecure parenting and schooling will build in ineffective, unrealistic and depressing systems of thinking into the system.

Clinical vignette 4

Both Claire and Steve (not their real names) were told on the same day that their surgery appointments would, regrettably, be delayed by a month. Claire, with optimal software, feels slightly disappointed but thanks the surgeon for giving her so much notice and starts planning what to do with the extra month. She trusts that the operation will eventually happen. Steve, whose parenting was suboptimal, partly due to a father who repeatedly lied, becomes flustered and angry and begins to shout resentfully at the surgeon because his software is programmed to believe that the operation will never really happen and that the surgeon is lying to him, just like his father used to.

Here we can see how an identical activating event results in different quanta of affect depending on the software or interpretive matrix that has been loaded, since birth, into the system, day after day.

Generally, patients with low quality parenting have low self-esteem, which engenders beliefs about themselves, other people and life itself, which are pessimistic and exaggerated, such as:

- Self: 'I'm no good', 'I'm not likeable', 'I get everything wrong'.
- Others: 'Other people can't be trusted', 'Other people don't care about me'.
- Life: 'Life is too hard and is a waste of time', 'Life is unfair and cruel'.

Patients with high self-esteem hold beliefs more akin to:

- Self: 'I'm as good as anyone else', 'I can do things well when I try'.
- Others: 'Other people are different to me but are generally safe'.
- Life: 'Life can be great if I put in the effort'.

The patient's interpretive matrix is essentially the sum total of all the beliefs that the patient holds. These beliefs determine how she or he will interpret all the events that life, in all its wonder, will provide. Life is not responsible for our emotions, it is responsible for providing trigger events. Our interpretive matrix is responsible for our emotions. As it took decades to develop, it cannot be easily changed. In fact, for change to take place, emotional experience as well as information needs to be internalized. A therapist can tell the patient that she or he does not despise the patient until she or he is blue in the face. It is not until the patient has the emotionally alive experience of the therapist's non-judgemental behaviour that she or he will register a change. This is why individual therapy and group work is so much more effective than reading books about therapy. The human emotional experience is what laid down these programs and only a new emotional experience will suffice both to delete the previous message and to record a new one.

It should be stressed that the therapeutic models that have been proven to be most effective at creating enduring change in the patient's interpretive matrix are cognitive–behavioural therapy and rational–emotive therapy. Fortunately, these models do not require the instructor to have been through a lengthy analysis or a long and complex training. For over half the dysphonics in a typical clinic, I believe that these models offer an opportunity for change. For cases where there has been either a gross disturbance of the mother–baby relationship or substantial trauma during the formative years, a more psychodynamic or Gestalt approach is indicated. If every voice clinic had a regular provision of group work of both cognitive and psychodynamic types, patients could be assisted not only to self-help their way out of their dysphonia but also to improve their level of everyday functioning and live happier lives. This, eventually, would save the NHS millions.

Clinical vignette 5

Jason (not his real name), 23, actor. Jason is a particularly successful case of referral to group work who not only obtained full relief from his dysphonic symptoms after surgical intervention, but also came to understand that his anger about his treatment at the hands of his mother was making his symptoms worse. This encouraged him to confront her, which built up his self-esteem and helped lessen his anger. This meant that he was able to significantly reduce the amount of illegal drugs he was ingesting and give up smoking. He was able to become less promiscuous and to start taking regular exercise. He left psychotherapy after a year with a considerably improved lifestyle.

The patient's cathartic techniques (PCT)

Once our patients find themselves with a quantum of affect, be it happiness, sadness, fear or anger, given the fundamentally homeostatic nature of the psyche-soma, that affect will crave release, or catharsis. If catharsis is not effectively and thoroughly provided, discomfort, both physical and mental, will ensue. A metaphor that I often use in clinical practice is that of the bladder. When the bladder is full, it craves immediate and thorough catharsis (which originally meant 'purging' or emptying). If the emptying is not done immediately, pain will ensue and will increase until catastrophe occurs, both mental (wetting oneself is embarrassing) and physiological (a stretched hypotonic bladder). If the bladder is half-emptied, this will leave the patient only half-relieved and continually needing another visit to the toilet. If the emotional reservoir is not adequately emptied, not only will the emotion endure ('tingling' all the while), but the patient will permanently be needing to 'leak' emotion. This usually manifests as the patient being permanently on the edge of tears, on the edge of rage or chronically anxious. Equally, clinical depression can ensue. As the muscles of phonation are the final common path of all dysphonia of psychogenic origin, they must be involved in the treatment. (Greer and Watson's work on breast cancer has shown that a significant proportion of women with carcinoma have great difficulty ventilating anger. They generate it, as we all do, but they do not allow it out of the body, often not even allowing it to manifest as a frown. Like Ruth in clinical vignette 1, they often wear an omnipresent half-smile and bury their emotions behind it. Eventually this emotional suppression can even produce disturbance of the endocrine system and (possibly) immunosuppression, which in turn produces an increased susceptibility to both exogenous and endogenous disease.)

Clinical vignette 6

Stefano (not his real name), 28, photographer. I recall the case of Stefano, a volatile Italian, whose interpretive matrix would generate large quanta of anger if he encountered red traffic lights when he was rushing to a photo assignment. He presented in psychotherapy because he was 'permanently angry – ready to tear people's heads off!' He revealed how he would panic about being late and therefore losing people's respect. He wanted to scream with rage in the car but felt he 'should not' as his father had dropped dead of a massive coronary thrombosis during a temper tantrum. Therefore he arrived at locations angry, as a way of dealing with his fear. Therapy revealed his lack of self-esteem regarding his job and his fear of dying as his father had done if he allowed himself to get really angry. Part of the work we did involved him screaming in the car, into pillows and experiencing the physical relief from the catharsis of the anger. We also discussed how his inhibition about ventilating anger was more likely to lead to coronary trouble than keep him clear from it!

Eventually he was able to scream in the car without anxiety. In fact, he took delight in catharting the rage from his body, safe in the knowledge that he was helping his health rather than hindering it. It is worth noting in this case how successful treatment involved:

1.   Analytic exploration (exploring the past).
2.   Practising cathartic technique (exploring the present).
3.   Technical discussion of psychosomatics as relevant to phonation.

I believe that successful treatment in this case depended on going beyond conventional therapeutic boundaries and combining the roles of analyst, anger-management coach and 'psychosomatics information provider'. This is indeed what we attempt to combine in the weekly treatment groups.

Often, a difficulty with the externalization of sadness will often lead to dysphonia as the musculature struggles to push down the sobbing and tears that need to come out. After a long time spent working with patients on dealing effectively with powerful feelings I have come to believe that there are two components in effectively catharting an emotion. As befits the concept of psychosomatics, one half is mental, the other physical.

The physical component

For those patients who have accumulated anger or sadness, the only way forward here is to facilitate them to release the shouting and the crying. In my experience, the louder they shout and cry, the more relief they will feel. Occasionally they need to be taught how to scream without damaging the vocal cords. It seems to assist them if I give them a large pillow or cushion and ask them to push it onto their face and scream into it. They will often need reassurance that we will not laugh at them or think them silly. I have found that the simplest way to do this is to take the pillow myself and demonstrate exactly what I want them to do. I have not found that this disturbs the patient–practitioner relationship adversely. Some, as they begin to scream, really 'find their voice' for the first time in years and experience a rush of energy in the upper arms. This happens because the unconscious is allowing the body to be really angry, and the body wants to hit, punch and flail about when it is angry. Patients will often hit the cushion a few times, some will hit the seat of their chair in order to cathart the muscular energy in the arms. Others may stamp their feet.

The communicative component

Clinical vignette 7

Gwillim (not his real name), 36, teacher. Gwillim was one of those who attended the first weekend workshop at Queen Mary's and entered weekly psychotherapy shortly afterwards. His dysphonia was connected to the fact that he was working with some-one with whom he had had a relationship and she had broken it off. He was still very emotionally churned up (sadness and anger) about this situation, which he found unbearable. He found that the scars were opened up every time he saw her and there was no time to heal. He felt unable to say a word to her about how he was feeling and he noticed that his consumption of cigarettes, alcohol and other drugs was on the increase. He was unaware that he needed to sob and scream with impotent rage and felt unable to allow himself to really express his feelings. He presented with self-disgust, depression and was constantly on the edge of tears in the counselling room. This man needed to be helped to cry loudly, scream with rage and communicate his thoughts, feelings and needs to the woman concerned, who had no real idea of what he was going through. He had not only 'gone quiet' regarding the expression of the emotion, he had also stopped communicating verbally with her. A double silence, both ideational and emotional. This body and mind were paying a double price.

Psychogenic dysphonics tend to have had an upbringing that has contained two covert messages:

(a) I must not tell people what I think, how I feel or what I need. When I disagree, the best way to get through life is to keep quiet about my dissent.
(b) I must not show my feelings of anxiety, sadness or anger. If I do, the results will be catastrophic for me.

Clearly, in both cases, the self-esteem of the parents has been so low that effective communications of thoughts, needs and feelings has been precluded. The truth is seen as dangerous rather than reparative. This is also indicative of a loss of faith in the world. The patient does not believe that the world is:

(a) interested in what they have to say;
(b) willing to accede to their requests;
(c) able to hear and contain their pain;
(d) able to withstand the forceful expression of their feelings.

The patient's beliefs, which nestle within their interpretive matrix, have boxed the patient into a way of living in which their thoughts, needs and feelings are almost never expressed. No wonder their psyche-soma is cluttered. It is quite typi-cal for the family and friends of our patients to have no real idea of what inner emotional pain the sufferer is in, just as the colleague in the above clinical vignette had no idea that her ex-boyfriend was in terrible pain.

Hopefully, by now, the psychosomatic aetiology of the symptom will be clear to the reader. This will raise the question 'What can be done about such patients?' and in the next section I hope to answer this question.

Running a group designed to assist psychogenic dysphonics to lessen and cope with their symptoms

The development of group work with dysphonics

I was invited in 1992 to make a contribution to the series of five consecutive Friday afternoon voice classes that were being offered to dysphonics at Queen Mary's. This invitation resulted in a collaboration that has produced a weekend workshop and a successful programme of group work during the last five years.

The voice classes were scheduled to last 2 hours, from 2 pm to 4 pm and I was invited to come along and give a presentation on the role of thoughts and feelings in dysphonia, in the hope that a talk might be useful to those patients in the group whose symptoms were either caused or exacerbated by their way of dealing with their thoughts and feelings. Neither of us was sure of whether my talk would meet with a frosty 'I'm not a nutcase' silence or a cooperative response. I can well recall my anxiety. During my first presentation, which was intended to be a one-off experiment, the response from the group was so positive that it became clear that the hour allotted to me was not going to give people a chance to have their questions dealt with in a useful manner. I agreed to return the following week and thus the regular psychological component in the voice group was born.

Over the following 3 years we refined the technique and now have a format, including paper-based exercises, with which we are happy. The voice group takes place over five consecutive Friday afternoons from 2 pm to 4 pm, and I am given an hour during weeks 2, 3 and 4 in which to offer my ideas. Our goal is modest, namely to make some of the patients aware of the role of the mind in the aetiology or exacerbation of their symptoms. We have no illusions of offering miracle insights leading to miracle cures. Our hope is merely to show them how they may be able to help themselves. We hope to set a process in action that will lead them to review the way in which they deal with their feelings. Ideally, those that need to enter counselling will make the choice so to do and will be helped to make the necessary arrangements.

I will now sketch out what it is that we actually do with the groups during the three afternoons when I am present.

The content of the three presentations

Each of the three hour-long presentations has a very specific goal and a specific handout. Copies of these are available from the voice clinic at Queen Mary's on written request.

1. Helping the group become aware of psychosomatic processes, the relationship between emotions and body states.
2. Helping the group see how their unique way of seeing the world (PIM) affects the way in which their voice works.
3. Helping the group assess the effectiveness of their ways of dealing with anxiety, sadness and anger (PCT). Looking at next steps if they wish to improve their emotional self-management and follow up this taster of self-exploration.

I shall now relate in some detail what we do in each of the presentations. My goal here is to be clear enough so that if you, the reader, wish to create a voice group treatment programme, the following pages will enable and empower you so to do. There is no suggestion that our format is the best way. It works for us and is a constantly evolving thing, benefiting from any ideas that we have. We hope that you will feel inspired to create groups that make the most of your skills as unique individuals.

First meeting: helping the group become aware of the relationship between emotions and body states

When I arrive on the second of the five afternoons, the group is already beginning to bond. They have spent 2 hours together and have been briefed that someone with psychological training is going to be joining them for the following three weeks. They are seated on armchairs in a circle. My approach is friendly and casual. Having been introduced by Sara, I say a few words about how I come to be there and about how I feel about sitting down with a new group of some 10 people. I make a point of mentioning that my anxiety manifests in specific physical ways: butterflies in the tummy, feeling warm, dry mouth, shortness of breath and tight throat. In this way I model what the next hour will be all about, namely helping them identify what body changes happen in them when they experience anxiety, sadness and anger. I ask the group to tell me their names and the nature of their voice problem, which gives me a chance to start formulating an idea of their basic personality type, their degree of self-esteem and the quality of their self-expression, voice-production and respiration. Then I ask Sara what she observed in her body and what thoughts and emotions she is aware of. After her answer, I then hand out the first handout, which is a sheet of A4 with four simple questions on it with large spaces in between so that they, with the pens provided, can fill in the gaps. The sheet is entitled 'Exploring the mind–body connection'. At the top of the sheet are the following words:

> All our human emotions are accompanied by body changes, some subtle, others highly noticeable. They range from the hair on your head to the soles of your feet. On this sheet you have a chance to become aware of some of the changes that are commonly reported. Hair standing up, headache, burning in the ears, feeling hot, feeling cold, feeling numb, flared nostrils, tearfulness, blushing, dry mouth, tight jaw, blood draining away from face, tight throat, voice loss, high voice, cracking voice, bizarre voice, breathlessness, pounding heart, butterflies, tummyache, tight muscles, need to go to the toilet, sweaty palms, cold hands, feel hot/cold all over, toes curl up in shoes, high energy, low energy, etc.

The questions are these:

(a) What changes do you experience in your body when you feel anxious, frightened, scared, nervous or terrified? Please try to list as many as you can.
(b) What changes do you experience in your body when you feel cross, angry, irritated, annoyed or pissed off? Please try to list at least six.

(c) What changes do you experience when you feel sad, down, low, depressed or blue? How many can you find?

(d) What body changes do you experience when you feel happy, glad, up, exhilarated or ecstatic?

We give the group a few minutes to fill in the form, during which we fill it in too, and then, taking one emotion at a time, we start by telling the group what changes we (Sara and I) observe in ourselves. We then turn to the group and ask 'How about you?' Responses are usually forthcoming within seconds and group members tend to spontaneously disclose the triggering events and situations that habitually mobilize them to emotional arousal. For example:

Patient: Well, I tend to blush terribly when I get angry and then my throat goes tight and I feel really hot. I get really tearful if my boss asks me a question in that angry voice of his because he sounds just like my father. This happens almost every day at work because he is a real pig to us women in the office and he treats us as if we were really stupid. None of us say anything because he would fire us. Sometimes he picks on me and I get so upset I have to go home.

Therapist: When did your voice problem start?

Patient: About 3 months ago.

Therapist: When did you start working for this man?

Patient: Four months ago ... gosh ... I'd never associated the two things before ... I thought it was just part of getting older.

Therapist: Interesting, eh?

In the first session I would not take the exploration any further than that. Pushing an individual too far, too soon, can act as a disincentive for other people to step forward with an anecdote from their lives. Other disclosures follow as we work through the four emotions and before we know it, it is time to begin to wrap up the first session. Normally I recap the principal ideas and ask them to begin thinking about next week's topic, by finding a situation in which they have responded to a situation by developing dysphonic symptoms.

Second meeting: helping the group see how their unique way of seeing the world (PIM) plays a role in how their voice works

In this session we start off by asking the group if they have had any thoughts on how their emotional states influenced their voice quality during the week since the last meeting. Usually some comments are forthcoming and these are used to begin to increase the group's awareness of how their interpretive matrix and cathartic techniques determine the number and intensity of their somatizations. For example:

Patient: I've noticed that my voice begins to 'dry up' when I start getting teased at work.

Therapist: Go on, could you give an example?

Patient: Well, often when I am at work one of my colleagues will start teasing me about something and I just <u>know</u> they <u>all</u> think I'm <u>stupid</u> and that I <u>should</u> be fired and I feel really <u>terrible</u> and start to blush and I want to say something but I know that it <u>wouldn't do any good</u> because <u>people never listen</u> once they start on a good tease so I just don't say anything and I *pretend* that I can't hear what they're saying. I don't even look at them. I can feel my throat going tight and I *want to cry, but I'd never let them see* that because I <u>know</u> that if they saw me crying they'd just <u>crucify me just like when I was at school</u>.

Therapist: What happens next?

Patient: Well, after about half an hour the tension in the room lifts and the subject gets changed but for the rest of the day *my throat hurts* and when I get home *I can hardly speak* and I'm *moody all evening*, which spoils the atmosphere for my whole family. *Instead of crying I tend to shout at the kids.* Then *they end up crying and everyone's hurt and cross!*

Therapist: That all sounds like a very painful pattern, does it happen often?

Patient: About once a week, sometimes when my sister is critical of me or when my father disapproves of something I've said or done. I hate it but I just don't know what to do about it.

The above paragraphs contain a fascinating insight into how a patient can melt her past and present together in such a way as to make a slightly difficult situation (being teased or criticized) very difficult indeed. I have underlined the sections where the patient's interpretive matrix is distorting the situation and put into italics the sections where the patient's cathartic techniques can be seen to be inadequate and problem creating (or somatogenic). Working with a piece of self-disclosure such as Mrs X's above, is quite challenging. Here is a suggestion of how to go about it in such a way that she learns something and the group learns something about how their interpretations and catharting techniques influence their voice. I would repeat at this juncture that all one can do in the confines of a total of 3 hours with such a group is to try to ask the right questions so that the process of reflection can commence. For a group of this nature to really influence the psychosomatic profile of a psychogenic dysphonic in an enduring way it would need to meet at least six times over six consecutive weeks. The alternative would be a weekend workshop offered by a team of speech therapist and a psychotherapist specializing in psychosomatic dysfunction.

Therapist: I would like to comment on several parts of what you just said and this would be easier if it were written on the board. Would that be all right? (Writes the paragraph on the board and underlines the problematic sections as above.) I notice that you said 'I <u>know</u> they <u>all</u> think I'm <u>stupid</u>'. Is this a fact or a belief that you are currently holding?

Patient: What do you mean?

Therapist: Well, have they all told you that they find you stupid?

Patient: No, of course not!

Therapist: Then how do you know that is what they think?

Patient: Well, I just assume it.

Therapist:	Why?
Patient:	I don't know.
Therapist:	Could it be because part of you believes that you are stupid because one of your parents called you stupid when you were a child?
Patient:	I suppose it could be. ...my brothers always called me stupid...
Therapist:	You also said that saying how you felt about being teased would not do any good. How do you know that?
Patient:	Well, it didn't when I was a child.
Therapist:	Does that mean that it definitely wouldn't work with the adults at work?
Patient:	No, I guess not.

For more information about how to challenge a polarized statement see any manual or textbook of cognitive–behavioural therapy or rational–emotive therapy. Sage Publishing produce appropriate books on both techniques. (See Appendix 9.2 Further Reading).

Third meeting: helping the group assess the effectiveness of their ways of dealing with anxiety, sadness and anger (PCT). Looking at next steps if they wish to improve their emotional self-management and follow up this therapeutic exploration

In this meeting we begin by asking the group if they have had any insights into the relationship between their emotions and their voice since the previous week. There are usually two or three comments and this helps get the hour off to a positive start. The previous session was essentially about how they think about situations and therefore how they create their emotions. This third meeting is about how effectively they deal with emotions once they are present in awareness. We start by splitting the group into pairs and asking them to spend 5 minutes discussing with their partner what they do or say when they are experiencing sadness, anxiety and anger. When the 5 minutes have elapsed, we ask for volunteers to tell the group what they do when they feel these feelings. We write the behaviour on the board and rate its effectiveness as a cathartic technique on a scale of 1 to 10. For example, one person might say 'When I'm sad I never cry because that's giving in, which is weak.' So, we would write, 'I never cry' on the board and the group will, hopefully by now, be sophisticated enough to realize that this technique is highly somatogenic and therefore scores very low in cathartic effectiveness, 0 out of 10 in fact. Someone else might say, 'I cry but only on my own', this might receive a 5. The highest score would be for something like 'I try to talk it through with someone that I trust and if I need to cry I let it out and ask for a hug afterward'. The emphasis, as we work through all the different things that people can do with the three dysphonias is on:

1. Talking the feeling through with another person.
2. Catharting the emotion through the larynx – crying or shouting.
3. If necessary, especially with anger, catharting the emotion through the body – hitting the bed, kicking a cushion around the room, going for a run, playing squash, etc.

In other words, doing the opposite of the 'stiff upper lip' technique of emotional self-management. Our goal for this third meeting is that we leave the patients with a clear idea of what their body requires, in terms of physical catharsis, in order to maintain balance and health.

At the end of the session we provide an information sheet that includes a reading list and a list of organizations and individuals that provide counselling and psychotherapy, these are to be found in Appendix 9.2. There is also a handout on self-esteem the text of which can be found in Appendix 9.1.

Appendix 9.1

Towards an understanding of self-respect

1. Self-respect is to do with how much we honour the self as a unique, valuable person. It is shown by the warmth, friendliness and fair treatment that we extend to ourselves. If our parents hardly ever treated us in this way, we won't know how to do it very well.

2. This honouring of the self needs to be consistently nurtured in the home environment during the first 15 years, at least. If it is not, the child will make judgements about him- or herself based on what he or she sees and hears. If we are treated as if we are worthless, we will start believing that we are worthless, even if the word is never actually spoken. If our schools fail to provide adequate encouragement, respect and support we will conclude, painfully and angrily, that we do not have value or deserve respect.

3. Even if self-respect is adequately fostered at home, it can become damaged by traumatic experiences, after which, for example, our mind tells us that we are somehow damaged, tainted or wrong. These traumas can come from the outside world, like a failed exam or a relationship break-up, or they can be generated from the inner world, as in the case of people who feel anger towards a sibling or a parent and then call themselves wicked, evil and bad. In some families, where 'difficult' personalities surround us, it is important to remember that feelings of anger and hate are understandable and inevitable. It does not mean that we are bad people, just that we felt hurt or frightened and then felt angry and hateful.

4. As we grow up, the mind creates a special collection of cruel names that other people have called us that we have believed are true. The only insults that will 'hurt' us are ones that *we* already believe are true. These are names such as 'stupid', 'evil', 'ugly', 'worthless', 'cowardly', 'bad', 'wrong', 'useless', 'unlovable', 'cold', 'idiot', 'failure', etc. These names are cruel, unfair exaggerations. They have a grain of truth but not more than that.

5. Because it is very painful to live under the weight of these names, we develop ways of being that try to prove that the opposite is true, for example people who secretly believe that they are cowardly failures may well become brash, aggressive, loud, confrontational people who love telling the world how successful they are. As a result, the scared and hurt child inside that person

never gets the nurture and reassurance that he or she needs and will continue to feel hurt inside, probably becoming louder and brasher as the anger regarding the unmet needs for warmth continues to increase.

6.   So what can we do if we have grown up with either inadequate nurture or our own special collection of cruel and hurtful names that we continue to call ourselves? We can learn to tell the truth to ourselves about ourselves and other people in a radical and responsible way. We can start to take responsibility for our own feelings, which means doing less blaming. We can learn to communicate our feelings effectively, honestly and respectfully. We can learn to become a good parent and best friend to ourselves. We can learn to ask for the honesty, warmth and support that we all need. Like learning to drive, these skills need to be patiently developed over time. Support will probably be necessary through books, group workshops or individual exploration with a trained professional.

7.   May you find the strength, courage and persistence to nurture your self-respect. It is a task that is demanding and that will bring out the very best and most lovable parts of you. Though an arduous task, there are few which can be more worth doing. With self-respect comes a new integrity, better psychosomatic health, satisfaction about the self and effectiveness in relationships, based on courage, clarity, honesty and love.

Appendix 9.2

Notes on terminology

Terms used in this chapter

ANORGASMIA – The inability to achieve orgasm.

ANXIOGENIC/ANXIOLYTIC – Describes something that increases or lessens anxiety. Holding one's breath may be anxiogenic, deep breathing may be anxiolytic.

CATHARSIS – The discharge of an emotion. We cathart sadness by crying, we cathart anger by shouting. We cathart fear by telling someone that we are afraid.

COGNITIVE BEHAVIOURAL THERAPY (CBT) – A form of counselling in which the patient's thoughts and subsequent actions are scrutinized. The past is not considered very important and results can be immediate.

DYSMENORRHOEA – Dysfunction of the menstrual cycle.

DYSPEPSIA – Difficulty with digestion.

DYSTHYMIA – A psychiatric term denoting mood-swing disorder.

HYSTERICAL PARALYSIS – An inability to use muscle(s) caused by the mind and its emotions.

IMMUNOSUPPRESSION – The reduction of normal functioning of the immune system.

PSYCHE-SOMA – A Greek expression for the mind-body system.

PSYCHODYNAMIC – Describes a way of understanding mental life and personality in which differing parts of the mind are in dynamic conflict with each other.

PSYCHOGENIC – This adjective is used to describe a symptom, such as a headache, which is caused by the mind (psyche) and its feelings rather than by a physical cause. Usually the cause will be the mismanagement of an emotion such as anxiety, anger or sadness.

RATIONAL EMOTIVE THERAPY – A variant of CBT in which more emphasis is placed on the patient's emotional world.

SOMATIZATION – The process by which an emotion, when inadequately discharged, takes up residence in the body. For example: an angry man who does not shout enough may somatize the anger as ulcers. Some people who handle stresses poorly may produce arytenoid granulomas. (Soma = body in Greek.)

VAGINISMUS – The mind-produced, involuntary contraction of the vaginal sphincter, rendering penetration painful or impossible.

Some other frequently encountered terms in the psychological assessment of voice disorder

PROJECTIVE IDENTIFICATION (PI) – A subtle and interesting psychological phenomenon mainly discussed by the psychoanalytic thinker Melanie Klein in the 1940s.) During PI the patient behaves in such a way as to get the other (teacher/spouse/therapist) to experience the emotion that they cannot themself experience. The emotion will be one of three: anger, anxiety or sadness. If the practitioner feels one of these and it has not been caused by what has been happening in his or her own private life, it is likely to be an emotion, identified projectively, (thrown forwards) into the practitioner and is experienced there, as if the patient has vomited it *into* the therapist.

PASSIVE AGGRESSIVE BEHAVIOUR – This is a variety of projective identification in which the patient behaves in such a way as to get the other person angry, not by shouting, but by quite passive behaviours such as sulking, stubbornness, avoidance, silence or non-cooperation.

SECONDARY GAIN – An emotional or relational benefit that the patient gains through their symptom(s), which can both reinforce and entrench the symptom(s).

SPLITTING – This is the name given in psychotherapy theory to the process in which someone reduces a complex situation to a simple 'all or nothing' split. For example, 'All French art is rubbish. There's nothing as good as Dutch art' or 'John's absolutely terrific but there's nothing good about Terry'. It is a primitive defence against anxiety. When a therapist hears someone saying something that sounds like a 'split', it is usually a sign that the person has a lot of buried feelings that he or she wishes to avoid. The giveaway words are: 'always/never', 'nobody/everybody/totally', 'absolutely', 'everything/nothing' and 'good/bad', and all their relations such as 'marvellous/terrible'. The person who is splitting is trying to avoid the painful greyness and complexity of the world – which demands thought – and is preferring to simplify and thereby distort reality. The Nazi holocaust is an example of splitting.

Psychotherapy: useful addresses for readers in the UK

Where an individual approach to psychotherapy or counselling is felt appropriate, the clinic is often asked how to go about finding help. The following alphabetical list is therefore included.

The British Association of Psychotherapists
37 Mapesbury Rd, London NW2 4HJ
Tel: 0181-452 9823

The British Guild of Psychotherapists
The Administrative Secretary
19b Thornton Hill, London SW19 4HU
Tel: 0181-947 0730

The Gestalt Centre
60 Bunhill Row,
London EC1
Tel: 0171-490-8274

The Lincoln Centre and Institute for Psychotherapy
19 Abbeville Mews, 88 Clapham Park Rd, London SW4 7BX
Tel: 0171-987 1545

The Tavistock Centre
120 Belsize Lane, London NW3 5BA
Tel: 0171-435 7111

You may also contact your local GP who will know of counselling services locally and Citizens Advice Bureaux will also know of local services.

References

Bridger MWM, Epstein R (1993) Functional voice disorders. A series of 109 patients. Journal of Laryngology and Otology 97: 1145–1148.

Freud S, Breuer J (1895) Studies on hysteria. Volume 1. In the standard edition of the Complete Psychological Works of Sigmund Freud. 24 volumes. London: Hogarth.

Gerritsma EJ (1991) An investigation into some personality characteristics of patients with psychogenic aphonia and dysphonia. Folia Phoniatrica 43: 13–20.

House A, Andrews HB (1987) The psychiatric and sound characteristics of patients with psychogenic dysphonia. Journal of Psychosomatic Research 31: 483–490.

Kinzl J, Bierl W, Rauchegger H (1988) Functional aphonia. A conversion symptom as a defensive mechanism against anxiety. Psychotherapy and Psychosomatics 49: 31–36.

Morrison M, Rammage L (1994) The management of voice disorders. San Diego: Singular Publishing Group Inc.

Further Reading

Clarkson P (1989) Gestalt counselling in action. Sage.
   This is especially for patients who interrupt the natural cycles of crying, shouting and breathing. Warmly written and fascinating.

Cleese J, Skynner R (1983) Families and how to survive them. Mandarin.
   A light hearted discussion of how we come to be the adults we become, between the famous comedian and a master of family therapy. Illustrated with great cartoons.

Lowen A (1958) The language of the body. Collier.
   On different personality types and the body shapes they tend to create. A good introduction to psychosomatic psychology.

Lowen A (1967) The betrayal of the body.
   How our way of seeing the world influences what we do with the self, the body, food, sex and behaviour patterns. How to reclaim the body from its defensive positions.

Lowen A (1975) Bioenergetics. Coventure.
   A comprehensive overview of the relationship between mind, personality, emotions and body states. Fascinating and transformational.

Yalom I (1989) Love's executioner. London: Penguin.
   A collection of ten tales of psychotherapy by a Professor of Psychiatry who specializes in philosophical therapy in the existential tradition. Informative, engaging and inspirational. This book may well assist patients to find the courage to enter counselling or psychotherapy.

CHAPTER 10

Drugs and the pharmacological treatment of dysphonia

TOM HARRIS

But know also that man has an inborn craving for medicine ... the desire to take medicine is one feature which distinguishes man the animal, from his fellow creatures. It is really one of the most serious difficulties with which we have to contend ... the doctor's visit is not thought to be complete without a prescription.

William Osler, 1894

Drugs that act on the vocal tract

Any disease, condition or symptom that affects the biomechanical function of any part of the vocal tract is of immediate concern to both the dysphonic patient and the phoniatrician treating them. Because of the social, professional and financial pressures that dysphonia places on many patients, clinicians are frequently persuaded to try pharmaceutical measures where, under other circumstances, only simple conservative measures would be undertaken. The sheer volume of propri-etary pharmaceuticals manufactured and sold, mostly without benefit of medical prescription, for 'the hoarse or tired voice' is enormous, and yet evidence that there is any therapeutic benefit is usually anecdotal at best. Most of the drugs prescribed for voicing problems are not even system-specific and are therefore liable to unwanted side effects. Many have more than one pharmacological mode of action and therefore produce a composite effect that is less than optimal. It is also appar-ent that in current clinical practice, many of the drugs prescribed are being used principally for placebo purposes. This chapter largely disregards cultural and national prescribing variations and considers only those drugs currently available that can be shown to have genuine applications in the treatment of dysphonias. The chapter is intended primarily for the medical reader, but clearly is of interest to other health professionals who may be faced with the consequences of inappropriate prescribing. We ask those without any background in pharmacology to bear with the inevitable use of terms to which they are not accustomed.

Most types of drugs used in current laryngological practice have been available for a number of years, and those in common use in Western, allopathic medical tradition may be summarized as:

- drugs that affect coughing and viscosity of mucus (cough suppressants; expectorants; mucolytics);
- drugs that modify allergic or asthmatic symptoms;
- anti-inflammatory drugs;
- bronchodilators;
- antibiotics;
- drugs that modify vocal performance are also occasionally prescribed. (These may act centrally, on the autonomic nervous system, on the endocrine system or peripherally on the motor end plates.)

Drugs that affect coughing and viscosity of mucus

The troublesome cough

Coughing serves a necessary, physiological function when it removes secretions, exudates or foreign material from the lower airways (the juicy cough that expels quantities of unpleasantness from the airways is usually referred to as a 'productive' cough). It is generally unwise to suppress this reflex as the lower respiratory tract is cleared less efficiently. 'Unproductive' or dry coughing has no such physiological function and may be treated symptomatically.

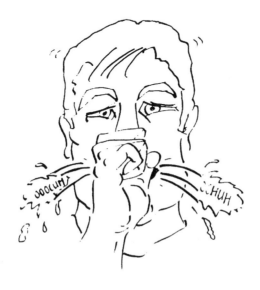

The most effective treatment for all coughs remains removal of the cause. In general, it is more effective (and more logical) to treat the irritation rather than the response (the resultant cough). For instance, where there is tracheobronchial irritation, stopping the cough is best achieved by soothing and reducing the swelling of the irritated mucous membranes with steam inhalations, thus reducing the input of nerve impulses indicating irritation on the afferent side of the cough reflex arc. Tincture of benzoin compound (Friar's Balsam) or other aromatics such as menthol may be added to the steam. The latter stimulates cold receptors in the mucosal lining of the airways. The brain interprets a 'cold' mucosa as one being exposed to a very considerable flow of air and thus a temporary illusion of a clear airway is produced. Steam inhalations should always be tried BEFORE using any other remedies to soothe an irritated vocal tract.

Treatment

As far as the voice clinic is concerned, the airway irritation is commonly most pronounced above the vocal folds, as in pharyngitis, for instance. In this case, simple demulcents or linctuses are soothing.

Demulcents are used in a similar manner to saliva substitutes (e.g. Salivart, Saliva Orthana) or tear substitutes (e.g. hypromellose); they coat an irritated or dry mucous membrane with a soothing low viscosity hydrophilic layer. The main constituents are water and carboxymethylcellulose, generally with additional sorbitol and electrolytes. There appear to be no harmful side effects in clinical practice.

All centrally acting cough suppressants (antitussives) will, to some extent, sedate patients. Sedation suppresses coughing, but may be disastrous if the patient is a performer. Antitussives fall into two main groups: the opiate-based cough suppressants acting in the medulla and on the higher cortical centres as a tranquillizer, and the antihistamine (H_1-receptor) suppressants that are used for their anticholinergic and sedating (but not their antihistaminic) actions. Both classes of drug also produce drying of the mucus blanket, which limits their value in the treatment of dysphonia. To complicate matters further, the latter group is commonly marketed in combination with a non-specific α-sympathomimetic agent such as pseudoephedrine (pseudepinephrine), which may cause a variety of side effects, ranging from insomnia, tachycardia (with occasional rise in blood pressure) and cardiac irritability, to urinary retention and rashes.

The therapeutic value of these medicines is limited, and although significant side effects are rare, the author feels that they have little place in modern phoniatry (see section on Drugs and the modification of performance below).

Caveat. Drugs that are known to have coughing as a side effect. Be aware of all the drugs a patient may be taking for other reasons, many may have problematic side effects on the vocal tract. Two examples known to cause refractory coughing are: ACE inhibitors used for treatment of hypertension and serotonin-selective reuptake inhibitors (SSRIs) such as fluoxetine (Prozac) used in the treatment of depression.

Stringy mucus

Respiratory mucus consists largely of water containing glycoproteins linked by disulphide bonds. Normally, around a litre is produced from the respiratory tract and swallowed every day. During respiratory infections there is an increase in 'normal' mucus production. In addition, protein-containing exudates from damaged membranes bind with the glycoproteins of the mucus, increasing their viscosity and producing thick, sticky accretions. A further problem associated with the period of recovery after upper respiratory tract infections is that, as a result of the damage inflicted to the cilia of the mucous membranes, they are no longer able to waft the thickened mucus blanket towards the stomach. The result is a build-up of the sticky accretions in the airway. To compound the problem further, the mucus has been in transit in a non-sterile environment for much longer than is normal in a healthy individual, and the increased time available permits much greater bacterial growth prior to its breakdown in the stomach. It is this bacterial overgrowth that colours the already stringy mucus and gives it its unpleasant taste and smell.

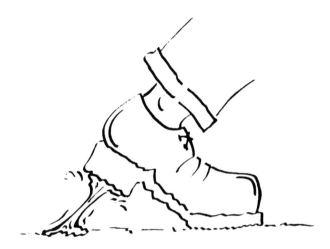

In Britain, these stringy accretions are traditionally attributed to 'sinusitis', and the doctor is likely to encounter considerable patient resistance to the idea that the offensive rubbish in their trachea or postnasal space is better treated by removal of the rubbish than by unhelpful courses of antibiotics.

Treatment

Whatever the cause of mucus stasis, it is effectively treated by nasal douching with a spray of normal saline. Modern buildings are frequently air-conditioned, producing artificially low levels of humidity; many homes now possess central heating, which also lowers levels of humidity – witness the level of drying out and damage to furniture or other wood when the heating is turned on when the weather turns cold. Most means of transport are also equipped with means of drying out mucous membranes, the most obvious examples being the car heater and the ventilation system in an aircraft that normally bleeds totally dry air from the compressor stage of the engine inlet to supply the cabin space. A portable spray of normal saline solution for the hand luggage is strongly recommended to those performers who have to travel long distances between performances.

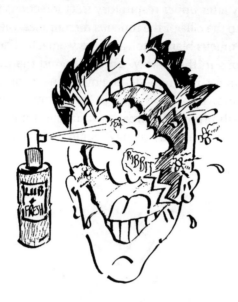

Further down the respiratory tract mucolytic drugs may be used to thin mucus. This makes clearance of mucus from the airways more effective, and by making the mucus act more like a lubricant and less like glue may, on occasion, improve an unreliable vocal attack. Acetylcysteine and methylcysteine have free sulfhydryl groups that can open disulphide groups in mucus, thus reducing viscosity. They are administered in aerosol inhalation, although acetylcysteine and the related carbocysteine may also be taken orally.

A small caution, however. All of these may from time to time produce gastrointestinal irritation or allergic reactions. Another mucus-thinning drug, bromhexine, may also be taken orally but is no longer universally available. Detergent aerosols, such as tyloxapol, are probably more irritant and not significantly more effective than the above.

Expectorant drugs cause hypersecretion of mucus, the rationale for their use being that a dry cough becomes productive and that the resultant expectoration is less viscous. Expectorant preparations may contain iodides, chlorides, bicarbonates, citrates, guaifenesin, ipecacuanha, creosotes or squill. They all have undoubted placebo value in clinical practice, although in high doses many exhibit emetic properties as well.

Caveat. Many drugs in common clinical use have enormous numbers of side effects as they are very non-specific in action. For example Largactil (chlorpromazine) is so named because it is a dopamine antagonist but has, in addition, anticholinergic and a-adrenergic blocking activity. Small wonder that the side effects range from (reversible) dry mouth and upper airways to (irreversible) tardive dyskinesia.

Drugs that modify allergic or asthmatic symptoms

It is impossible to produce good voice with inadequate air support if the chest cannot release its reservoir of air. Histamine is an inflammatory mediator that occurs widely in the surface membranes of the body in bound form in mast cells. It is released either in response to noxious stimuli, immunoglobulin (IgE) activity in anaphylactoid (Type 1) allergy, or by precipitating antibodies in the slower Type 3 reaction. Histamine release is accompanied by other inflammatory mediators such as peptides (kinins) and arachidonic acid derivatives (leukotrienes and prostaglandins). These mediators act on intracellular cyclic AMP and GMP and produce the changes found in asthma – constriction of bronchial smooth muscle, production of bronchial mucosal oedema and excessive mucus production.

There are at least two different receptor types. The H_1-receptor sites, which are found in the respiratory tract, are associated with production of symptoms such as asthma, and the H_2-sites, which are found chiefly in the alimentary tract, are associated with the control of digestive activity. Recent generations of antihistamine drugs have been designed to be specific for each receptor type.

Treatment

The most successful treatment of allergic symptoms remains avoidance by identification and exclusion of identifiable allergens from the patient's environment. Taking a medical history usually identifies probable candidates, and this is confirmed by skin prick testing with known allergen preparations. Blood tests can detect a rise in the general level of serum IgE globulin, which indicates the probability of an allergic reaction but not the implicated allergen.

Raised allergen-specific IgE levels in type 1 allergies are (more expensively) identified by RAST testing the patient's serum. In asthmatic conditions, allergens may be identified by provocation testing, getting the patient to inhale minute quantities of the suspected allergen, although this test is not without risk.

Antihistamines are competitive inhibitors at receptor sites and are most useful if administered prior to allergen exposure in, for example, hayfever. They generally have associated anticholinergic effects, and while they are useful in the prevention and treatment of allergic manifestations in the nose, eye and larynx, they are also commonly associated with an increase in the viscosity of the mucosal blanket and sedation. Insomnia, nervousness and tremor are also common. Astemizole, terfenadine and ketotifen are relatively recent examples among many that are relatively free from side effects. They are not useful in the treatment of intrinsic, delayed type asthma (Laurence and Bennett, 1987).

Mast-cell stabilizers such as sodium cromoglycate inhibit release of mediators from sensitized mast cells. Aerosol preparations are useful in the prevention of allergic symptoms of the respiratory tract as they have minimal side effects. Sodium cromoglycate is not nearly so effective in the prevention of food allergy.

On occasion, singers complain of performance-related vocalization problems due to increased bronchial reactivity, a vocal equivalent of exercise- or cold-induced asthma (Cohn et al., 1991). As in the case of asthma, any alteration in the characteristics of a vocalist's lung function can significantly alter their technique for breath support. These patients respond satisfactorily to treatment with bronchodilators. A small practical difficulty may arise from the administration of this drug as an aerosol into the airways; although the drug itself is remarkably free from side effects in the larynx, from time to time patients may complain that the aerosol leaves a rather porridgy layer on the mucosa, which can interfere with normal voicing patterns.

Bronchodilators in current clinical practice come in two categories: β_2-adrenoreceptor agonists eg salbutamol, rimiterol, terbutaline, fenoterol and reproterol, and xanthine derivatives e.g. theophylline, aminophylline. The first group have limited activity at the (cardiac) β_1-receptor, but act mainly on bronchial tissue at the mast cell and smooth muscle by increasing intracellular cyclic AMP, which diminishes mediator release (see below) and produces bronchodilatation. The second group reduce the breakdown of cyclic AMP, achieving a similar effect by a different route. Unsurprisingly, the actions of the two groups are additive. The most troublesome side effect that may occur in vocalists is an occasional increase in reflux oesophagitis with the use of xanthines.

Glucocorticoid steroids have enjoyed a place in the laryngologist's armamentarium since the 1950s, when the first semi-synthetic preparations were marketed. They produce their anti-inflammatory effect in the delayed allergic response by entering mast cells passively and inducing production of the protein lipocortin. This in turn inhibits the enzymatic production of arachidonic acid, the precursor of the prostaglandin and leukotriene mediators. They also have anti-inflammatory effects by reduction of the vascular response and inhibition of the cellular component of the inflammatory response, together with diminution of capillary proliferation and fibrin deposition of chronic inflammation.

All this may be of clinical benefit to the dysphonic patient in the short term. Other effects of steroids are less desirable in phoniatry: muscle bulk is reduced by most steroids through gluconeogenesis, and associated fat redistribution. Immunosuppressive actions and mineralocorticoid water retention cannot be entirely avoided. Dysphonia is a common complication of inhaled steroid therapy and it has been suggested that steroids produce dyskinesia of the intrinsic laryngeal musculature, and that this in turn may produce bowing of the vocal folds (Williams. et al., 1983; Toogood, 1990). Inhaled steroids may also exacerbate many dysphonias associated with stress or clinical hypothyroidism and can, on occasion, precipitate oesophageal candidiasis, especially where frequent maintenance doses are required (Toogood et al., 1980). Steroids are also prone to exacerbate reflux oesophagitis, especially when used in conjunction with bronchodilator xanthines, such as theophylline.

Delivery systems affect where the drug is deposited in the airway (Moren, 1978; Dolovich et al., 1983). Where it is necessary to treat asthma in a performer, the routine use of a spacer with the inhaler and post-inhalational breath holding maximize the steroid deposited in the lower respiratory tract and minimize deposition in the laryngopharynx (Newman et al., 1982). In general, there are fewer side effects associated with inhaled steroids than with therapeutically equivalent doses of systemic steroids, such as prednisolone (Toogood, 1987). However, laryngologists contemplating rechallenging patients with a history of inhaled steroid induced hoarseness should be aware that one study found a 60% recurrence rate (Settipane et al., 1987).

Pharyngo-oesophageal acid reflux and dysphonia

During the last decade it has often been reported that dysphonia may be concomitant with oesophageal acid reflux (Jones et al., 1990). If asked directly whether they are suffering from 'heartburn' in the clinic, very few patients will answer 'yes'. However, further direct questioning as to attributable symptoms noticeably increases the incidence. There has been considerable work done on the objective measurement of what is, at best, a very intermittent phenomenon, and careful history-taking plus fibreoptic oesophagoscopy to indicate significant oesophagitis will only identify around 42% of refluxers. Twenty four-hour ambulatory pH monitoring provides much greater specificity (Jenkinson et al., 1989), but even then there will remain a quorum of patients whose symptoms are not confirmed by endoscopy or monitoring but who improve dramatically with a course of treatment to reduce acid exposure.

There is still controversy as to whether the dysphonia reported in some patients with acid reflux arises as a direct result of mucosal irritation from laryngeal overspill onto the posterior third of the larynx, or from (possibly protective) reflex hyperkinetic activity of the vocal tract. In one trial (Jones et al., 1990), over 50% of patients with hoarseness who reported symptoms of reflux more than once per week were proven by ambulatory pH/manometry monitoring and fibre endoscopy to have significant reflux. Treatment with H_2-blockers, e.g. cimetidine or ranitidine, coupled with antacids, over a period of 6 weeks produces an improvement in voicing in approximately 65% of patients. Where control of symptoms from proven acid reflux is poor with H_2-blockers, proton pump inhibitors such as omeprazole or lansoprazole are highly effective. Where long-term maintenance is required, however, we are not happy to leave dysphonic patients on drugs inhibiting acid secretion. Twenty four-hour manometric monitoring of gastro-oesophageal acid reflux seems to suggest that nocturnal reflux, when the patients are lying flat in bed, while not necessarily producing more oesophagitis, still presents the biggest problem. There is still no irrefutable evidence of which we are aware, but it seems that when lying flat there is a higher incidence of acid coming back as far as the pharynx, producing episodes of paroxysmal nocturnal coughing

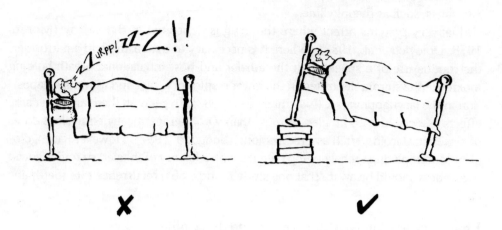

and/or laryngospasm as well as hoarseness. We therefore prefer to try those patients whose symptoms are improved by proton pump inhibitors on a regimen involving elevating the head of the bed on blocks and treating them with a prokinetic agent, cisapride.

Antibiotics

Despite the universal awareness that antibiotics are intended for the treatment of bacterial infection, there is still a widespread tendency to administer them 'prophylactically' to vocal performers suffering from (usually viral) upper respiratory tract infections, even where there are minimal dysphonic symptoms. The usual justification of this practice is that it allays the patient's anxiety. Among the conditions they are used to treat are the following.

Sinusitis

Doctors are frequently guilty of prescribing antibiotics for 'sinusitis' when a patient complains of a small quantity of mucopus in the nose, together with a sensation of reduced nasal airway and an altered sensation of resonance. Genuine sinusitis, with pus present in one or more of the normally air-filled sinuses, is only satisfactorily proven by a coronal CAT scan of the sinuses showing uniform thickening of the mucosal lining of the involved sinus, a fluid level or total opacity. Puncture of a maxillary antrum (the sinus found in the cheek) and washing out the cavity may be required in order to prove the presence of pus. Thickening of the mucosal linings of the nasal cavities and sinuses may alter a patient's perception of resonance, but the change is subjective rather than objective. Very frequently the patient may complain of 'sinusitis' when they have in fact got a degree of vasomotor rhinitis, which does not respond to antibiotics or antiallergic treatments.

Tonsillitis

Tonsillitis is a much abused term that is used by patients and doctors alike to cover all forms of oropharyngeal infection. Routine use of a throat swab for culture would diminish the prescription of antibiotics considerably. If a patient is apyrexial and has had a sore throat for less than 24 hours, then, in the author's view, commencing antibiotic cover is very unlikely to improve vocal performance within the next 48 hours. There is, therefore, no justification for initiating antibiotic cover until the bacterial nature of the infection has been demonstrated. If, on the other hand, there is a bacterial infection that requires treatment, then prescription of a 5-day course of antibiotics will render the patient apyrexial but may well be insufficient to prevent the infection recurring.

Laryngotracheobronchitis

Many of the antibiotics prescribed for this condition are broad-spectrum. This practice does not obviate the risk of superinfection, but instead increases the likelihood of laryngopharyngeal candidiasis. It is to be hoped that in future, the use of antibiotics for their placebo value will decline.

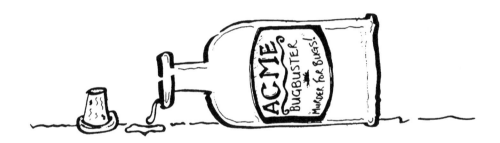

Drugs and the modification of performance

Laryngologists today are in a privileged position when it comes to the pharmacological modification of voicing. It is not an illegal act for a medical practitioner to prescribe a steroid, a strong opiate analgesic or a sympathomimetic amine for a performer, whereas if the performance was to be regarded as athletic and subject to international rules of competition, then the use of such drugs could lead to a lifetime ban from competition.

Bodies such as the International Olympic Committee seek not only to prevent athletic competitors from gaining an unfair advantage, but also to prevent athletes from seriously damaging themselves by their inappropriate use of drugs in their pursuit of excellence (IOC, 1989; British Sports Council, 1989). It is therefore useful to be aware of those drugs that are banned by the IOC and to compare them with those commonly prescribed for voice-users. More than 40 sympathomimetic amines or respiratory stimulants such as ephedrine, pseudoephedrine and phenylpropanolamine, many of which are freely available in 'cold cures' and hayfever preparations, are all banned drugs.

Athletes with asthma may only use one of four aerosols of the β_2-adrenorecep-tor agonists: bitolterol, orciprenaline, rimiterol, salbutamol and terbutaline. Of the narcotic analgesics, only dextromethorphan is acceptable as an antitussive. Diuret-ics for the purpose of weight loss are banned, as are peptide hormones and β-blockers. Anabolic steroids that have a structure and activity related to testosterone are, of course, banned. It is worthwhile for the clinician to remember that anabolic steroids have a variety of side effects, ranging from psychological to liver and cardiovascular damage, which may be lethal. Even in the dose range that phoniatri-cians might be tempted to use, there may be subfertility in males and virilization in women with its attendant and irreversible alteration in pitch range and timbre (Beckford et al., 1985). The author feels that there is no place in clinical practice for the treatment of 'vocal fatigue' by steroids.

Centrally-acting benzodiazepine tranquillizers and peripherally acting β-block-ers are banned from competition requiring fine motor control. They might be thought to provide a legitimate advantage if applied to vocalists. They do not. The only dysphonia transitorily amenable to a (high) dose of benzodiazepine is a true hysterical conversion. Vocal performance after low-dose tranquillizers may suffer in a similar manner to preperformance alcohol ingestion.

'The Pearlies' (lack of accustomed muscle control with or without tremor, brought on by extreme stress associated with live performance) β-blockade appears to reduce symptoms of abnormal anxiety in musicians, and may actually improve performance (James et al., 1977), but the same is sadly not true of young singers whose performance is not improved (Gates and Montalbo, 1987).

'Recreational drugs'

The great majority of drugs taken to modify performance are not on the prescrip-tion of the doctor, they are simply 'recreational drugs'. The majority of recre-ational drugs do not enhance performance, but are likely to alter the taker's perceptions of events. In most countries, apart from those products found in liquor stores and tobacconists, they can only be purchased illegally. Most have significant mental and physical side effects. A glass of port has been suggested as being 'good for the performer' before a performance, a half bottle of scotch is certainly not. Alcohol irritates, anaesthetizes and then pickles mucous membranes, it impairs judgement and motor control, and, in the last resort, audiences are not amused by unscripted accidents into the orchestra pit. Similarly with cannabis-related substances; their smoke is very irritating to the larynx, and the loss of motor control greatly diminishes performing skills. The affected person will probably find the loss of skill and the hoarseness hilarious; unfortunately audiences generally won't. 'Sniffing a line' of cocaine will make the user feel alert and brilliant, it will also be liable to precipitate psychotic activity, especially when the use becomes habitual. Sigmund Freud was initially an advocate until he saw what it was doing to himself and to others. It will also irretrievably damage the mucosa where it is deposited because of its very powerful vasoconstrictor activity. Psychotropic drugs (e.g. LSD and 'angel dust') are potentially extremely damaging to the mind if not the body. Greed and the nature of availability ensure that doses and contents of 'illegal substances' are unreliable at best. To see just one performer with a career destroyed by 'a couple of bad trips' is enough to persuade most clinicians that the price for 'seeing the pretty lights' is too high. Even drugs with recognized pharmacological value become hazardous when used inappropriately. Benzodiazepines and barbiturates become 'downers', outdated slimming pills become 'Es', and so on. There is no control in relation to addiction, and the users of substances such as 'Ecstasy', which the subculture has deemed 'safe', are generally unaware of idiosyncratic effects, ranging from hyperthermia and cardiovascular collapse to acute drug-induced paranoia, until they become the victims.

Drug treatment of the dysphonia of ageing

Ageing of the human vocal tract produces perceptual, acoustic and anatomical changes, many of which are apparent to the patient and observer alike. Proposed mechanisms for ageing abound: free radical oxidation due to loss of mixed-function oxidases; covalent and hydrogen bond cross-linkage between molecules and genetically programmed cell death have all been postulated (Chodzko-Zajko and Ringel, 1987) and may all occur in nature. Age-related changes in the larynx include structural modifications, such as calcification, banana-like remodelling of the arytenoid vocal processes, muscle atrophy with fewer but larger motor-pools (nerve–muscle connections), fewer 'fast-twitch' muscle fibres and degeneration of the vocal ligament (Hirano et al., 1983). These changes make the ageing subject much more susceptible to the stretching, thinning and bowing of the vocal folds that may be a late result of persistent vocal hyperfunction. Workers such as Biever and Bless (1989) have tied acoustic and aerodynamic measures to videostroboscopic findings in the elderly and have identified the most striking stroboscopically observed changes in vocal function: greater aperiodicity, incomplete glottal closure, mucosal wave alterations and reduced amplitude of vibrations. Acoustic and aerodynamic measures exhibited greater shimmer and more intersubject variability in F_o and mean airflow rates. Baken suggests that the activity is increasingly chaotic (R. Baken, personal communication, 1994).

Age-related changes in the body's metabolism and function are at present irresistible, although in the short term, many patients with characteristically ageing voices may seek help in delaying the change. From the pharmacological viewpoint there is little to offer the patient with early phonasthenia other than hormonal support. At the present time, only hormonal support in women in and after the climacteric has been adequately researched to the point where it may be offered in clinical practice.

Oestrogen and the larynx

Research has demonstrated that the epithelial cells of the human larynx have high affinity membrane receptors for 17-ß-oestradiol (Aufdemorte et al., 1983;

Fergusson et al., 1987). The numbers of these receptors are comparable with those found in breast, ovary and uterine tissue (Abramson et al., 1983). In 1961 it was suggested that oestrogen could affect the quality of the mesenchymal extracellular matrix or 'ground substance' by causing a breakdown of mucopolysaccharides into smaller units, thus shifting the normal sol–gel equilibrium towards the sol state. Fergusson's work (1987) has suggested that surface sites, when triggered, induce changes in calcium equilibrium, which in turn triggers cytoplasmic synthesis and nuclear breakdown. The biochemistry of the stimulation of the oestrogen receptor, which was originally researched in primary breast carcinoma, has shed some further light on the mode of action of the oestrogen receptor (Parker, 1991). Parker states that binding of the oestradiol ligand primarily favours dimerization and hence DNA binding, and secondarily activates the oestrogen-dependent transcription activation factor (TAF-2).

Clinical considerations

From a clinical standpoint, Abitbol et al.'s series (1989) found that the cyclical changes in cytological smears taken from the vocal folds followed *pari passu* the menstrual changes found in cervical smears. These findings support the clinical observations of vocal changes noted in the female voice in the premenstrual period and during the climacteric. Abramson et al. performed a detailed evaluation of a large group of trained singers' subjective impressions of premenstrual changes in vocal quality in 1984 and commented that the findings confirmed the clinical impression that there is a small drop in fundamental frequency together with a loss of vocal quality in the premenstrual period. They added that the changes could not be accounted for in terms of absolute oestrogen levels, but seemed more dependent on changes in level, especially where there was a small sharp drop (Abrahamson et al., 1984).

Hormone replacement therapy (HRT)

Cardozo has nicely summarized the current state of management of post-menopausal symptoms (Cardozo and McPherson, 1991). The menopause now occurs in European women at an average of 51 years, as judged by the last monthly period. The symptoms of oestrogen withdrawal may become apparent during the five or more pre-menopausal years or 'climacteric'.

In addition to a perceived loss of timbre and loss of the top of the vocal range, phoniatricians should be aware of other age-related findings in the following broad categories:

- Vasomotor dysfunction (hot flushes, night sweats). This is an immediate manifestation of oestrogen withdrawal.
- Psychosocial troubles (mood changes, depression, insomnia, loss of memory etc.) are implicated by association, but no causal link has yet been established with hormonal depletion.

- Urogenital dysfunction (vaginal dryness, etc.) typically sets in within a few years of the menopause.
- Osteoporosis and cardiovascular disease are late complications of lack of oestrogen support.

Oestrogen replacement is generally successful in the symptomatic relief of the first three categories. It also reduces osteoporosis and the death rate from cardio-vascular disease. Its disadvantage is that it can also affect the breast and other sensitive tissue. Although HRT is not contraindicated in cases of benign breast disease, and its short-term use does not seem to have any increased risks attached, with long-term use (10–20 years) there is an increased level of risk of 50% of devel-oping breast cancer. This risk is much reduced if a combination HRT dose of oestrogen plus progestogen is given. It should be noted, however, that in 10% of women progestogen causes either premenstrual tension syndrome (PMT) or migraine. HRT is contraindicated where there is a history of breast or endometrial cancer. Some women may find it 'unacceptable' because of continuing cyclical withdrawal bleeds.

HRT may be administered orally, or by implants, patches or vaginally. Contrary to popular belief, it does not in itself lead to an increase in blood pressure or to weight gain. Little research has been done to date to demonstrate the changes in vocal function that may be produced by long-term administration of HRT.

Between 7 and 8% of postmenopausal women in Britain are on HRT and then usually only for a brief period. The percentage in the United States is much higher.

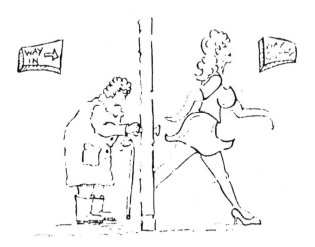

Drugs affecting neurological problems

Spasmodic dysphonia was first described as a clinical entity in a paper by Traube in 1871. Unfortunately, further research into this affliction virtually ceased for the next 70 years as the disorder was held to be an hysterical phenomenon on the grounds that most sufferers were women, that many of them could associate the problem with stress, that their vocal folds looked 'normal' on examination and their singing voice was affected less than the speaking voice. As hysteria became a less popular diagnosis, the cause of the condition was relabelled 'psychoneurosis', and it is only in the last 15 years that the underlying organic factors have begun to be generally recognized.

Spasmodic dysphonia is a condition that has been described as 'trying to talk whilst being choked' (Critchley, 1939). More recent work suggests that the condition properly belongs to the group of focal dystonias, and it is now frequently referred to as laryngeal dystonia (Blitzer and Brin, 1988) This is a neurological disorder of central motor processing characterized by action-induced spasms of the vocal folds that are poorly controlled by the patient and exacerbated by stress. Related focal and segmental presentations of dystonia may include blepharospasm, oromandibular dystonia and hemifacial spasm, spasmodic torti-collis, cranial–cervical dystonia (Meige's syndrome), writer's cramp and other task-specific dystonias. These syndromes may be dominated by involuntary sustained (tonic) or repetitive patterned muscle contractions. Tremor often accompanies dystonia (Blitzer et al., 1988; Jancovic and Brin, 1991)

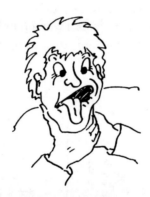

Seventeen per cent of the series of patients with primary laryngeal dystonia described by Blitzer and Brin had a family history of dystonia. Family studies have identified an autosomal dominant inheritance with incomplete penetrance, and a recent development is the identification of a gene locus marker in the q32–34 region on chromosome 9 (Bressman et al., 1989; Ozelius et al., 1989). This finding may open up the possibility of reduction in the incidence of dystonias in the future by genetic means.

Treatment of laryngeal dystonia

Psychotherapy, biofeedback and speech therapy rarely improve voicing objectively by more than a modest and unreliable margin. Occasionally marked relief of dystonic symptoms may be achieved pharmacologically, but results are likewise not reliable. The most useful drugs in current clinical practice at the present time are muscle relaxants and anticholinergic drugs such as benzhexol (known as trihexyphenidyl in the USA) (Artane) (Burke et al., 1986) either singly or in combination with other drugs. Drugs suggested as adjuncts in more severe cases are: dopamine receptor-blocking drugs such as pimozide (Orap), an antipsychotic of the diphenyl-butyl-piperidine group; reserpine-like drugs such as tetrabenazine (Nitoman), which acts on amines such as serotonin and noradrenaline (norepinephrine) and which depletes dopamine and blocks dopamine receptors in the brain (Jancovic and Orman, 1988).

Examples of other drugs currently used in attempts to relieve dystonic and tremulous symptoms are:

- Clonidine (Dixarit), which in low dosage is sometimes useful in the treatment of 'tics'. Clonidine is an alpha-blockade agent, usually associated with the treatment of hypertension and migraine. It has more recently found a place in the treatment of neurological problems such as Gilles de la Tourette syndrome, in which dystonic 'tic' features are apparent. Its mode of action is not known.
- Benztropine (Cogentin), a drug with powerful anticholinergic effects mostly used to treat Parkinsonian tremor.
- Ethopropazine (in the USA), a phenothiazine derivative developed for the symptomatic relief of Parkinsonism.
- Benzodiazepine tranquillizers/anticonvulsants, e.g. clonazepam (Rivotril) and carbamazepine (Tegretol).
- Levodopa and related dopa-decarboxylase inhibitors, e.g. Sinemet and Larodopa, developed to treat Parkinsonian rigidity/spasticity.

Treatment of focal or segmental dystonias with any of the above drugs is directed at symptomatic relief, and none deal precisely with the underlying neurological problem.

Caveat: All these drugs are accompanied by significant side effects and interactions. Good control of symptoms without the development of (occasionally severe and irreversible) attendant problems, e.g. tardive dyskinesia, is unusual, hence the recent interest in treating the problem at the site where it is being expressed as a loss of normal motor control.

Surgery to interrupt motor nerves supplying dystonic muscle groups provides one such solution. In 1976 Dedo published results of recurrent laryngeal nerve section for spasmodic dysphonia (Dedo, 1976) and produced satisfactory improvement in many cases of poor voicing. The principal advantage of recurrent laryngeal nerve section is that surgical treatment is usually required once, and the vocal result is, in most cases, permanent. The obvious disadvantage is that the treatment produces a gross 'all-or-nothing' qualitative change, without any means of control to produce a quantitative incremental response. Other surgical variants have been published since then, but still suffer from the problem that any return of innervation is accompanied by a return of dysphonia.

It was for these reasons that chemical means of highly selective denervation were sought, which would preferably be permanent and could be used to produce a subtotal response. The most effective agent introduced into clinical practice to date has been purified botulinum toxin A, a neurotoxin consisting of a light and heavy protein chain linked by a disulphide bridge. Experiments were begun in 1973 in rhesus monkeys (Scott et al., 1973), and first applied in clinical practice in 1980 for the treatment of strabismus (Scott, 1980). The toxin works preferentially on peripheral cholinergic motor end plates, and has the great advantage over many other neurotoxins that it is extremely specific to this site. Blockade of acetylcholine release is produced by the light chain fraction within the nerve end, the heavy chain fraction being necessary for selective binding to the motor end plate and the disulphide bridge for internalization of the toxin into the nerve. The two most important sources of purified toxin at present are: in the UK, Dysport (Porton Products), and in the USA, Occulinum (Allergan Corp.). These products are, of course, not generally available, and are only for use in laboratories on a 'named patient' basis.

Treatment is commonly carried out by direct injection under electromyographic control of diluted toxin into the laryngeal musculature, using a Monopolar hollow 26 gauge Teflon-coated needle electrode. Ford et al. (1990) have suggested that an alternative indirect laryngoscopic approach and placement of the injection under visual guidance is more accurate. The normal site of injection is one (or both) vocalis muscle(s) for adductor dystonia. Attempts have been made to treat abductor dystonia by injecting the PCA muscle. The results are less satisfactory. We would suggest that, in cases of adductor dystonia, it may be more logical to inject the lateral cricoarytenoid rather than the vocalis. This would allow for approximation of the folds for speech while reducing the subject's ability to seal the folds totally with their dystonic activity.

The principal drawback to this current means of treatment of laryngeal dystonia is the temporary nature of the induced paralysis. Many patients may require further injections at intervals ranging from 3 months upwards. In the search for a more permanent solution, laboratories in Britain and the USA have synthesized a conjugate of the heavy chain of botulinum toxin with another potent and permanent toxin, ricin. This substance has not as yet undergone any laboratory trials for receptor specificity or clinical applicability, but might, in the future, provide a more permanent pharmacological solution in the treatment of dystonias.

What of the future?

Pharmacological treatment of voice disorder is always going to be most usefully applied when the symptom has a distinct, single pathological process underlying it. Possible avenues for future research are therefore as wide and numerous as ever, and research will undoubtedly bring new groups of drugs into the arena of clinical treatment of voice disorder. It is already possible to reduce myxoedematous thickening of the vocal fold cover with thyroxine supplements, but what about properly conducted trials of tretinoin and its derivatives in the treatment of dysplasia of the vocal fold mucosa? Even more dramatic are the possibilities offered by current research into the role of the telomeres of the chromosomes. Might it be possible in future to arrest the, until now, inevitable ageing process that finishes careers? In future there may be a larger and more useful place in the voice clinic for pharmaceuticals than we have seen so far.

The place of medication in multimodality treatment

In general, voicing is a biomechanical activity involving many body systems, and the present ability of a doctor to alleviate the symptoms of dysphonia by pharmacological means is limited either to the treatment of discrete pathological processes or to non-specific modification of mood or metabolism. With few exceptions, modification of vocal symptoms precipitated by inefficient vocal behavioural patterns remains outside the remit of pharmacological treatment alone.

We find that modification of inefficient vocal gestures in combination with appropriate pharmacotherapy may be much more effective than drug therapy alone (Harris and Lieberman 1993). Indeed, in the great majority of pathological processes producing dysphonia, where drug treatment is applicable, the result is improved if vocal rehabilitation therapy is also part of the treatment plan.

References

Abitbol J, de Brux J, Millot G (1989) Does a hormonal vocal cord cycle exist in women? Study of vocal premenstrual syndrome in voice performers by videostroboscopy-glottography and cytology on 38 women. Journal of Voice 3: 157–162.

Abramson A, Essman E, Steinberg B (1983) Membrane receptors for 17-ß-oestradiol in the human larynx. Transcripts of the 12th Symposium Care of the Professional Voice II, pp. 292–294.

Abramson AL et al. (1984) Estrogen receptors in the human larynx: clinical study of the singing voice. Transcripts of the 13th Symposium Care of the Professional Voice II, pp. 409–413.

Aufdemorte TB, Sheridan PJ, Holt GR (1983) Autoradiographic evidence of sex steroid receptors in laryngeal tissues of baboon (papiocynocephalus). Laryngoscope 93: 1607–1611.

Beckford NS, Rood SR, Schaid D (1985) Androgen stimulation and laryngeal development. Annals of Otology, Rhinology and Laryngology 94: 634–640.

Biever DM, Bless DM (1989) Vibratory characteristics of the vocal folds in young adult and geriatric women. Journal of Voice 3: 120–131.

Blitzer A, Brin M (1988) Laryngeal dystonia: a series with botulinum toxin therapy. Annals of Otology, Rhinology and Laryngology 100: 85–89.

Blitzer A, Brin MF, Fahn S, Lovelace RE (1988) Clinical and laboratory characteristics of focal dystonia: study of 110 cases. Laryngoscope 98: 636–640.

Bressman SB, de Leon D, Brin MF et al. (1989) Idiopathic dystonia among Ashkenazi Jews: evidence for autosomal dominant inheritance. Annals of Neurology 26: 612–620.

British Sports Council Doping Control Information Pack (1989) Drugs and sport: a comprehensive guide. Media Medica (UK); MIMS (Australia).

Burke RE, Fahn S, Marsden CD (1986) Torsion dystonia: a double-blind, prospective trial of high-dosage trihexyphenidyl. Neurology 36: 160–164.

Cardozo L, McPherson K (1991) Medicalising the menopause; hormone replacement therapy – solution or problem? Journal of the Royal Society of Medicine 84: 567–569.

Chodzko-Zajko WJ, Ringel RL (1987) Physiological aspects of aging. Journal of Voice 1: 18–26.

Cohn JR, Sataloff RT, Spiegel JR, Fish JE, Kennedy K (1991) Airway reactivity-induced asthma in singers (arias). Journal of Voice 5:332–337.

Critchley M (1939) Spastic dysphonia ('inspiratory speech'). Brain 62: 96–103.

Dedo HH (1976) Recurrent laryngeal nerve section for spastic dysphonia. Annals of Otology 85: 451.

Dolovich M, Ruffin R, Newhouse MT (1983) Clinical evaluation of a simple demand inhalation device. MDI aerosol delivery device. Chest 84: 36–41.

Fergusson BJ, Hudson WR, McCarty KS (1987) Sex steroid receptor distribution in the human larynx and laryngeal carcinoma. Archives of Otolaryngology and Head and Neck Surgery 113: 1311–1315.

Ford CN, Bless DM, Lowery JD (1990) Indirect laryngoscopic approach for injection of botulinum toxin in spasmodic dysphonia. Otolaryngology, Head and Neck Surgery 103: 752–758.

Gates GA, Montalbo PJ (1987) The effect of low-dose ß-blockade on performance anxiety in singers. Journal of Voice 1: 105–108.

Harris TM, Lieberman J (1993) Integrated pharmacologic, therapeutic and manipulative approach to treatment of granulomatous based dysphonias. The Pacific Voice Conference, San Francisco.

Hirano M, Kurita S, Nakashima T (1983) Growth, development and aging of human vocal folds. In Bless DM, Abbs JM (Eds) Vocal fold physiology. San Diego: College Hill Press, pp. 22–43.

International Olympic Committee (1989) List of doping classes and treatment guidelines. Doping control information booklet No. 2. British Sports Council.

James IM, Pearson RM, Griffith DNM et al. (1977) Effect of oxprenolol on stage-fright in musicians. Lancet 2: 952–954.

Jancovic J, Brin MF (1991) Therapeutic uses of botulinum toxin. New England Journal of Medicine 324: 1186–1194.

Jancovic J, Orman J (1988) Tetrabenazine therapy of dystonia, chorea, tics and other dyskinesias. Neurology 38: 391–394.

Jenkinson LR, Norris TL, Watson A (1989) Symptoms and endoscopic findings – can they predict abnormal nocturnal acid gastro-oesophageal reflux? Annals of the Royal College of Surgeons of England 71: 117–119.

Jones NS et al. (1990) Acid reflux and hoarseness. Journal of Voice 4: 355-358.

Laurence DR, Bennett PN (1987) Clinical pharmacology (6th Edn). Edinburgh: Churchill Livingstone.

Moren F (1978) Drug deposition of pressurised inhalation aerosols. I. Influence of actuator tube design. International Journal of Pharmacology 1: 205–212.

Newman SP, Pavia D, Garland N (1982) Effects of various inhalation modes on the deposition of radioactive pressurised aerosols. European Journal of Respiratory Diseases 63 (suppl) 119: 57–65.

Ozelius L, Kramer PL, Moskowitz CB et al. (1989) Human gene for torsion dystonia located on chromosome 9q32-q34. Neuron 2: 1427–1434.

Parker M (1991) Oestrogen receptors in breast carcinoma. Presentation at 73rd annual meeting of the Endocrine Society, Washington DC, USA.

Scott AB (1980) Botulinum toxin injections into extraocular muscles as an alternative to strabismus surgery. Ophthalmology 87: 1044–1049.

Scott AB, Rosenbaum A, Collins CC (1973) Pharmacological weakening of extraocular muscles. Invest. Ophthalmol. 12: 924–927.

Settipane GA, Kalliel JN, Klein DE (1987) Rechallenge of patients who developed oral candidiasis or hoarseness with beclomethasone dipropionate. New England and Regional Allergy Proceedings 8: 95–97.

Toogood JH (1987) Efficiency of inhaled versus oral steroid treatment of chronic asthma. New England and Regional Allergy Proceedings 8: 98–103.

Toogood JH (1990) Complications of topical steroid therapy for asthma. American Review of Respiratory Disease 141: S89–S96.

Toogood JH, Jennings B, Greenway RW, Chuang L (1980) Candidiasis and dysphonia
    complicating beclomethasone treatment of asthma. Journal of Allergy and Clinical
    Immunology 65: 145–153.
Traube L (1871) Spastische Form der nervosen Heiserkeit. In Gerammelte Beitr. Pathol. Physiol
    vol. 2. Berlin: Hirschwald, p. 677.
Williams AJ, Baghat MS, Stableforth DE, Cayton RM, Shenoi PM, Skinner C (1983)
    Dysphonia caused by inhaled steroids: recognition of a characteristic laryngeal abnormality.
    Thorax 38: 813–821.

CHAPTER 11

Phonosurgery – the cutting edge?

TOM HARRIS

...the most unkindest cut of all

William Shakespeare, *Julius Caesar*

This chapter is addressed primarily to the surgeons and speech therapists reading this book. However, we believe that it is important for all professionals with an interest in voice to know something of the advantages and, occasionally, perils of surgery to improve the laryngeal function of anyone who habitually uses their voice – potentially more than 99.9% of the world's population. It is not intended to be a comprehensive 'how to' description. For full and careful descriptions we would highly recommend acquaintance with the interactive video book of Guy Cornut and Marc Bouchayer (1994), which gives instruction on microsurgical techniques for the management of benign laryngeal lesions, and we recommend reading the publications on laryngeal framework surgery, especially those of Nobuhiko Isshiki (Isshiki et al., 1974; Isshiki, 1989) and James Koufman (1986).

There are two very different reasons for contemplating laryngeal surgery: the first is in keeping with the doctor's traditional role as a person charged with the curing of disease. If a patient, even a professional voice-user, has a disease of the larynx that threatens life or health, then there is no question that treatment designed to cure the condition, even if it damages the voice, is of primary importance. Surgeons have no business risking their patients' lives by undertreating potentially serious conditions.

The second, much newer, role for the surgeon is the challenge of improving vocal function by correcting structural abnormalities in such a way that the biomechanical function of voicing is improved. The majority of patients with lumps on their vocal folds are not sick, they just want a better voice, and it is therefore incumbent on the surgeon to act more like the motor mechanic whose job it is to repair and tune an engine in order that it works more efficiently rather than the coach-builder who makes the car's bodywork look very nice but who does nothing for its performance.

It is very difficult for a surgeon who has spent the greater part of a working life tidying up bits of anatomy to leave things alone, even if they look untidy. When a surgeon undertakes a reduction procedure on the cover of the vocal fold for Reinke oedema, if, after sucking or rolling out the fluid and removing a little of the by now redundant mucosa, there seems to be a flap or tear or other problem, removing it merely adds insult to (functional) injury. Making sure that the mucosal edges of the incision meet edge to edge without tension is a better option than making the operative field look tidy but denuded.

Phonosurgery is surgery to correct dysfunction, and superficial laryngeal examination may not reveal the whole truth about the reasons for dysphonia. Visual assessment of the proper production of mucosal waves **must** be made prior to any surgery. This is normally done by inspection in stroboscopic light. Historically, this has not been done routinely, and is the single biggest reason for poor functional results following surgery. It is certainly the reason why many professional voice-users still quite rightly fear that any laryngeal surgery spells the end of a career, in much the same fashion that some cancer patients fear that surgery will only spread disease.

If the surgeon is used to preoperative assessment of vocal fold function by means of a stroboscope, it rapidly becomes clear that, regardless of the actual lesion, the most important single factor on which a successful outcome depends is the preservation or restoration of an intact superficial layer of lamina propria (Reinke's space) (see the section on the microanatomy of the vocal fold, Chapter 2 p. 33). For normal voicing, in addition to the horizontal vibration of the vocal folds, normal patterns of glottal opening and closure depend absolutely on the vertical component of vibration supplied by the generation of mucosal waves. It follows that any operation that deprives the vocal fold of the superficial layer of the lamina propria and effectively 'nails' the vocal fold cover to the body of the fold, also deprives the owner of any possibility of normal voicing thereafter.

As far as surgery and the voice are concerned, we are at a crossroads. Most ENT surgeons were taught in their youth that gross swelling of the vocal fold cover (Reinke oedema or polypoid degeneration) was associated with an inappropriately low-pitched voice, and that a sensible treatment might therefore be to strip all the swelling off the folds and let the surface heal over. This teaching was, of course, catastrophic. It is true that the vocal folds look immaculate after such surgery, but unfortunately they cannot, nor will they ever again, work normally. It would seem that our surgical forebears were generally guilty of very **un**self-critical follow-up postoperatively. Fortunately, the instruments for assessing voice dysfunction now available in some clinics make crass mistakes increasingly rare (Hirano, 1981).

The other side of the coin is that there are many benign conditions of the vocal folds that will only resolve with surgery. There is absolutely no point in a singer taking a year's enforced 'rest' because they have a vocal polyp hanging from a small pedicle, when its careful surgical removal would enable them to be back on stage inside 3 weeks.

Surgery to correct vocal dysfunction is divided into two parts. The first is endoscopic correction of the structure and function of the vibrating structures, the vocal folds themselves, and the second is external surgery to adapt the laryngeal framework that suspends, positions and tensions the folds. The endoscopic procedures are carried out by means of a speculum placed in the patient's throat at microlaryngoscopy, and could be more accurately described as surgery of the cover of the vocal fold (meaning the surface epithelium and the underlying superficial layer of the lamina propria or Reinke's space). The surgery of the laryngeal framework is performed via an open operation on the neck.

Microlaryngoscopy

Laryngoscopy came of age with the advent of the operating microscope. This instrument revolutionized surgical abilities in ear and eye work, and has latterly become indispensable to other specialities, such as neurosurgery and vascular surgery. The microscope offers a binocular view of the larynx, and, when using a 350 mm focal length objective lens rather than the 400 mm lens that has been frequently used in the past, a comfortable operating distance can be maintained between the surgeon and the vocal folds. One can also decrease the distance a little more by resetting the eyepiece lenses from 0 to +4 prior to the start of the procedure. Some microscopes, for example the Storz Urban (USA), do not require a beam-splitter attachment to acquire a television image, as they use an alternative system working through the light inlet. This, too, permits a reduction of the distance between the surgeon's eyes and the operating field. Yet another way to acquire video images of microsurgery without adding a beam splitter to the microscope is to use a laryngeal speculum fitted with a rod telescope, such as those manufactured by Storz (Germany).

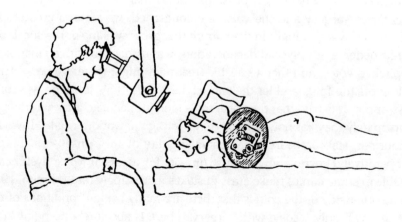

Instruments

Once laryngologists were enabled to work with a greatly enlarged view of the operating field, it rapidly became apparent that much finer surgical tools were necessary to achieve further improvements in technique. Professor Oscar Kleinsasser was the first surgeon to develop a full set of instruments (largely by extending the shafts of instruments for middle ear surgery). These have been used around the world for approaching two decades. Nothing stands still for long, however, and a second generation of instruments specifically designed for direct endoscopic laryngeal work has been developed by surgeons such as Marc Bouchayer and others (Bouchayer and Cornut, 1992).

These instruments recognize that the vocal folds are not conveniently set at right-angles to the operator's line of view and are accordingly offset, so they work precisely along or across the line of the vocal ligaments. This makes them extremely easy to use. If the laryngologist becomes involved in frequent micro-laryngeal surgery, he or she may also wish to consider additional instruments, such as a Jako-style needle-holder for manipulation of extremely small needles (e.g. 4.5–6 mm neural anastomosis needles swaged to 8/0 Vicryl) for mucosal repair or flaps. They may also experience difficulty in keeping arrowhead knives extremely sharp after repeated sterilization, in which case a Bouchayer-style Harris microknife with disposable blades will be helpful.

The author's personal choice of instruments for suspension microlaryngoscopy depends largely on the ease of access to the patient's larynx. Where there is no problem at all, then the optimum view with least distortion of the vocal folds and the entire supraglottic larynx is afforded by the series of Lindholm specula. For general purposes, a Kleinsasser anterior commissure speculum is satisfactory. Where the larynx is really difficult to visualize, the Dedo-Pilling speculum is much the easiest to position. The general rule seems to be that the easier it is to place any given operating laryngoscope, the less good will be the view and access for instruments. Finally, if prolonged microsurgery causes the arms to tire, and the instruments (when viewed with the microscope at least) to shake, then consider leaning the wrists on a neurosurgeon's bar placed over the patient's face. This is much more satisfactory than trying to kill the shake by resting the instruments on the side of the speculum.

For those surgeons interested in documenting their surgery, there is a choice between two systems. The microscope can be fitted with a beam splitter and small video camera, enabling the field of view from one or other eye to be recorded. The other, slightly more recent technique, is to use a laryngoscope fitted with a channel for a Hopkins rod telescope and video coupler. The latter technique gives a greater depth of focus and great stability of the image, but necessarily there is some obtrusion of the telescope tip into the operative field.

The choice of laryngoscope naturally dictates the choice of suspension arm used for keeping the laryngoscope in the optimum position. Early suspension arms were attached to the laryngoscope while the other end was placed on the patient's chest. This provided a satisfactory view, but by virtue of the pressure on the chest it was bound to impair chest movement for respiration. An early practical answer to this was to place the chest support end on a Mayo table above the patient's chest. Problems arose because most Mayo tables were never designed to support heavy weights and so do not provide adequate structural rigidity for this application. A better solution is to use a purpose-built rigid gantry arm support over the patient's chest, which is attached to the operating table beneath, and which is, in addition, adjustable for height. Of these, the most widely used is the Stange table, although other excellent variants are undoubtedly available. The extra freedom of vertical movement, in addition to the rotation of the laryngoscope already permitted by the suspension arm machine head, makes the description of the operation 'suspension microlaryngoscopy' a little more accurate. If only sagittal rotation of the laryngo- scope by the machine head is available, a more accurate or honest description would be 'neck hyperextension microlaryngoscopy'.

Anaesthesia for microsurgery

Modern anaesthesia provides several methods for maintenance of the patient's airway, and each has its own advantages and disadvantages. The two styles to contrast are closed methods, where a small diameter cuffed endotracheal tube is inserted through the vocal folds to seal the trachea with the tube, and air entrain- ment methods, where anaesthetic gases are injected via a venturi tube through the vocal folds at high speed in order to inflate the lungs. The venturi tip may be placed above or below the vocal folds; in either case, air is dragged into the airway by the small high-velocity gas stream.

The principal advantage of the closed endotracheal tube school is that the vocal folds on which the surgeon wishes to operate are motionless throughout the (microscopic) procedure. The patient is paralysed and the vocal folds are splinted by the presence of the tube lying in the posterior commissure. It is also possible to pack the subglottis with heat-absorbent materials if laser surgery is being contem- plated. Herein also lies the main disadvantage of this style of anaesthetic. The tube does restrict the view of the posterior glottis, and the vocal folds are splinted so that the position in which they naturally lie may be somewhat different to that seen down the microscope at operation.

The principal advantage of air entrainment techniques is the freedom of access afforded by the absence of a relatively large bore tube lying in the lower part of the operating field. This technique is ideal for endoscopic procedures where the micro- scope is augmented by inspection of 'hard-to-get-at areas', such as the ventricles and subglottis, by means of angled telescopes. It is also excellent for operations where medialization or lateralization of a vocal fold is part of the procedure. It is, however, suboptimal where operations on the vocal folds involve elevation of very small and delicate mucosal flaps and/or microsuturing of such flaps. There is a significant risk that the entrained breeze will simply rip up your most delicate handi- work during the operation. (This risk may of course be contrasted with the alterna- tive hazards of careless extubation by an unthinking anaesthetist after a closed venti- lation procedure has been completed.) Some surgeons find it somewhat frustrating to have to make frequent stops at critical points in surgery so the patient can be ventilated if a venturi system is being used. It is for these reasons that, on balance, the author routinely asks for a standard microlaryngeal tube in a paralysed patient for the most common phonosurgical procedures on the vocal folds.

Use of lasers in microsurgery

Lasers have only been mentioned in passing so far. The acronym 'laser' stands for 'light amplification (by) stimulated emission (of) radiation'. Laser light is mono-chromatic and coherent. This means that all the light has only one wavelength and all the waves are oscillating synchronously in an identical phase and that their paths are exactly parallel to one other. In a surgical context, it is a tool for the intense heating of very small areas of tissue, which results in local coagulation and subse-quent vaporization of tissue – cauterizing or cutting by intense cooking. This is somewhat akin to the effect of focusing the sun's rays on a piece of paper by means of a magnifying glass. At the time of writing, the laser's big advantage lies in its ability to leave a clean and virtually bloodless operating field because of the simul-taneous cautery of blood vessels (how much haemostasis depends on the type of laser and the power used. Both these factors affect the penetration of tissue and the amount of devitalization that results. The CO_2 laser commonly used in ENT surgery has little penetrating ability and will cauterise blood vessels up to 0.6 mm in diameter). Its main disadvantages are that it acts like a knife of slightly indeter-minate length and so cuts across tissue planes very easily; it offers no propriocep-tive feedback (no 'feel') to the surgeon; the path of an incision made by laser is always wider than that made by a sharp microknife; and tissue surfaces heal more slowly than when cut by knife or scissors. All instruments need to be minimally reflective and strict precautions need to be taken if inadvertent reflections of the beam are to be prevented causing accidental burns in the wrong place. Technology is improving all the time, and the surface area 'spot size' of the target gets steadily smaller. It is probable that increasing numbers of surgeons will use the laser more frequently for phonosurgical procedures. The author, however, feels that at present, the laser has no very clear advantages over conventional 'cold steel' and cautious microdiathermy in the field of phonosurgery with one single exception: the endoscopic ablation of laryngeal papillomatosis, where a dry operating field and minimal spread of contamination are of great importance. The great majority of cases where a laser seems appropriate are to do with the ablation of disease rather than improvement of phonatory function.

> *If it ain't broke, don't fix it.*
>
> Bert Lance

Before any phonosurgery is undertaken it is absolutely **essential** to have performed a full videostrobolaryngoscopic examination. For those who do not routinely use a stroboscope while examining voice patients, it is respectfully suggested that the chapter following this one should be read. It is not always possi-ble to tell the difference between a nodule or polyp and a mucus or epidermoid cyst by simple inspection alone. It may not always be possible to identify a sulcus vocalis or vergeture (the French word for 'stretch mark') without benefit of apparatus to visualize vocal fold movement. Just as it is now considered mandatory to have a preoperative audiogram indicating the degree and nature of the deafness prior to any surgical exploration of the middle ear in order to improve a conductive hearing loss, so it should also be the rule for phonosurgery. It is the author's view that surgery to correct laryngeal dysfunction without any preoperative assessment of the function will soon be regarded as being unacceptable from a medicolegal standpoint.

Microsurgery for benign vocal fold lesions

Epithelial lesions with limited/partial involvement of Reinke's space superficial layer of the lamina propria (SLLP)

Nodules and pedunculated polyps

Nodules are a mucosal lesion probably produced by damage to the basement membrane zone. Reinke's space (the superficial layer of the lamina propria) may also show some inflammatory/fibrous reaction, but scarring does not generally involve fibrous adhesions through to the intermediate and deep layers of the lamina propria. As a general rule, it is safe to excise lesions of the mucosal cover directly. The lesion is merely grasped with fenestrated tissue-holding microforceps, so that the smallest possible ellipse of mucosa that encompasses the lesion is produced in a direction parallel to the vocal fold-free border. The lesion is lifted away from the vocal ligament lying underneath, slightly stretching the mucosa, and is then excised with either curved microscissors or a sharp (disposable) arrowhead microknife, so that the edges are clean and the absolute minimum of normal mucosa accompanies the lesion. Provided that there has been minimal damage to the underlying Reinke's space, then the mucosa will heal over with negligible tethering to the vocal ligament. The same technique is used to remove pedunculated vocal fold polyps.

Lesions of the epithelium and the whole of Reinke's space (SLLP)

Reinke's oedema and polypoid degeneration

If the pathological change principally involves the superficial layer of the lamina propria (Reinke's space), then it is no longer appropriate to leave an incisional scar on or near the free border of the vocal fold, as this will inevitably lead to synechial tethering between layers with resultant inhibition of mucosal wave generation. A so-called 'superior cordotomy' should be performed for access to the space. In fact, this cordotomy should not under any circumstances be allowed to damage the vocal ligament underneath. The resultant adhesions from mucosa to the ligament will obliterate Reinke's space between the damaged layers.

If the rule about preservation of the superficial layer of the lamina propria is obeyed, it follows that the surgical treatment of Reinke's oedema or polypoid degeneration will be to make an incision in the mucosa on the superior aspect of the fold, a superior cordotomy, and then to develop a flap of mucosa downwards and medially over the free border, and roll or squeeze surplus thin fluid out of the space via the incision. Do not damage more of the structure of Reinke's space than necessary. Any and all microhaemorrhages will increase the amount of postoperative scarring across the superficial layer of the lamina propria. Note that not all Reinke oedema is semifluid. Sometimes it will resemble thick pseudomyxoid material and may be so stiff that it actually requires cupped forceps to remove. (It may also mimic a true mucous cyst if the material is very thick – the surgeon approaching such a lesion may be surprised not to find a capsule.)

Having reduced the contents of the space to levels approaching 'normal' quantities, the thin and somewhat atrophic mucosal cover is once again draped over the free border of the vocal fold. It is then apparent that there is a variable degree of redundant tissue overlying the original cordotomy line. The excess mucosa is then trimmed with the disposable arrowhead knife or microscissors taking only enough to permit neat edge-to-edge positioning of the mucosal margins. No denuded areas of vocal ligament must be left exposed.

Closure of mucosal incision margins: fibrin glue versus microsutures

In some centres the flap is held in place using fibrin glue, e.g. Tissucol® or Tisseel®. Other surgeons prefer to ensure that flaps remain in position with microsutures. A word of warning – suturing mucosal flaps is slow. Add at least an extra 20 minutes to the operation time. It is suggested that 8/0 suture material such as Vicryl® is used with a specialized Jako laryngeal needle-holder. The needle you will require is the absolutely shortest specimen that your supplier can furnish – the double-ended 45 cm sutures for micro-ophthalmic work with 6 mm micropoint spatula needles, swaged to 8/0 coated Vicryl® are preferred by the author (Ethicon W9559). Larger needles tend to become jammed against the speculum at inconvenient moments. The knots are more conveniently tied outside the speculum and slid down to the vocal fold. The author's personal preference is to use an assistant to immobilize one end by holding it against the speculum while he uses two hands to advance the throw toward the mucosa. Other centres where this type of surgery is performed prefer to use an endo-knot suture technique (Woo et al., 1995).

Sewing up or 'glueing' mucosa may not be necessary at all if removal of mucosa has not been overenthusiastic, and flaps are not to be advanced or rotated. The patient's own clotting mechanisms will suffice if mucosal edges sit closely together without any tendency to retract.

Caveat. There is an underlying reason for restricting the use of fibrin glue that has not been prepared from the patient's own blood – in the UK at least, there is the possibility that any patient who, at any later stage in life, subsequently develops a degenerative disease that has been deemed 'transmissible' might be in a position to take legal action against the laryngologist unless the surgeon was in a position to **prove** that the infection could not have been the result of using fibrin glue.

Lesions involving epithelium and more than one layer of the lamina propria

Life gets much more complicated when the epithelium and fibres of the vocal ligament are bound together. The two functional layers may be in direct contact, as in a sulcus vocalis, vergeture or previous stripping, or they may be indirectly anchored by an epidermoid or mucus cyst that has attachment to both layers. Lesions may be either congenital in origin (such as the sulcus and epidermoid cyst) or acquired, such as the vergeture and the mucus cyst. In either case, in order to avoid tethering of the layers of the free border it is essential that the minimum of scarring is produced. For this reason all these problems are approached via a mucosal incision sited away from the free border, either a superior cordotomy incision or a mini-flap of mucosa. Some surgeons distend the layers a little with a small injection of steroid before incising. This is not as useful as it might at first appear, as the areas that require surgery remain closely adherent.

Epidermoid and mucus retention cysts

Both these types of cyst can vary greatly in appearance. If the lesion is large and prominently situated in the superficial layer of the lamina propria, then there will be no difficulty in making the diagnosis. More commonly, however, the possibility of an intrafold cyst is only raised when the vibration of the folds has been viewed strobo-scopically and the absence of a mucosal wave has been observed. The patient comes to theatre for a microlaryngoscopy and exploratory superior cordotomy with a 'probable' diagnosis. In theatre, the vocal fold mucosa is first gently explored for deep tethering and for the presence of a cyst punctum using fine forceps or a slightly curved elevator. To remove a cyst is a matter of meticulous dissection. Either type of cyst is approached via a superior cordotomy and exposure from Reinke's space. A superior cordotomy is performed with a sharp arrowhead knife. The incision is made parallel and lateral to the free border of the fold, and the mucosa is then carefully elevated away from the vocal ligament towards the free border.

In the case of a mucus cyst, the close attachment of the cyst to the epithelium is first gently freed, and then the deeper attachments to the vocal ligament. By contrast, it is often easier to dissect out the deep surface of an epidermoid cyst from its nidus within the fibres of the vocal ligament, before dealing with the super-ficial epithelial attachments. There may be a punctum connecting the cyst with the surface of the mucosa, and this will require careful isolation and division. When both superficial and deep layers have been fully separated, the remaining anterior and posterior fibrous adhesions can be safely divided with curved scissors and the cyst (hopefully still intact) removed from its nidus.

Now check the resultant space that you have created to see that it is clean and that there is no remaining scar tissue or other pathology before laying the mucosa back in place over the ligament. It is not obligatory to anchor the flap back in place, but if you do not, there is a small risk that postoperative retraction of the incision borders will produce a significant denuded vergeture on the fold. If you decide to fix the flap in position, the two alternative methods available for closure are, once again, fibrin glue or microsutures. In this case, the author has a strong preference for precise suturing of the mucosal edges as this gives better postoperative results than simply laying back the cut mucosal edges in contact with each other.

Caveats. (i) Watch out for the occasional punctum. A small track capable of inter-mittent discharge of some of the cyst contents may from time to time be responsible for the 'now you see it, now you don't' type of problem that is sometimes encoun-tered by laryngologists confronted by patients with variable dysphonia. Even when you have looked, always roll the mucosa gently under a blunt instrument, such as an elevator. It may provide the only clue as to what is lurking underneath the mucosa even when the inspection is being performed under the operating microscope. (ii) If you successfully and cleanly remove a cyst, always check to see there are no others before closing. Nowhere is it written that there will only ever be a single epidermoid cyst in a vocal fold that is solely responsible for the dysphonia.

Sulcus vocalis and vergeture

Authors such as Bouchayer have suggested that sulci vocalis are congenital in origin, and that they are a variety of epidermoid cyst whose ostium has been stretched wide open (Bouchayer et al., 1985). This may seem unlikely at first, but any surgeon with fairly wide experience in phonosurgery becomes increasingly aware that there does appear to be a continuum between true cysts, cysts with wide ostia, sulci vocalis which are more like pockets, and the classical furrow-like sulcus along the free border of the fold. It may be hypothesized that the broad ostium of an open epider-moid cyst is elongated into a furrow along the fold because the points where maxi-mal shearing stresses are applied when the folds vibrate will be at the boundaries between normally mobile fold layers and layers ablated by the cyst, i.e. the anterior and posterior margins of the ostium. It is suggested that these boundaries may, as a result of the constant stretching and shearing, become adherent to the ligament, causing progressive elongation of the ostium into the characteristic sulcus.

Exactly how an open-mouthed cyst or sulcus is treated depends to a degree on the size of the deficit in the mucosa produced by the cyst ostium or sulcus. While a small track from a cyst may simply be divided, a wide mouth cannot be ignored. The superior/lateral margin of the pocket or sulcus has already been elevated away from the vocal ligament, but the inferior/medial margin usually consists of the mucosa reflected back on itself around a small band of tight fibres to form a tight lip to the lower margin of the sulcus. It can be very difficult to incise accurately along this tight margin and then divide the two layers of mucosa, and yet this is what must be achieved if a pocket is to be ablated. When the pocket lining is entirely freed up via the superior cordotomy and lower lip dissection, it can be everted. The thin epithelium of the lining may then be appropriately trimmed at its freed lower margin by cutting it along a line to match the edge of the mucosa at the lip of the inferior border. Ensuring edge-to-edge contact will prevent exposure of the vocal ligament at the end of the operation.

'Vergetures' are a little different. It is suggested that they are an acquired lesion, commonly the result of chronic laryngitis (Garel, 1923) or even of colleagues' 'fold-stripping' activities. A vergeture is an area of vocal ligament covered by a little scar tissue and a thin layer of atrophic-looking epithelium. There is no clearly defined lower margin nor a pocket of mucosa invaginated inwards, just an area in which the normal structure of the lamina propria has been destroyed. Surgically, they are very difficult to treat.

Once again a superior cordotomy is performed superolateral to the lesion, and the mucosa is dissected free from the ligament fibre by fibre. When the area has been fully mobilized, hopefully to margins where there is 'normal' Reinke's space, the developed mucosal flap is laid back. In the author's experience the best functional results have been achieved by continuing to mobilize past the vergeture in the Reinke's space plane in order to create a small advancement flap which is then held in place with sutures. It is usually not possible to recover the whole area of denuded ligament, but if enough advancement can be achieved to cover the edge of the free border once stitched in place, then the results can be (acoustically) very satisfactory. Very small pieces of autogenous fat may provide a 'filler' where there is only the elevated vergeture mucosa to play with. It does not make a substitute Reinke's space, but may usefully fill out atrophic notches to improve vocal fold closure.

Mucosal bridges

A sulcus may have developed from a cyst or cysts with more than one ostium. Bouchayer suggests (1985) that if both ostia elongate along the fold, and communicate beneath the mucosa, this may produce a mucosal bridge. The surgery of a sulcus with an associated bridge is little different from that required for the straightforward structure. The sulcus is elevated as per normal via a superior cordotomy, and the bridge is treated as a bipedicled lesion and is merely excised at its attachments at both ends. Many surgeons have attempted to divide, unroll and flatten out mucosal bridges; it is extremely difficult to do, and the results using this 'salvaged' mucosa rather than the epithelium elevated from the floor of the sulcus show no objective improvement in postoperative function.

Webs at the anterior commissure: endoscopic versus open surgery

Before the advent of the operating microscope, **most** surgery of the vocal folds requiring more than a 'simple avulsion' of a lesion used to be undertaken using an external approach to the larynx. The thyroid cartilage was split in the midline to produce a so-called laryngofissure. This was accompanied by careful separation of the folds by extending the incision through the anterior commissure. This approach now offers little advantage over endoscopic microsurgery with the sole exception of surgery to divide thick webs or other lesions at the anterior commissure. The problem with division of any but the very smallest microwebs is the inevitable postoperative readherence of the tissue at the site of the division. If there is no covering mucosa on at least one side, then synechiae will form and the web will reform, quite possibly thicker than before. The methods available to avoid this consequence are to swing miniflaps of healthy mucosa over the denuded vocal ligament either at laryngofissure or endoscopically. In the author's hands the formal external approach is much the easier exercise.

Stent placement: endoscopic versus laryngofissure

If, as is often the case, there is not enough remaining mucosa locally available to create a mucosal rotation flap, then a stent or keel to keep the denuded folds physically apart becomes essential. There is a considerable body of opinion that states that the endoscopic route is the modern, acceptable way to do things. The problem with endoscopically-placed stents, however, is the variable but generally unavoidable blunting of the anterior commissure. Many surgeons achieve reasonable results with endoscopically-placed stents with only anchoring sutures being passed through the epiglottic petiole/thyroid notch superiorly and the anterior cricothyroid ligament inferiorly, which are then brought out through the skin. Indeed, the patients like it and it used to be the author's preferred method of stenting. Relatively poor phonatory results, however, have since persuaded us that a formal endoscopic division of the web and (damaged) Broyle's ligament should then be followed by a formal laryngofissure and insertion of an 'umbrella' stent, which is both technically easier to perform and produces better postoperative functional results.

To operate or not to operate

Nodules

There are different codes of practice in different centres. In some units you will hear that most nodules are excised whereas in others the stated management of nodules is that they should all be left to the speech therapist. We try to maintain a pragmatic approach to the different groups of patients. For example, we do not remove 'screamer's nodules' in young children because the risk of misdiagnosis and of excessive postoperative scarring is, in our view, unacceptably high. In centres with expertise in the field it may be deemed reasonable to operate on prepubertal children over the age of nine if phonation is greatly impaired. In adults, if the nodules are recent or soft and are not causing any great phonatory problems, e.g. preventing full fold closure or inhibiting generation of mucosal waves on stroboscopy, then there is no indication for surgical interference. If, on the other hand, the nodules are long-standing, hard and interfere with phonation in a manner that the patient finds unacceptable, then it is sensible to remove them surgically as part of a surgery/speech therapy package. The patient can be voicing normally in a fortnight if the nodules have been very precisely removed with minimal damage inflicted on the underlying Reinke's space. The waste of speech therapy time and the protracted period of many months before there is any possibility that firm fibrous nodules will resolve precludes the simple 'therapy only' treatment regimen from our practice. The same attitude applies to polyps that are pedunculated.

Cysts, sulcus vocalis and vergeture

The decision for or against surgery is less contentious here. The time taken for successful postoperative vocal rehabilitation is much greater than for primarily epithelial lesions. If the patient cannot give you a minimum of 2 months between professional commitments involving voice use, don't be tempted to operate (Bouchayer et al., 1992 and 1994). It would be wise to double that figure if he or she is a classical singer. In the author's experience, improvements both in strobo-scopic appearance and in voicing may continue over a span as long as 2 years.

Caveats. (i) The biggest 'sins' in occasional errors in diagnostic judgement come when a genuine vocal fold cyst is labelled either a 'nodule' or a pseudocyst of poly-poid degeneration, especially after inadequate or absent stroboscopic examination. The golden rule for phonosurgery is 'play it safe'. Be pessimistic – it is perfectly reasonable to approach either a cyst or a pseudocyst via a superior cordotomy, it is a grave offence to try to excise a 'nodule' directly, only to find that you have scalped a true cyst thereby guaranteeing a scar though all layers of the lamina propria. (ii) Always check when you stretch a soft bleb of polypoid degeneration away from the fold prior to excising it, that there is no fibrous scar tissue tethering the mucosa to the ligament above the swelling. It is probable that the polypoid damage has arisen because the tethering has prevented even deformation of the vocal fold cover on phonation. This means that the travelling mucosal waves are suddenly obliterated, the energy being dissipated in the cover medial to the adhe-sion as shearing stresses that eventually produce the structural damage. (This is broadly analogous to the travelling wave set up in a whiplash suddenly running out of rope down which to travel – the energy is all lost suddenly at the tip.) Similarly, more extensive swelling may be found, probably for the same reasons, along the inferior border of a true sulcus vocalis (see below).

Laryngeal framework surgery

We have so far mostly attended to the vocal folds, but the most complex problems lie in the operative adjustment of the laryngeal cartilaginous skeleton, so-called 'framework surgery'. Many people have devised operations to modify the laryngeal airway or vocal fold position or thickness, but the man who has done most to systematize the types of modification and what can be expected by way of postop-erative results is Professor Nobuhiko Isshiki, whose book *Phonosurgery* (1989) is a very readable work of reference.

Procedures to alter the fixed position of the vocal folds

Vocal fold lateralizing procedures, such as Woodman's operation or laser endoscopic or external arytenoidectomy, used to be employed to improve the patient's airway after bilateral vocal fold paresis or other problems that produce an inadequate airway due to persistent narrowing of the glottis. That these operations work is indisputable. What is also indisputable is that the quality of phonation is always worse postoperatively. Of these procedures it is the author's experience that the laser arytenoidectomy gives the best compromise results. In our clinic, patients are usually encouraged to try to use a long-term tracheostomy with a speaking valve, which, although it gives an inferior cosmetic result, leaves the patient both with a good airway and a passable voice.

Fold-medializing procedures

These procedures bring the vibrating portion of a paralysed, weakened or fixed fold into a midline position where it can close against a 'working' fold. They are used to improve a breathy or whispery voice, usually after a vocal fold paresis. If the patient is suffering from paresis of non-malignant aetiology, it is appropriate to wait for a period of 6 months after the onset before undertaking a surgical procedure. By that time it is generally possible to make an accurate assessment as to whether there will be a clinically satisfactory reinnervation on the paretic side, or, indeed, if the compensatory activity is satisfactory on its own.

Injected implants

There are basically two approaches to fold medialization and both are exemplified in the German literature of the early part of the century. The first approach is to inject foreign material lateral in to the vocal process of the arytenoid and lateral to the vocalis muscle. Brünings wrote about injecting paraffin wax thus in 1911. He stopped doing it because of foreign body reaction to the implant material, and the story has been much the same ever since. All the materials tried so far are either not inert enough, are not entirely biocompatible and/or resorb after a short period. Recent examples include Gelfoam® suspended in saline, silicone, Teflon® paste and stabilized (GAX) collagen in solid or paste form (Phonogel®) or the patient's own fat. Most of these may be injected successfully with some short-term improvement in voicing. None can be relied on not to produce a severe inflammatory reaction that will be impossible to excise without further damaging the voice.

The second approach is to implant a piece of material (originally the patient's own cartilage) deep (lateral) to the vocalis muscle/conus elasticus. Payr devised an operation for this in 1915, cutting three sides of a brick of cartilage into the thyroid lamina. The fourth, anterior, side was left uncut, and the wedge was simply pushed inward at the posterior end in order to displace the vocal fold medially. This technique has some obvious limitations: the displacement of the fold is likely to be inadequate and more often than not, the thyroid cartilage may have calcified in parts, making bending of the cartilage impractical.

The concept, however, is sound, and in recent times Isshiki and subsequently Koufman and others have developed the thyroid window approach into a reliable and relatively simple procedure, usually described as an Isshiki type I thyroplasty (Isshiki et al., 1974; Isshiki, 1989; Koufman, 1986; Bielamowicz et al., 1995).

Thyroplasty

A transverse skin incision of approximately 3 cm is made over the thyroid lamina of the patient's larynx at a level midway between the thyroid notch and the lower margin of the thyroid cartilage. This should be extended over the midline to the opposite side by a further 1 cm.

The perichondrium of the thyroid cartilage is exposed from the notch to the lower margin of the cartilage and approximately three quarters of the lamina is exposed posteriorly. (The posterior margin must be palpable for purposes of sizing.) A point in the midline, midway between the notch and the lower border is established, and a horizontal line is drawn posteriorly. (NB This is more or less perpendicular to the posterior margin, rather than the line between notch and lower margin.) The line corresponds to the upper margin of the vocal fold within, and the superior margin of the window will, therefore, form part of it.

The window itself will be approximately 6 x 12 mm in large male larynges (pronounced '5 x 10 mm' if you are anxious) or 4 x 10 mm in women. Its length is limited by its ability to override the cricoid arch – cut too far posterior, and the window cannot be displaced medially enough. For those of a mathematical turn of mind, Koufman (1986) has suggested a formula for devising correct window size:

$$\text{window height} = \frac{\text{thyroid alar height} - 4}{4}$$

$$\text{window width} = \frac{\text{thyroid alar width} - 4}{2}$$

The anterior margin of the window should be 5–7 mm behind the mark you made at the midline. It extends inferiorly to the line previously marked out to represent the upper limit of the fold. The window can be cut with a No. 11 blade or with a fine-cutting burr if the cartilage has calcified. More recently, a semi-disposable 6 x 10 mm box-shaped punch blade has been developed by Messrs J. Weiss, and this may be tapped through the cartilage regardless of any calcification.

Originally, the intent was for the window fragment itself to form the prosthetic wedge in the larynx. In practical terms, however, it seems that it is easier to create the entire medializing wedge from Silastic®. Proposed shapes abound, but it seems to the author that the most practical shape within the thyroid is a wedge configuration tapering to nothing anteriorly, and whose theoretically optimum posterior depth is identified by half the angle subtended by the thyroid cartilage at the midline. A flanged wedge configuration was proposed by Godley in 1992, but was intended to lock in the brick of cartilage as originally described by Isshiki et al. (1974).

It seems to us that there is better control of the final medialization if the small cartilage brick is first removed, and a deeper wedge of Silastic is created that will lie directly lateral to the vocalis/conus. Although this is the 'right' shape, the angles are far too sharp to fit snugly behind the vocalis muscle, and the final configuration must be a compromise between this and the 'safest' shape – that of a rounded, smooth elliptical button of similar dimensions anteriorly and posteriorly. Whatever the final shape of the internal wedge, it will be slightly longer antero-posteriorly than the window, it will require a small flange (approx 1 mm high) superiorly and inferiorly, and, if carved as a 'one-off' from a block of Silastic, will require a brick-shaped base whose dimensions are the same as the window. Koufman recommends two incisions in the brick-shaped window segment, allowing the front and back ends of the prosthesis to be folded through the window. If flanges have been carved on the superior and inferior aspects of the midsegment, they too can easily be pushed through the window with an instrument such as a Freer's elevator. The author has suggested a range of trial sizing instruments that may simply be pushed into a standard-sized window should this procedure be performed under local anaesthic. This allows the patient to try voicing to establish the appropriate size and configuration for the Silastic prosthesis before it is inserted.

Caveat. It has recently come to the author's attention that Dow-Corning, the manufacturers of Silastic, are no longer going to manufacture block Silastic themselves. This may of course mean that the one reasonably convenient material that does not appear to elicit much of a tissue reponse will not be generally available for much longer. The hunt is on for yet another suitable material with which to produce implants for thyroplasty.

Another technique employed to medialize a paralysed vocal fold is known as *arytenoid adduction.* The arytenoid is rotated antero-medially about the joint axis, increasing medial compression (Bielamowicz et al., 1995). Earlier versions advocated opening the joint capsule and rotating the arytenoid about the posterior crioarytenoid ligament (Isshiki, 1989). The rotated position is maintained by passing a suture through the muscular process of the arytenoid and anteriorly through the thyroid cartilage. The suture approximates the activity of the LCA muscle.

Pitch-changing procedures

There is interest in a few specialized centres in pitch-changing procedures. These are rarely required in the general population, but there is a consistent demand for them. The most common request is for a pitch-raising procedure in male-to-female gender reassignment. At the moment there is little that can be done to the vocal folds that will actively reduce the mass of the fold free border, while at the same time reducing the antero-posterior length of the vibrating fold and maintaining or even increasing the tension in the vocal ligaments.

Many procedures have been proposed by experienced phonosurgeons, such as Tucker and Isshiki, but most have the disadvantage that initially satisfactory results deteriorate as the folds stretch to their original length and bow in the process. Attempts to counter this by shortening the antero-posterior width of the thyroid lamina and broaden the anterior angle are difficult surgically and not entirely reliable. The combination procedures of choice that currently appear to produce reasonable (and at least partially) sustainable results are closure of the cricothyroid visor (Isshiki type IV procedure) performed at the same time as an endoscopic plication of the anterior 1/4 of the vibrating vocal folds. The surgical locking of the visor is interesting in that it is almost exactly the reverse of what we try to achieve in our voice clinic every week.

What of the future?

There are many avenues to explore that will improve functional results, especially at the hands of ENT surgeons who may not have a specialist interest in voice. To take a few examples, ranging from the mundane to the theoretical. The first is further improvement in instrumentation, e.g new purpose-built systems for simplifying the Isshiki type I medialization thyroplasty. Using these instruments it is hoped that it will, in future, be possible to do most operations under local anaesthetic without causing the patient any anxiety or discomfort and allowing them to phonate on request to assess the optimum medialization.

A second avenue, improving reimplantation or reinnervation procedures, still has rather further to run before it becomes an approach of excellence. It is not simply the technical difficulty of implanting myoneural pedicles that is the problem; achieving an excellent functional outcome will be harder than that. The built-in difficulties with these procedures stem both from our currently imperfect understanding of the patterns of muscle use in the whole complexity of laryngeal function, and from the seemingly scattered distribution of efferent nerve fibres to different laryngeal muscles within the recurrent laryngeal nerves.

Yet another avenue is in the field of predictive assessment. Some of the most recent advances in programming, computer and imaging technology have made it possible to process large amounts of data very quickly. There is at least one multi-centre university project investigating stereo video strobolaryngoscopy and generation of virtual reality models of the function of individual patients' vocal folds. Work is also under way in the construction of a 'chaotic' mathematical model of the glottal sound source. It is hoped that one of the outcomes of these projects will be to make it possible to perform 'what if' exercises on an individual patient's phonation waveform, predicting exactly what the outcome of any proposed surgery will be before the operation takes place. Clearly, such a tool would enable design of surgical procedures for the correction of laryngeal function to be undertaken much more precisely than ever before to the enduring satisfaction of the surgeon and patient alike.

References

Bielamowicz S, Berke GS, Gerratt BR (1995) A comparison of Type I Thyroplasty and Arytenoid Adduction. Journal of Voice 9:4 466–472.

Bouchayer M, Cornut G (1994) Phonosurgery for benign vocal fold lesions: an interactive video textbook. Gibraltar: The Three Ears Co. Available through the British Voice Association, London.

Bouchayer M, Cornut G, Loire R, Roch JB, Witzig E, Bastian RW (1985) Epidermoid cysts, sulci and mucosal bridges of the true vocal cord; a report of 157 cases. Laryngoscope 95: 1087–1094.

Cornut G, Bouchayer M (1992) Microsurgical treatment of benign vocal fold lesions: indications, technique, results. Folia Phoniatrica 44: 155–184.

Garel J (1923) Vergetures des cordes vocales, sesquelles de laryngite chronique. Rev. Laryngol. 44: 206–211.

Godley FA (1992) A simple implant design for vocal cord medialization. Laryngoscope 102: 824–826.

Hirano M (1981) Clinical examination of voice. Wein: Springer-Verlag.

Isshiki N (1989) Phonosurgery. Theory and practice. Tokyo: Springer-Verlag.

Isshiki N, Okamura H, Hiramoto M (1974) Thyroplasty as a new phonosurgical technique. Acta Otolaryngologica 78: 451–457.

Koufman JA (1986) Laryngoplasty for vocal cord medialization: an alternative to Teflon. Laryngoscope 96: 726–731.

Woo P, Casper J, Griffin B, Colton R, Brewer D (1995) Endoscopic microsuture repair of vocal fold defects. Journal of Voice 9: 332–339.

CHAPTER 12

Visual Observation of the Laryngeal Sound Source and Supraglottic Vocal Tract: an Outline Guide to the Equipment and Its Use

TOM HARRIS

'Curiouser and curiouser!' cried Alice.

Lewis Carroll, *Alice's Adventures in Wonderland*

There are two important reasons why a clinician may wish to observe either the vocal folds or the supraglottic vocal tract (SGVT). The first is to study the vibratory behaviour of the sound source (the vocal folds), and the second is to study the shape and characteristic configurations of the SGVT, the collective term for the supraglottic larynx and the hypopharyngeal, pharyngeal, oral, nasal and palatal structures, which make up the resonating tube above the vocal folds. In the voice clinic there are generally two means of observation available: the rigid laryngoscope and the flexible fibreoptic nasendoscope. Both have advantages and disadvantages: we find that the rigid instrument gives better quality pictures than the flexible instrument, but the flexible instrument causes less disturbance in the SGVT during observation. These instrumental observations are the only ones that it is essential to make prior to organizing a treatment plan, and they are performed during the initial consultation when all the clinic members are present. For this reason they are discussed in the clinical part of this book.

Observing the sound source

The larynx may be considered as a converter of a 'direct current' source of mechanical energy – the airstream exhaled from the lungs – into an 'alternating current' waveform of (also mechanical) energy. It does this by chopping up the airstream passing through the glottis extremely rapidly by means of the rapid and repeated opening and closure (oscillation) of the vocal folds. The larynx is therefore the sound source of the vocal instrument, just as the double reed in the end of an oboe or the player's lips in the embouchure of a trumpet perform the same function. The larynx is just as prone to dysfunction as any other mechanical oscillator and therefore close inspection of the function of the glottis is required if a proper diagnosis of a mechanical problem is to be made.

Laryngoscopy

At the end of the first half of the nineteenth century an interest developed in attempting to view the larynx in live patients. To identify disease, physicians such as Czermak devised systems of mirrors to look at the vocal folds indirectly, although the outstanding achievement in observation was certainly that of Manuel Garcia, a Spanish singing teacher, who, using laryngeal mirrors, taught himself autolaryngoscopy, to observe the gestures made by the larynx during differing activities. He presented his work to the Royal Society in 1855 and subsequently all over Europe. His basic technique and tools for observation (laryngeal mirror, light source and head mirror) were so simple and robust that they remain the baseline method of viewing the folds to this day.

Recent modifications to the technique of indirect laryngoscopy include the use of the binocular operating microscope in conjunction with the laryngeal mirror to produce a magnified, binocular view of the larynx. The picture thus provided is excellent, but the limitations and difficulties in performing this endoscopic observation are no different to those using the mirror alone.

There has also been an enormous improvement in the quality of telescopes for indirect endoscopic viewing of the larynx in recent years. They too produce considerable magnification of the image, but until very recently, there have been no suitable instruments available for clinical applications that could produce good stereoscopic images.

The choice of methods for observing vocal fold activity is, therefore, between indirect microlaryngoscopy and telescopic laryngoscopy. Each method has its protagonists, and we decided early on that, on balance, the telescopic rigid laryngoscope was the most suitable for routine use. The reasons for this decision are because it is possible to use a single size of laryngoscope for all patients from adults right down to children of approximately four years of age, and also that all VCR recording machines that are within the realms of financial possibility for a clinic record a single channel of video. What you see is what you record/is what you are able to play back.

We use Machida and Storz laryngoscopes with the objective field of view angled to 70°. There are, however, several other excellent instruments to choose from. Some practitioners prefer instruments that provide a 90° viewing angle, but in our hands at least, a higher percentage of patients are able to tolerate the examination when using the 70° instruments, which are slightly less likely to interfere with the soft palate and posterior pharyngeal wall.

Moving pictures

The chief difficulty with observation of vocal fold vibration is the speed with which the movements occur. The human eye/brain is unable to assimilate any useful visual information about cyclical events that, in the case of the voice, are usually produced more than 80 times per second; the motion is simply reduced to a blur. If the vibratory movements can be apparently slowed down to five or less cycles per second, however, then all sorts of observations may be made about the nature of the vibration of the folds: amplitude (size), regularity (or lack of it), the proportion of the whole cycle during which the folds are actually closed, whether the closure is complete, and the nature of the waves generated in the 'cover' of the folds – the mucosal waves.

How then may we slow up an activity that, in 'real time', is taking place faster than we are able to observe it? We owe a great deal to the enthusiasm of the Victorians who developed the techniques of photography, in particular, Fox Talbot, for the development of light-sensitive emulsions that did not require several minutes of exposure, and subsequently the Lumière brothers for popularizing the 'moving pictures' of cinema.

A further significant contribution was that of another pioneer of the time named Eadweard Muybridge. He realized that to record an event accurately it is necessary for the event itself to trigger the recording device(s). If one is able to record an image of an event, taken at a predetermined, precise moment in time, then it is possible to study that event at leisure (see Figure 12.1).

If many images of an event are recorded in rapid succession, they too can be studied at length, and the movement characterized. If the images are shown one

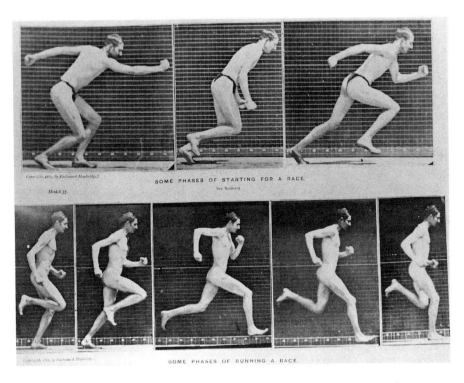

Figure 12.1 Muybridge's moving pictures (Courtesy of the British Film Institute)

after another in rapid sequence, the retina of the human eye retains each image for around 0.2 seconds after the actual image has been removed. This persistence of an image within the retina allows a sequence of subsequent images to fuse with the previous ones to produce an apparent continuous motion, provided that the progressive alteration of the image takes place in a smooth and regular manner throughout the sequence of exposures. This is termed *correspondence*. For a fuller description see Hirano and Bless, (1993). If alterations occur in an irregular manner then the illusion of motion is lost and the image appears jerky or seems to flicker.

The most precise means to date of recording the rapid movements of the vocal folds is high-speed photography. This technique accurately records the features of the regular vibrations of the folds, as well as the irregularities and cycle-to-cycle variations. It is, however, time-consuming and very expensive as an investigative modality. Another problem is that the sheer volume of data gathered makes proper analysis either during or immediately after recording impossible, even for the most dedicated of clinicians. To take one second of film of a patient's voice at eight frames per cycle while they are singing, say, a middle C, would generate over 4000 frames of film. Clearly this is not practical in the voice clinic! To take just eight pictures of a single cycle, on the other hand, risks losing all information about irregular beating as well as offering no guarantees that the particular cycle captured on film or video is typical. How then may one set about retrieving 'enough' information about the vibratory cycle without risking throwing the baby out with the bathwater? The current most practical solution for the clinic is to use the technique known as stroboscopy.

Laryngostroboscopy

A stroboscope is defined as 'an instrument for studying periodic movement seen by flashes (of light)' (from the Greek στροβος, strobos = a whirling). The object of the exercise is to flash-illuminate only a small fraction of each occurrence of the cycle of movement, and then, by viewing all the successive images thus obtained (much like the sequence of images on a piece of movie film), to produce an impression of greatly slowed rate of movement. The beginning of each cycle is detected electronically and the onset of every cycle triggers the discharge of a flash of light. This causes the sequence of images obtained to appear stationary. If an

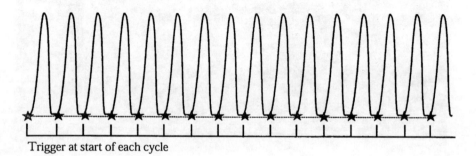

Trigger at start of each cycle

Figure 12.2 Stroboscopy; freezing cyclical motion

identical small delay is added to every triggering, then different parts of the cycle can be viewed, apparently motionless. Exactly which bit of the cycle is seen is dependent on the amount of delay which has been added to each triggering.

If the triggering is synchronized with the cycle, then assembling the series of pictures will apparently produce a 'freezing' of motion (see Figure 12.2).

How to (apparently) slow a movement down eightfold (See Figure 12.3). The beginning of each cycle is detected electronically as before. The time taken for a single cycle (the period) is calculated automatically, and a small fraction of this time is then added incrementally to the period of each successive cycle in order to progressively delay the discharge of flashes over a given number of cycles. In the example given, an eighth of a period is being added to each cycle, so the sequence recurs after eight cycles.

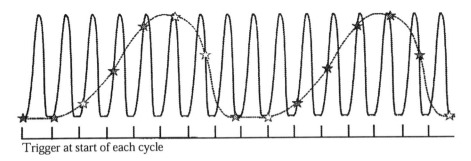

Trigger at start of each cycle

Figure 12.3 A 'slowed down' movement. Please note the configuration of the movement in the aggregated 'slowed' image is the same as that of a single wave as if it were simply spread out over the same time scale

Oertel devised a stroboscope as early as 1876, using a mechanical rotating disc to 'chop up' the light beam into flashes (Oertel, 1895). He and other contemporary researchers of the day became so familiar with vocal fold activity that, incredibly, by 1898 it was possible for Musehold to publish his paper on the photographic appearance of vocal fold movement in chest and falsetto registers. At the time it was not possible to get the vibration itself to trigger the light flashes, and these researchers had to match the rate at which the machine produced flashes to the pitch of the subject's phonation or vice versa.

Modern stroboscopes are much simpler to use, as they are now triggered by the patient's phonation, either by means of a 'tracking filter' monitoring the acoustic signal or by means of an electroglottograph tracking the electrical impedance of the glottis. This obviates the need for the patient to be able to sustain a given pitch for any length of time, and frees the observer to concentrate on the pattern of the images rather than the control of the rate of flashing. Schönhärl provided a description of contemporary stroboscopic techniques and findings as long ago as 1960.

Characteristics of the beating vocal fold

Slowing down the apparent rate of vibration of the vocal folds when they are beating allows the observer to view the characteristic configuration of the folds during successive phases of the vibratory cycle. The stroboscopic illusion will pick up much, but by no means all, qualitative visual information about wave activity on the superior and medial surfaces of regularly beating folds during the open and some of the closed phase. For further reading about the nature of fold oscillation, see the overview by Titze (1994). The configurations differ with the vocal register and pitch depending on physical factors within the fold itself and the air pressure driving the vibration:

(i)   *Within the fold itself* The actual size and length of the fold, the tension in the vocal ligament and the stiffness of the underlying vocalis muscle of the body of the fold. The condition of the mucosal cover of the vocal folds, whether or not it is thickened or stiffened, or tethered to other layers.

(ii) *Subglottic air pressure and airflow volume* These will in turn be modified by the resistance and resonating characteristics of the supraglottic vocal tract and the viscosity of the air itself.

Much work has been done in the past to characterize the beating vocal fold. Not only is there a horizontal component of abduction/adduction, there is also a vertical component of fold movement initiated by fluctuating subglottal pressure and airflow pulsing. In chest or heavy register particularly, one can identify two distinct free edges to the beating fold, an upper and lower, the chief difference between them being the phase difference in their opening and closing. (The lower margin appears to open and close earlier in the vibratory cycle than does the upper.) This might be expected empirically as the lower border is exposed to fluctuations in subglottal pressure and flow slightly earlier than the upper margin, but detailed knowledge of mechanical rules governing the amplitude and characteristics of the vibration, its mode and the phase relationship of the components are not mandatory for the beginner. For those readers who wish to read further, we would highly recommend Titze's *Principles of Voice Production (1994)*.

Several mathematical models that attempt to characterize the activity observed have been proposed. Figure 12.4 illustrates a simple and sufficiently accurate (for clinical purposes) version known as the 'Two Mass Model', originally suggested by Stevens (see also Kitzing, 1985). There are many other more sophisticated models, but most are beyond the scope of this book. Of course it depends on the purpose of the model: is it a wire model for illustration, is it a finite element model for description or does it involve particle tracking for research? Sadly, using complex models to demonstrate vocal fold motion requires more time and computation power than is generally available to voice clinics.

What to look for

The simple 'Two Mass Model' illustrated in Figure 12.4 indicates that there will be phase difference between the opening and closing of the lips of the free border superiorly and a second wave that is developed beneath it during vibration, and this is exactly what is seen on strobolaryngoscopy. These so-called 'mucosal waves' are best demonstrated by the subject phonating in a firm steady tone in the lower part of their vocal range, in modal voice. Waves are still visible at higher pitches,

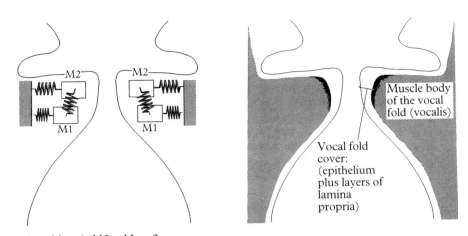

Key: M1 = Mass 1, M2 = Mass 2

Figure 12.4 Two Mass Model

but are much smaller, especially when in falsetto voice, above the 'break' known as the passaggio. A nice steady 'Heeeeee' will prevent the tongue position from becoming too 'backed', thereby preventing complete exposure of the laryngopharynx (Figure 12.5).

This is, of course, what is supposed to happen. The purpose of a voice clinic is to identify the nature of a problem when phonation does not occur exactly as it is supposed to. The findings on stroboscopic examination should therefore be recorded. We suggest that for practical purposes this could be combined with the other physical findings on a proforma such as the one illustrated in Appendix 12.1.

Caveats

1. If there is any asymmetry, reduction in size or local loss of waves, then there **must be a reason**, whether or not you can identify it at the time.
2. While you may wish to observe what happens to the folds when a subject phonates in a high pitched falsetto, this particular gesture produces very small mucosal waves, and is of little value in assessing the closed phase of the vibratory cycle.
3. Be aware that a weakness of stroboscopic assessment of fold activity is that the effective reduction by filtering of the quantity of visual information tends to reduce information about irregular (chaotic) beating or beating outside the range of frequency preordained by the electronic filter. There may be additional vibratory patterns but they will be 'ironed out' by the method of observation (see Švec et al., 1996). It is to be hoped that computer techniques such as the construction of 3-D 'phase portraits' of beating will prove clinically useful in future.
4. It is recommended that the observer palpates the subject's neck to identify the height of the subject's larynx and the state of the laryngeal cricothyroid visor both at rest and when voicing the notes to be observed before viewing the stroboscopic motion of the folds. This greatly aids interpretation of the observed findings (see also Chapter 5).

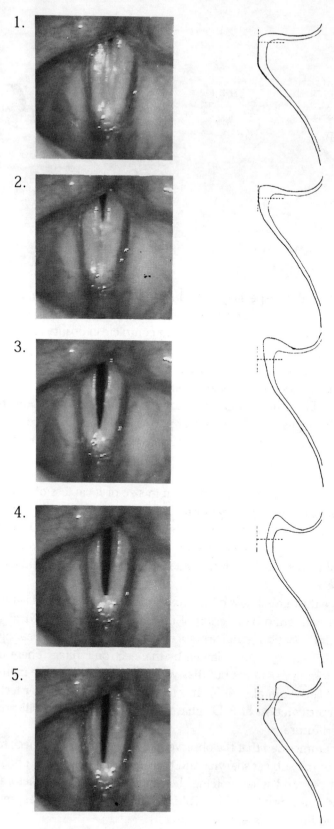

Figure 12.5 Vocal fold motion in sequence

6.

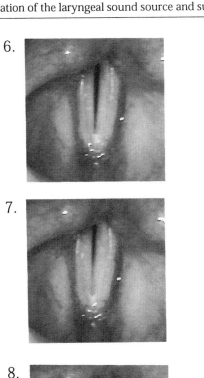

7.

8.

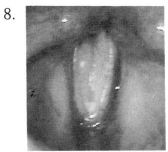

9.

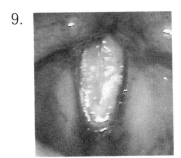

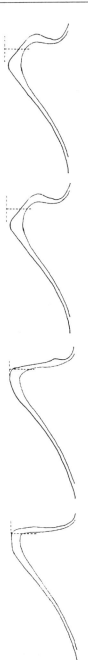

Videostrobolaryngoscopy

We now live in an age of evidence based medicine. It is always a good idea to back up your opinion with evidence, just as it would be considered routine to produce audiological evidence prior to any surgery to improve the hearing. Small, extremely light-sensitive television cameras are now relatively inexpensive; one can buy a very good single-chip CCD for under £2000. 'Three-chip' cameras give improved colour quality and more lines, but they are, in general, slightly less light-sensitive than their single-chip equivalents, and will require the purchase of an expensive laryngoscope to compensate for this. They also more than double the price. (At the time of writing, a Teli model CS 5850 three-chip camera with a resolution of 600 lines costs approximately £5000.)

Preserving the image

Video

The video recorder (VCR) that you select for your clinic is inevitably going to be chosen with price as a major factor in the decision. If money were no object, we should all be using machinery with grand-sounding titles such as 'High Band One-Inch Beta' format VCRs, but this is not a problem for the real world. Sony lost the war of the formats to National Panasonic, and the better, Beta, format is now only found in major television centres; the rather less good but by now ubiquitous VHS format is, in effect, the standard. VHS is ageing as a format, however, and was never really intended for re-editing. The heir to the VHS line, 'son of VHS', is cunningly titled S-VHS. This does not signify 'super' anything, but rather a system in which recording of light values (luminance) and colour values (chrominance) are performed separately. The result is an improvement in picture definition and a very considerable improvement in quality of edited clips of video. It is for this reason that increasing numbers of clinics now have S-VHS-based recording systems. Approximate price indications at the time of writing are between £1000 and £3500. We would urge readers to save up to buy into the high quality professional end of the range, as the freeze-frame capability and the time-coding systems are greatly superior when it comes to editing. There will inevitably be a considerable change over the next decade or so with the introduction of high definition television, and it goes without saying that as soon as you buy equipment it is already on the road to obsolescence – there is never going to be an ideal moment to buy, as technology moves relentlessly on.

Some centres, often the ones with better funding, are currently suggesting that it is time to abandon the VCR altogether. If the laboratory is already the proud possessor of a recent and fairly powerful computer, it is fairly easy to install a frame grabber card. With this card, video input is digitized and stored to disc or to a read-write CD ROM. This is clearly going to be the way to go about things in future, but at present the major problem is in storing the torrents of data generated by video. If the user of this system feels that very short clips of movement are adequate, then a digital compression system such as M-PEG will be the answer to their prayers. Manipulating the images is slow, however, and storage of longer clips of video will very soon occupy gigabytes of storage space. This does not yet seem like an ideal solution, even though there are obvious advantages in the archiving and retrieving of material.

Stills

For general purposes it is impractical at the present time to disseminate pictorial information about a patient's vocal folds, or even to keep a video cassette with the patient's notes. A still frame is not as informative as a moving picture, but is none the less far better than the artistic efforts of the majority of surgeons or therapists.

How then to get a selected frame of video onto paper? The choice at present is really between three types of technology. A Mavigraph® (Sony) is a machine that downloads the selected electronic image or images and prints them onto PVC 'paper'. Alternatively, the lab with a computer fitted with a frame grabber can keep the image in the disk or CD memory, or can print it out on plain paper using a colour printer such as an Inkjet®. It is also possible to add other varieties of technology to the video system. For example, Polaroid™ offers systems for image capture, but beware, although the systems are versatile, the top of the range is required for maximum image definition. We have these systems available and our preferred system is the Mavigraph, although others feel that the printout quality of most colour printers when used with the (more versatile) image grabber is quite satisfactory.

Storing dynamic aspects of vibration as a still photograph

The weakness of stroboscopy as a means of gathering information about cyclical activity is that irregular patterns of vibration may not be picked up. In the future, a technique known as **videokymography** may prove extremely useful to voice clinics, especially those with an interest in research. The technique developed by Švec and Schutte (1996), involves the use of a high-speed video camera operating at around 8000 images per second and selection of a single horizontal line from each complete image. Instead of building an image from 625 separate lines of scanned information, as is the norm for a conventional television image, the same line is scanned the same number of times and the whole is then displayed, the lines being redisplayed one under the other to build a complete picture as in a conventional television picture. The image is no longer representative of glottal appearance; instead, as each line from each scaning sweep is separated from the next in time only, the image will give a detailed record of the vibratory activity as if through a slice across the vocal folds.

Like conventional high-speed photography it will pick up details of asymmetry and irregularity of beating, subharmonics and other findings that stroboscopy might lose. It has the great advantage over storage of other 'high-speed data' that the valuable output can be reduced to an image stored as a single composite photograph, which can be analysed/interpreted at leisure.

Observing the resonators (the supraglottic vocal tract)

Although a rigid laryngoscope produces an excellent image of the activity of the vocal folds, the requirement for the tongue to be protruded and grasped before an examination can take place means that it is not possible to observe what a patient is doing in the supraglottic vocal tract to change resonance characteristics. Ideally, a totally non-invasive method must be used, and many research projects have used techniques such as high-speed X-rays and Xeroradiography to obtain these images. The problem for the clinician is that they mostly involve significant doses of radiation, generally demand that a patient is able to sustain a vocal gesture for a significant length of time and are not available actually in the clinic for use in a 'real-time' outpatient setting.

The clinical alternative is to use a minimally invasive technique such as is found in a great many general ENT clinics, fibreoptic nasendoscopy. Most modern nasendoscopes have a diameter of between 3.5 and 4.2 mm and have a tip that is manoeuvrable in a vertical plane (viz. instruments by Olympus, Machida, Pentax, Storz and others). With technological advances, a new generation of fused silicon fibreoptic bundles is being produced that offers greater picture definition and a smaller bundle diameter (viz. instruments by Omega). The obvious advantages of this are sadly somewhat offset by the increase in rigidity that their construction requires.

The most exciting new development in endoscopy of the upper aerodigestive tract seems to us to be found in the new rhinolaryngeal video endoscopes produced by Olympus and Pentax. A small monochrome camera chip is placed distally at the tip of the endoscope so that the picture is no longer dependent on fibre bundles. The field to be viewed is then very rapidly illuminated by a repeating sequence of red, green and blue light flashes from a special stroboscopic light generator. The camera input is reconstructed into high definition full colour pictures in a video processor. (Olympus EVIS 200 series; endoscope ENF 200; Pentax EPM-330P and VNL-1530 endoscope)

These systems are not, as yet, capable of producing stroboscopically slowed down pictures of vocal fold vibration. The price at the time of writing will put these systems beyond the reach of all but the best endowed centres.

We do not intend to give advice as to which model to buy, as it would almost certainly be out of date by the time this is read. We would, however, strongly recommend that anyone wishing to buy such a nasendoscope tries several instruments before parting with departmental money. There are always trade-offs between ease of use, image quality, peripheral distortion, field of view and diameter of the fibre bundle, to name but a few. In our clinic, for example, we seem to be able to cope with a larger diameter fibre bundle without distressing the patients unduly, and so an Olympus OES series instrument seems overall most satisfactory for our needs.

The most important thing to bear in mind is that in the construction of the fibrescope there are a finite number of glass threads each carrying a small fraction of the total image. This means that the resolution of the image, although good, is by definition never going to be quite as good as that of a lens-based instrument.

Endoscopy

Once organic disease has been excluded by inspection in a general ENT clinic, there are other clinical considerations about voice production to take into account. To get a reasonable view of phonation patterns the fibrescope is inserted into the nasal cavity horizontally, it is then advanced posteriorly, always under direct vision, and the tip is allowed to rise a little (usually it rests comfortably between the supero-medial aspect of the inferior turbinate and the septum). In mid-cavity, the anterior border of the middle turbinate drops in to view superiorly. The largest passage to the postnasal space is generally through the triangle between the inferior and middle turbinate laterally and the septum medially. The occurrence of bony septal spurs towards the back of the cavity (whose sole purpose seems to be to obstruct the passage of a nasendoscope) occurs more frequently in the left nasal cavity. Having negotiated the nasal cavity and passed through the choanae into the post-nasal space, a useful and repeatable position for viewing vocal manoeuvres seems to be to angle the tip of the fibrescope down at the level of the pharyngeal tubercle so that the free border of the palate is just visible at the bottom of the picture, and the base of tongue, lateral pharyngeal walls, entire hypopharynx and larynx are all visible. The shaft of the fibrescope is immobilized against the base of the skull, and it is thus possible to make judgements about the rise and fall of laryngopharyngeal structures. From this position it is possible to see most of the supraglottic vocal tract activity that takes place at a level behind and below the tonsils. Where appro-priate, in singers for instance, the clearest view is still afforded by the sustained vowel /i/ (Eeeeeeeeee), whatever the register or pitch. Be aware though, that at the highest frequencies, the formants of vowels change to accommodate the rise in pitch, and both the perceived sound and the pharyngeal gesture will change.

Appendix 12.1

Videostrobolaryngoscopy assessment form

A. PHARYNGEAL CHARACTERISTICS

Pyriform inlets   ☐ Dilated   ☐ Neutral   ☐ Constricted

A–P dimension between posterior pharyngeal wall and posterior aspect of arytenoids

☐ Dilated   ☐ Neutral   ☐ Compressed

B. SUPRAGLOTTIC GESTURE

Shape of supraglottis   ☐ Narrow   ☐ Open   ☐ Compressed

Stretched - lateral narrowing   A–P narrowing

Tilting of arytenoids on phonation
☐ Posterior   ☐ Neutral   ☐ Mod. anterior   ☐ Extreme anterior
☐ R > L   ☐ R = L   ☐ L > R

Apex of arytenoid rotated over midline? (scissoring)
☐ Yes   ☐ No   ☐ R round L   ☐ L round R

Vocal processes overriding one another?
☐ Yes   ☐ No   ☐ L over R   ☐ R over L

Ventricular bands   - In contact? (DPV)   ☐ Yes   ☐ No

Part exposing vocal ligament?   ☐ Yes   ☐ No
☐ L > R   ☐ L = R   ☐ R > L

Wholly exposing vocal ligament?   ☐ Yes   ☐ No
☐ L > R   ☐ L = R   ☐ R > L

Is either band apparently hypertrophic?   ☐ Yes   ☐ No
☐ L > R   ☐ R > L

Rotation of the larynx?   ☐ Yes   ☐ No
☐ If Yes, Clockwise   ☐ Anticlockwise

Any apparent dystonic activity?   ☐ Yes   ☐ No

Appendix 12.1 Videostrobolaryngoscopy assessment form

C. PHYSICAL CONDITION OF THE LARYNX

Please indicate if present:	Yes	No
Interarytenoid mucosal pachydermia	☐	☐
Inflammation of mucosa of medial aspect of arytenoids	☐	☐
Oedema of mucosa of the posterior laryngeal inlet	☐	☐
Granuloma of arytenoid	☐	☐

Condition of the vocal folds: ☐ Normal   ☐ Abnormal

☐ Atrophic	☐ Left	☐ Right	☐ Both
☐ * Minimal	☐ Slight	☐ Moderate	☐ Severe
☐ Oedematous	☐ Left	☐ Right	☐ Both
☐ * Minimal	☐ Slight	☐ Moderate	☐ Severe
☐ Inflammation	☐ Left	☐ Right	☐ Both
☐ * Minimal	☐ Slight	☐ Moderate	☐ Severe
☐ Telangiect.	☐ Left	☐ Right	☐ Both
☐ * Minimal	☐ Slight	☐ Moderate	☐ Severe
☐ Haematoma	☐ Left	☐ Right	☐ Both
☐ * Minimal	☐ Slight	☐ Moderate	☐ Severe

D. VOCAL FOLD OPENING/CLOSURE

Abduction	☐ Full	☐ Reduced	
	☐ L > R	☐ R > L	☐ Symmetrical
☐ * Minimal	☐ Slight	☐ Moderate	☐ Severe

Adduction	☐ Full	☐ Reduced	
	☐ L > R	☐ R > L	☐ Symmetrical
☐ * Minimal	☐ Slight	☐ Moderate	☐ Severe

Posterior glottic chink gaps (Södersten and Lindestad Category 1)

☐ None   ☐ Small intercartilag.   ☐ Wide intercartilag.

☐ Posterior third gap   ☐ Post. two thirds gap   ☐ No closure

Anterior and complex membranous gaps. Vocal processes closed.
(Södersten and Lindestad. Category 2)

☐ Spindle-shaped bowing   ☐ Post. third gap   ☐ Ant. third gap

☐ Both ant. and post. gaps (hourglassing)

E. STROBOSCOPIC FINDINGS

Mucosal waves

Symmetrical in amplitude? ☐ Yes   ☐ No
                         ☐ L > R   ☐ R > L

Degree of reduction   ☐ L > R   ☐ Minimal reduction   ☐ R > L
                         ☐ Absence of waves

Symmetrical in phase?   ☐ Yes   ☐ No

Degree of phase lag   ☐ L > R   ☐ Minimal delay   ☐ R > L
                         ☐ Independent vibration

Closure   ☐ Full   ☐ Incomplete
                         ☐ Absent

Closed phase   ☐ Absent   ☐ Short
                         ☐ Normal   ☐ Prolonged

Gap, if present   ☐ Interarytenoid   ☐ Hourglass
                         ☐ Bowing   ☐ Anterior

Irregular beats   ☐ None observed   ☐ Occasional
                         ☐ Many noted

Localized inhibition?   ☐ Yes   ☐ No   ☐ Left   ☐ Right   ☐ Both

Is the inhibition apparently due to :

	Yes	No	Left	Right
Polypoid degen.	☐	☐	☐	☐
Nodule(s)	☐	☐	☐	☐
Mucus cyst	☐	☐	☐	☐
Dermoid cyst	☐	☐	☐	☐
Sulcus	☐	☐	☐	☐
Vergeture	☐	☐	☐	☐
Scarring	☐	☐	☐	☐
Other lesion	☐	☐	☐	☐

Notes relating to the observation proforma

See also Chapter 7. During connected speech, in both trained singers and the population at large, the following should be looked for.

Rotation and/or positioning of the laryngopharynx away from the midline

This observation should always be correlated with the postural findings in the neck (see Chapter 6). Is one pyriform fossa more voluminous than the other? This is often associated with vocal fatigue.

Tongue backing

The larynx is covered by the back of the tongue for much of any piece of connected speech. There is obvious reduction in the normal A–P diameter of the pharynx. This produces a 'darker' or more 'plummy' sound.

Laryngeal height for speech

When speech commences, does the larynx rise or fall to a set position that is significantly different from the position at rest?

Constriction of the supraglottis during phonation for speech

When used in normal speech, this appearance is generally associated with hyper-valving and the narrow definition of hyperkinetic dysphonia. It produces variable vocal results depending on the associated subglottic air pressure, and whether or not the cricothyroid visor is held in a closed position or is allowed to relax.

For further details about the different characteristic patterns of vocal fold gesture, see the section on Patterns of isometric muscle activity in Chapter 7.

While singing, the following should be looked for. They are usually more obvious in trained voices.

Constriction of the supraglottic vocal tract at the level of middle constrictor

This is thought to be the constriction that is required for the maintenance of the 'singer's formant', the amalgamation of the third and fourth formants, to produce the ringing quality to a classically trained voice. The appearance is like an inverted blunt 'V' shape part concealing the pyriform inlets. It is best seen when notes are being sung moderately loudly in the upper part of the range in all but the highest sopranos.

Maintenance of open pyriform fossae

This is necessary to protect the absolute volume of the SGVT as a resonating tube. It is most clearly seen in males throughout their vocal range; in females this gesture may be abandoned for physical reasons when singing high vowels. It is not seen in 'belt' voice quality.

Constriction/deconstriction of the supraglottis

Whether this is a 'good' or 'bad' thing depends on the vocal quality desired. It is perfectly possible to deliberately train singers to use the muscularis and vocalis portions of the thyroarytenoid muscles independently. It is akin to the difference between a 'sob' and a (pre)-cough gesture. The position of the aryepiglottic folds is a useful marker.

References

Garcia M (1855) Observations physiologiques sur la voix humaine. Proceedings of the Royal Society 7: 13.

Hirano M, Bless D (1993) Videostroboscopic examination of the larynx. San Diego: Singular Publishing Group, Inc.

Kitzing P (1985) Stroboscopy – a pertinent laryngological examination. Journal of Otolaryngology 14: 151–157.

Musehold A (1898) Stroboskopische und photographische Studien über die Stellung der Stimmlippen im Brust und Falsett-register. Archiv für Laryngologie und Rhinologie (Berlin) 7:1–21.

Oertel MJ (1895) Das Laryngostroboskop und die laryngostroboskopische Untersuchung. Archiv für Laryngologie und Rhinologie (Berlin) 3:1–16.

Schönhärl E (1960) Die Stroboskopie in der praktischen Laryngologie. Stuttgart: Georg Thieme Verlag, pp. 64–65.

Södersten E, Lindestad P-Å (1990) Glottal closure and perceived breathiness during phonation in normally speaking subjects. Journal of Speech and Hearing Research 33: 601–611.

Svec JG, Schutte HK (1996) Videokymography: high-speed line scanning of vocal fold vibration. Journal of Voice 10: 201–205.

Svec JG, Schutte HK, Miller DG (1996) A subharmonic vibratory pattern in normal vocal folds. Journal of Speech and Hearing Research 39: 135–143.

Titze IR (1981) Biomechanics and distributed mass models of vocal fold vibration. In Steven KN, Hirano M (Eds) Vocal fold physiology. University of Tokyo Press.

Titze IR (1994) Vocal fold oscillation. In Principles of voice production. New Jersey: Prentice-Hall, Inc., pp. 80–109.

Part 3. Equipment for Measuring Voice: Uses and Limitations

Instrumental voice measurement: uses and limitations

DAVID M HOWARD

Vorsprung durch Technik
(Taking the lead through technology)

Advertisement

Introduction

The huge increase in the number of powerful desk-top personal computers in the past 15 years or so has widened the range of application areas in which they are employed. More recent developments in the area of multimedia applications, where sound and video are being added to text and graphics, have meant that sound and video processing capability are becoming a standard part of any modern personal computer system. One consequence of this is the increasing range of relatively inexpensive sound- and image-processing tools available for such systems, which were once only seen in large research laboratories.

The incorporation of sound-processing tools in personal computers, either as part of the multimedia capability of the machine or as special purpose hardware connected either internally or externally, offers the possibility of practical voice measurement in the clinic or laboratory. Such tools are available to an ever increasing number of users, many of whom will have little or no background in the theory of the signal processing techniques employed, which can often be highly complicated – in some cases involving assumptions about the nature of the input signal that are not always made clear to the user. Given the abundance of equipment now available in a voice clinic, it is becoming all too easy to make measurements. The potential for an unsuitable voice analysis technique to be applied with inappropriate parameters exists now more than ever before, with the resulting potential for

Footnote: The main part of this chapter is in normal print, but for those wishing for more detail, this is supplied in the sections in the smaller (sans serif) print.

erroneous conclusions to be reached, and this is often exacerbated by often very poor manuals.

This part of the book explores practical voice measurement techniques, thus providing an awareness upon which a well-founded understanding of commonly employed voice analysis techniques can be built so that: (a) an informed choice can be made of an analysis technique for a particular situation (e.g. clinical set-up, voice disorder, speaking environment), and (b) user-adjustable parameter values that are often available (e.g. threshold, gain, filter setting, smoothing, window size) can be adjusted appropriately.

Voice data are often used to corroborate objectively perceptual judgements regarding voice pitch and/or voice quality. The results may be represented on a computer screen in the form of visual feedback, or as part of a scientific investigation of some aspect of voice. A wide variety of signals can be measured to give insights into the dynamic processes that occur during normal, pathological and professional voice production as well as a number of other sounds produced by the normal voice, such as coughing, snoring, laughing and crying. All are analysed using essentially the principles outlined here, but even the most objective data require subjective interpretation that is informed by both the circumstances surrounding the origin of the data and the analysis techniques that have been employed. Informed practical voice measurement, therefore, requires knowledge of the human speech production process before the nature of commonly employed analysis techniques can be introduced, and this is the purpose of the next section.

Acoustics of speech production

Producing any sound acoustically involves three elements: a power source, a sound source and sound modifiers. Human voice production is no exception. Figure 13.1 shows these elements in human voice production for voiced sounds such as vowels, that are perceived as having a pitch associated with them that may vary with time. Sounds that do not have a clear pitch associated with them are described phonetically as unvoiced.

The key elements in the production of sounds are the action of the lungs to provide the power source. This causes air to flow past the vocal folds, which oscillate to provide the sound source in voiced sounds, or some other constriction in the vocal tract to provide the sound source during voiceless sounds. The sound source is then modified by the acoustic properties of the vocal tract, the sound modifiers. These are shown diagrammatically in Figure 13.1 during the production of a voiced sound and the right hand section of the figure shows the system further stylized into an idealized form to represent the lungs as a piston, the mouth as a flexible cavity and the soft palate as a valve that connects and disconnects the nasal cavity from the airstream. The arrows illustrate those elements that are adjustable and require appropriate control during the production of voiced sounds: lung action (power source), the position of the vocal folds (sound source) and the shape of the vocal tract (sound modifiers).

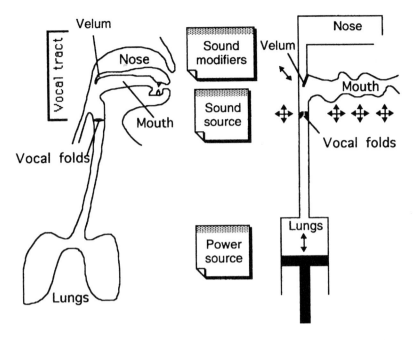

Figure 13.1 The power source, sound source and sound modifiers during the production of voiced sounds

Power source

The main function of the power source in voice production is to provide and sustain an air pressure that is higher than atmospheric. This will result in an outward flow of air or egressive airstream, as it is known in phonetics, from the mouth and/or nose depending on the position of the soft palate, otherwise known as the velum or velopharyngeal port. The vocal folds have to be apart for there to be such an airflow; for air to flow via the lips (oral airflow) there must be no complete constriction in the mouth; and for air to flow via the nostrils (nasal airflow) the velum, indicated in Figure 13.1, is lowered. The reservoir of lung air is depleted during voice production, and to maintain an air pressure higher than atmospheric, voice production must pause to enable the reservoir to be replenished by breathing in. In situations, particularly of heightened stress, where, for example, it may be absolutely imperative to convey a message very fast, voice production can also occur while breathing in, on an ingressive airstream (see for example, Wells and Colson, 1971; Ladefoged, 1975). Some languages other than English include voiced sounds that are ingressive.

Sound source

The sound source during speech or singing production is either: (a) voiced, as a result of the vibration of the vocal folds (e.g. the vowel sounds of 'bead', 'bard', 'booed', 'bed' and 'bud'); (b) voiceless, as a result of air being forced past a constriction in the vocal tract (e.g. the initial consonants in 'sin', 'chin' and 'fin'); or (c) mixed, as a result of vocal-fold vibration and air being forced past a constriction in the vocal tract (e.g. the initial consonants in 'zoo', 'gin' and 'vet'). In Figure 13.1, only the voiced sound source is represented. A voiceless sound source occurs at the point in the vocal tract where the constriction is formed, and a mixed sound source involves both a voiced and a voiceless sound source. The acoustics of both voiced and voiceless sound sources are introduced below.

The voiced sound source arises as the acoustic result of the vibration of the vocal folds. The basic mechanism by which they vibrate can be described with reference to a physical principle known as the Bernoulli effect. To initiate vibration, the vocal folds are brought closer together horizontally, or adducted. Air expelled from the lungs passes between the adducted folds via the glottis (the gap between the folds). The velocity of airflow must increase as it crosses the glottis due to the narrowed airway at this point, reducing the pressure exerted on the surrounding structure (the Bernoulli principle), which for the glottis is the vocal folds themselves, and this tends to pull the folds towards each other. This is illustrated in Figure 13.2. This action narrows the glottis still further. The air now flowing through this increasingly narrowed glottis must increase further in velocity, causing the pressure exerted on the vocal folds to reduce further (a positive feedback system), and therefore the force pulling the folds together increases incrementally. The result is that the folds are accelerated towards each other until they meet at the midline of the larynx where they snap together, closing the glottis and causing a very rapid reduction in the flow of air through the glottis and a local pressure drop immediately above the vocal folds. This rapid pressure change produces an instantaneous pulse-like acoustic excitation to the vocal tract.

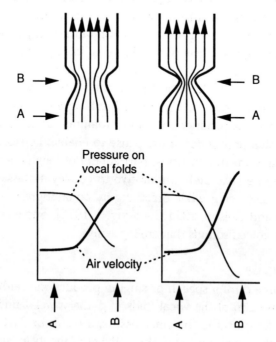

Figure 13.2 Stylized laryngeal tube in vocal fold region showing changes in air velocity and pressure on the vocal folds due to an egressive airstream

From this state in which the folds are in contact, there are two effects that contribute to the parting of the folds and the opening of the glottis: (1) subglottal pressure is higher than supraglottal pressure, tending to push the folds apart; and (2) the natural pendulum-like action of the folds that has the same effect. The folds thus tend to accelerate away from each other, passing through their rest or equilibrium position, decelerating due to their pendulum-like action until they reach a maximally open position. The oscillatory motion then causes the folds to accelerate back towards their equilibrium position. The Bernoulli principle again comes into play and the cycle repeats. The repeated cycles of vocal-fold vibration produce a rapid and more or less regular sequence of vocal-fold closures, each resulting in an acoustic pulse-like excitation.

Hitherto, vocal-fold vibration has been described in two dimensions. However, during the vocal-fold vibration sequence the lower edges of the vocal folds meet and part before the upper edges, due to the structure of the larynx and the direction of airflow. Thus the movement of the bottom edges of the folds is out of phase with the movement of the upper edges, as illustrated in Figure 13.3.

Vocal-fold vibration in a healthy larynx is, therefore, a cyclic sequence whose period is related to the natural frequency of the pendulum-like action of the folds themselves. *The myoelastic aerodynamic theory of vocal-fold vibration* (Van den Berg, 1958) suggests that their fundamental frequency of vibration (f_0) is determined by the mass, tension and elasticity of the folds. Greater mass, lesser tension or lesser elasticity of the folds will tend to reduce the f_0 of vibration, and the converse also holds true. The mass of the vibrating vocal folds can be altered by supporting a greater or lesser portion of the folds in an immobile position, and their tension and elasticity can be adjusted by stretching and releasing the vibrating tissue. The myoelastic aerodynamic theory of vocal-fold vibration does not provide a full explanation of the situation when the folds do not fully snap together, as in some examples of breathy voice production. Valuable insights into such situations and other more recent work on vocal-fold vibration can be found in Titze (1994).

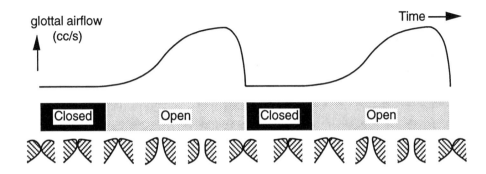

Figure 13.3 Schematized pattern of glottal airflow and cross-sections of healthy vocal fold vibration for two cycles, showing closed and open phases

In summary then, the acoustic excitation provided to the vocal tract by the vibrating vocal folds consists of a sequence of pressure pulses, each being a consequence of a vocal-fold closure. The number of closures per second gives the f_0 of the voice, which relates to the perceived pitch: a higher pitch is perceived when there are more vocal-fold closures per second and vice versa.

The sequence of pressure pulses input to the vocal tract by the vibrating vocal folds is essentially periodic, but as the period of each successive cycle tends to vary slightly it is usually described as quasi-periodic. The time taken for one complete cycle of vibration–excitation is known as the period (T_x), and the reciprocal of the period $(1/T_x)$ gives the **fundamental frequency** (f_0), which equates with the number of cycles per second and is measured in Hertz or Hz. In the case of healthy vocal-fold excitation, an idealized plot of the variation of acoustic pressure against time, or acoustic pressure waveform, of the acoustic excitation to the vocal tract is shown in idealized form on the left-hand side of Figure 13.4. Note the large negative-going pressure pulse resulting from each vocal-fold closure as they very rapidly cut off the flow of air from the lungs.

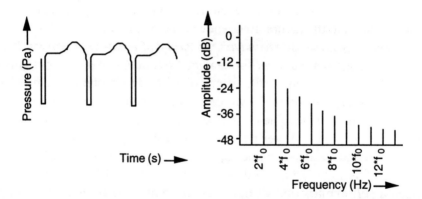

Figure 13.4 Idealized pressure waveform (left) and spectrum (right) for the acoustic excitation to the vocal tract produced by a healthy larynx. This is the sound source in voiced sounds

The pattern of vibration is, however, complex and a complete description of the vibrating sound source involves frequency components in addition to f_0. It turns out that any periodic waveform can be considered in terms of its mathematically defined frequency components, or Fourier components after the French natural philosopher Joseph Fourier (1768-1830).

Fourier postulated that: 'any periodic waveform can be built up from a series of simple vibrations whose frequencies are harmonics of a fundamental frequency, by choosing the proper amplitudes and phases of these harmonics'. Each harmonic represents a sinewave (the pure tone produced by a struck tuning fork is essentially a sinewave) and they are the basic building blocks from which a waveform of any shape can be synthesized. In the case of periodic waveforms the frequencies of the components are harmonically related as integer (1, 2, 3, 4...) multiples of f_0 (i.e. $1*f_0$, $2*f_0$, $3*f_0$, $4*f_0$...). The integer in each case is known as the harmonic number; thus the $(2*f_0)$ component is the second harmonic, and the $(3*f_0)$

component is the third harmonic. (An earlier system for describing the frequency components of a periodic waveform was in terms of overtones, where the first overtone refers to the first frequency component that is over or above f_0, and is therefore the second harmonic. The second overtone is the third harmonic, the third overtone is the fourth harmonic, and so on. This can sometimes be a source of confusion and we shall use the harmonic system here. Further discussion can be found in Howard and Angus (1996).) The $(1*f_0)$ component is the first harmonic, but it is more usually referred to as the fundamental frequency, or f_0. Note that f_0 is also the interval between successive harmonics. Any waveform that is periodic is therefore either: (a) simple, in which case it is a sinewave and therefore has just one frequency component which is the f_0; or (b) complex, in which case it has a number of components that are harmonically (integer multiples of f_0) related.

The idealized frequency components for the idealized pressure variation for the acoustic excitation to the vocal tract produced by healthy vocal fold vibration are shown on the right-hand side of Figure 13.4. A representation such as this, which shows the frequency and amplitude of the sinewave components of a waveform, is known as a **spectrum**. The important aspects to note are that all the frequency components that could exist, in this case they are harmonics (integer multiples of the fundamental) because the waveform is periodic, are present, and that their relative sizes or amplitudes, measured here in terms of pressure, reduce by a quarter as their frequency doubles. A more common way of expressing this is to note that a change of one octave (which contains 12 semitones) up or down is equivalent to a doubling or halving in frequency respectively, and that the amplitude of the components shown in Figure 13.4 can be said to fall by a quarter for a doubling in frequency, or more commonly by 12dB per octave (see Note 1).

During voiceless sounds the vocal folds do not vibrate. A narrow constriction is made somewhere in the vocal tract, for example by the tongue being positioned just behind the top teeth for the consonant in the word 'see'. If air flows gently past such a constriction, no sound is heard. As the airflow is increased, however, there comes a point where a noise-like sound is heard, which is the acoustic excitation during voiceless sounds. This noise, or friction, arises as a result of the airflow becoming turbulent at the point of constriction, and speech sounds with such an acoustic excitation are referred to phonetically as *fricatives*. The presence of acoustic noise can be readily confirmed by forming the constriction for the consonants (fricatives) in either 'see' or 'fee', and adjusting the airflow while listening to the acoustic result. It is also worth noticing that such voiceless sounds have no definite pitch associated with them (musical notes cannot be sung on the consonants of either see or fee).

Unlike the waveforms for voiced (pitched) sounds, which have a repeating pattern and are periodic, the waveforms for voiceless (non-pitched) sounds do not have a repeating pattern and are non-periodic. A non-periodic waveform does not have harmonics associated with its spectrum, which is represented as a continuous line, indicating that all frequencies are present (see Note 2). A spectrum of a sound whose waveform is non-periodic is known as a continuous spectrum. In particular, the spectrum of the acoustic excitation during unvoiced sounds is a horizontal line as shown in Figure 13.5, known as a flat spectrum. The signal itself it known as *white noise*, because all frequencies are present with equal amplitude as a corollary with white light, in which all colours are present in equal proportions. The amplitude of the frequency spectrum of the sound source during unvoiced sounds therefore falls off at 0 dB per octave.

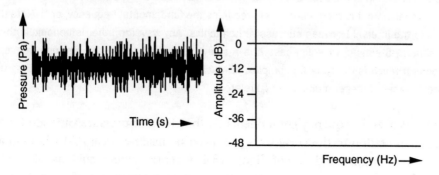

Figure 13.5 Idealized pressure waveform (left) and spectrum (right) for the acoustic excitation to the vocal tract produced by air being forced past a constriction in the vocal tract. This is the sound source in unvoiced sounds

During sounds whose sound source consists of a mixed excitation, both sound sources are used together. Turbulent airflow is produced at a point of constriction (the fricative part) while the vocal folds are vibrating (the voiced part). Such speech sounds are known as *voiced fricatives*. The airstream during these sounds is regularly interrupted by the closing and opening of the vocal folds and the acoustic noise thereby produced at the point of constriction is pulsed on and off. This occurs, for example, during the production of the non-vowel part of 'zoo', 'the' and 'vee'.

Sound modifiers

The acoustic excitation produced by the sound source, whether voiced, voiceless or mixed, is changed acoustically by the sound modifiers (see Figure 13.1) during speech or singing. The sound modifiers have an acoustic effect on the sound source due to the acoustic properties of the oral and nasal cavities between the sound source and the outside world. These cavities together form the vocal tract.

Figure 13.6 shows the parts of the vocal tract that can be moved, or articulated, during speech production: the tongue, jaw, lips and soft palate (or velum). The soft palate acts as a valve to include or exclude the nasal cavity with respect to the rest of the vocal tract. As the shape of the vocal tract is changed its acoustic properties are altered. The acoustic frequency responses for the three non-nasalized vowels, in 'bee', 'baa' and 'boo', are illustrated in Figure 13.6. Each is characterized by a series of peaks in its vocal tract frequency response curve, which are referred to as **formants**. Three are shown in the frequency response corresponding to each vocal tract configuration, and they are labelled first formant (F1), second formant (F2) and third formant (F3) in order of ascending frequency in the response curve. The different articulator positions for these vowels is illustrated in the figure. Notice that the velum is raised to shut off the nasal cavity

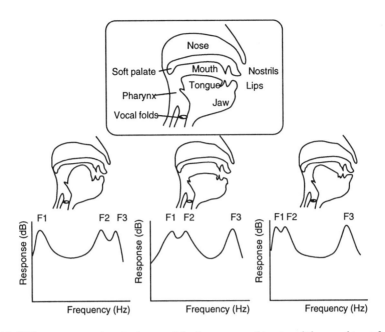

Figure 13.6 The main speech articulators of the human vocal tract and the vocal tract frequency response for the vowels in 'bee' (left), 'baa' (centre) and 'boo' (right)

during isolated vowels, and that the tongue and jaw adopt different positions for each vowel illustrated. These vocal tract shapes result in the variation in acoustic response characteristics of the vocal tract shown in the lower part of the figure.

It is important to note that the *formants themselves refer to acoustic properties of the vocal tract rather than those of particular sounds,* so that the 'same' vowel may be uttered with a whisper (no vocal fold vibration), or with an electrolarynx (used by some after tracheostomy). Although formants are most often associated with descriptions of vowel production, they are relevant to all speech sounds to a greater or lesser extent.

A more complete description of formants may be found in Ladefoged (1975), Pickett (1980), Baken (1987) and Kent and Read (1992). Typical average f_0 means and ranges and first three formant ranges for men, women and children are given in Table 13.1.

Table 13.1 Typical first three formant frequency ranges and f_0 mean and ranges values for conversational speech of men, women and children.
(f_0 values from Fry, 1979; F1, F2 and F3 ranges from Kent and Read, 1992)

Parameter	Men	Women	Children
f_0 mean	120 Hz	225 Hz	265 Hz
f_0 range	13 semitones	13 semitones	12 semitones
F1 range	270-730 Hz	300-860 Hz	370-1030 Hz
F2 range	850-2300 Hz	900-2800 Hz	1050-3200 Hz
F3 range	1700-3000 Hz	1950-3300 Hz	2150-3700 Hz

Three formants are generally considered when analysing speech, the first two being 'critical' in vowel production. Higher formants tend to remain relatively invariant during speech production, – however, the fourth, fifth and sixth formants are thought to perform an important function during professional operatic singing, and F3 has been shown to carry information regarding speaker individuality.

Speech output

The overall average *spectral trend* imparted onto the sound source during voiced and voiceless speech is illustrated in Figure 13.7. It is important to understand the nature of the average spectral trend in speech and singing as it is directly relevant to practical voice measurement.

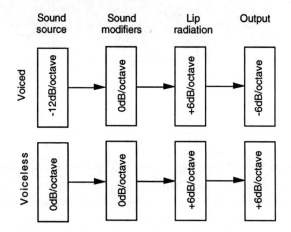

Figure 13.7 Average spectral trends of the sound source, sound modifiers and lip radiation during voiced (upper) and voiceless (lower) speech

The sound source during voiced speech exhibits an average spectral trend of -12 dB per octave (see Figure 13.4). That during voiceless sounds is 0 dB per octave (see Figure 13.5). The average spectral trend of the sound modifiers is 0 dB per octave. The effect of the lips radiating the acoustic signal to the outside world is +6 dB per octave. Therefore the overall average spectral trend per octave for voiced speech in decibels is equal to: (-12 dB + 0 dB + 6 dB) = -6 dB per octave, and that for voiceless speech is equal to: (0 dB + 0 dB + 6 dB) = + 6dB per octave.

The average spectral trends observed in the professional voices of trained singers and actors tend to deviate from these as different demands are placed on the sound source and the sound modifiers to enable both more efficient projection and a greater f_0 range to be used.

In practical voice analysis, the formants can be measured from the output spectrum of a vowel by looking for peaks in harmonic amplitudes, and the f_0 of the vowel can be measured from the harmonic spacing.

Figure 13.8 gives a spectral representation of the sound source, sound modifiers and output for the vowels in 'baa' and 'bee' spoken at the same pitch. Both here and in Figure 13.9, the effect of lip radiation is assumed in plotting the output spectra. The sound source is

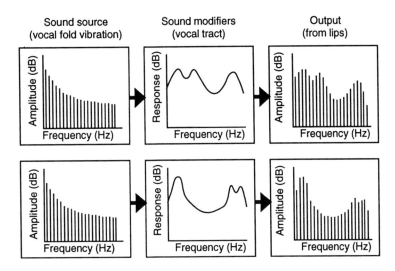

Figure 13.8 Spectral representation of the sound source, sound modifiers and output for the vowels in 'baa' (upper) and 'bee' (lower) spoken at the same pitch. The effect of lip radiation (see Figure 13.7) is taken into account in the output spectrum

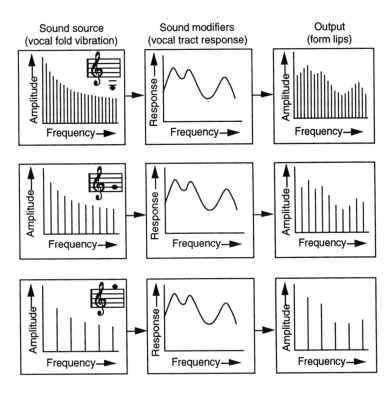

Figure 13.9 Spectral representation of the sound source, sound modifiers and output for the vowels in baa sung on three notes an octave apart as indicated on the inset staves. The effect of lip radiation (see Figure 13.7) is taken into account in the output spectrum. (From Howard and Angus, 1996)

voiced and consists of harmonics whose amplitude changes by -12 dB per octave with increasing frequency (see Figure 13.4). The f_0, and therefore the spacing between the harmonics, is identical in each example because the same pitch is used for the two vowels. The output from the lips is the result of each harmonic of the sound source being modified by the vocal tract response at the frequency of that harmonic frequency. This has the effect of imparting the formant pattern of the sound modifiers, or vocal tract response, for each vowel onto the harmonic spectrum of the acoustic excitation provided by the vibrating vocal folds.

Figure 13.9 illustrates the effect when the same vowel is sung at three different pitches. The different pitches result in a different f_0 (the note G spaced in this example by octaves as indicated by the inset staves). The harmonic spacing doubles for a pitch rise of one octave, and the spacing halves for an octave fall in pitch shown by the different values of f_0 and resulting different harmonic spacings. The note with the more closely spaced harmonics has the lowest f_0. The formant frequencies can be observed in the output spectra, but it can be seen that the formant peaks are less well defined in the output spectrum of the vowel sung with the higher pitch. Thus *it may be harder to identify formants in the output spectrum of a sound when it is sung or spoken on a high pitch.* This is particularly important when analysing sounds with high values of f_0 such as children's speech and higher notes sung by sopranos. It can be seen from Figure 13.9 that the formant peaks for the vowel sung at the highest pitch plotted are indiscernible in the output spectrum. It turns out that for sung notes with an f_0 of approximately 512 Hz (the C above middle C), the formant peaks are poorly defined in the output spectrum and the vowel being sung becomes increasingly difficult to determine as notes higher than this are sung (Howard and Collingsworth, 1992).

Practical fundamental frequency measurement

Appropriate control over the rate of vibration of the vocal folds is an essential aspect of phonation during both speech and singing. The number of vibrations per second of the vocal folds gives the f_0 of vocal fold vibration, and changes in f_0 manifest themselves perceptually as *changes in pitch*. Pitch variation in speech is heard as intonation patterns, as stress within sentences or words, or as different tones in languages such as Cantonese, and in singing as different notes. Variation during individual sung notes is perceived as *vibrato* (e.g. Dejonckere et al., 1995) while non-voluntary variation during speech is known as '*jitter*'.

The pitch we associate with a sound relates to the manner in which our hearing system processes the sound (psychoacoustics), and the pitch of any sound is therefore based on a subjective judgement made by a human listener, or subject, on a scale from low to high. The formal definition of pitch offered by the American National Standards Institute (1960) is: 'pitch is that attribute of auditory sensation in terms of which sounds may be ordered on a scale extending from low to high'. This contrasts with the measurement of the f_0 of vocal fold vibration which is an objective measurement.

It should be noted that small changes in pitch can also be perceived, albeit to a very much lesser degree, when the intensity (loudness) or the spectral content (timbre) of the sound are varied and the f_0 is kept constant (e.g. Howard and Angus, 1996). Many vocal disorders result in a perceived pitch that is considered to be inappropriate, and traditional clinical analysis based on informed listening might aim to assign a subjective rating of voice pitch for example, on a scale from low to high. Such techniques are likely to be unreliable due to inter-listener variation, unrepeatable (hence not scientifically rigorous) and unable to compensate for any pitch change that is brought about by changes in loudness or timbre. On this matter, Baken (1987) concludes that: *'perceptual judgements alone may well mislead the clinician' and that 'while it is important for the therapist to judge vocal pitch acceptability, it is vital that the fundamental frequency be measured'*. Any reliable analysis technique must therefore be based on a clearly defined objective measurement that is reliable, repeatable and not subject to the variability in the listening judgement between (and within) individuals.

Research into the measurement of speech f_0 began in the 1920s and still continues today. The reason for the continuation of this research is that no single device or method for f_0 measurement exists that works reliably for any speaker in any acoustic environment. It turns out that the choice of an f_0 measurement technique should be made with direct reference to the particular demands of the intended application in terms of: (i) the expected speaker population to be analysed (e.g. adult or child, male or female, pathological or non-pathological); (ii) all material that might be analysed (e.g. read speech, conversational speech, shouting, sustained vowels, singing); (iii) recording noise (e.g. mains hum, tape hiss); (iv) the likely competition from acoustic background or foreground noise (e.g. classroom, clinic, external noises); and (v) measurement errors that can be tolerated (e.g. f_0 doubling, f_0 halving, smoothing of the f_0 results, f_0 jitter due to the analysis).

There are many fields in which f_0 estimation is potentially important, for example:

- voice pathology
- speech and hearing research
- speech and singing synthesis
- forensic phonetics
- speech recognition
- linguistic research
- communications research
- music technology
- experimental phonetics
- professional voice production.

In practice, there are usually a number of f_0 estimation techniques available, even within a single analysis package. This field is often referred to in the literature as pitch extraction, but as pitch is a subjective judgement (which none of the algorithms to be discussed is making), the term 'f_0 estimation' is preferred. In order that a user is in a suitable position to make an informed choice of technique, it is vital that the advantages and limitations of the various f_0 measurement strategies are understood, based on an awareness of the principles behind each of the analysis methods themselves.

Techniques available

The operation of f_0 estimation devices or algorithms can be considered in terms of those that measure from:

(a) the input pressure waveform, which are said to work in the *time domain*;
(b) the spectrum of the input signal, which are said to work in the *frequency domain*;
(c) a *hybrid measurement* working in the time and frequency domains; and
(d) *direct measurement of laryngeal activity*. An extremely large number of algorithms have been proposed for f_0 estimation and it is not the purpose of this book to review all of them (a comprehensive and rigorous review is given in Hess, 1983). What is important here is to understand the basis on which f_0 estimation can be made in terms of how speech is represented in the time and frequency domains. Figure 13.10 illustrates the representation of a voiceless sound /s/ (A and B) and a voiced sound /a/ (C and D) in the time (A and C) and frequency (B and D) domains.

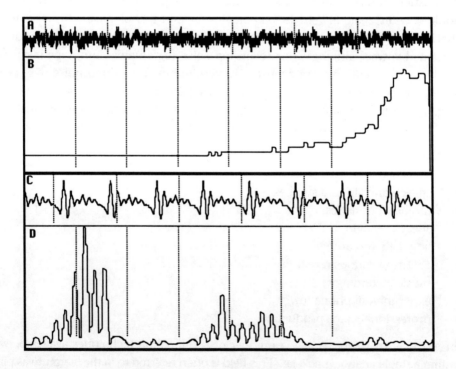

Figure 13.10 Waveform (A) and long-term average spectrum (LTAS) (B) for /s/, and waveform (C) and short-term average spectrum (D) for /a/. (Waveform x-axis calibration: 10 ms per division; spectrum x-axis calibration: 700 Hz per division.)

Time domain f_0 estimation techniques exploit the fact that the waveform of a periodic sound is repetitive (compare plot A with plot B in Figure 13.10) and they detect features that occur once per cycle during voiced sounds, such as the major positive (or negative) peak, positive- (or negative-) going zero crossings, the slope changes associated with major peaks or any readily identifiable feature on the waveform that can be identified as occurring once per cycle. Quite often the input signal is preprocessed to eliminate most of the effects of the vocal tract resonances, or formants, and voiceless energy before applying the period detection processing. Problems with time domain f_0 estimation occur when the shape of the speech pressure waveform changes as the formant positions move during the articulation of running speech. Such changes affect the definition of the repeating features in the waveform, such as peaks, troughs and zero crossings.

The changing shape of the waveform for the diphthong /ai/ is illustrated in Figure 13.11 as the formant structure of /a/ is changed to that of /i/. It may be seen that the nature of the major peaks and the zero crossings in the waveform change during the formant movement of /ai/. Rabiner et al. (1976) note that the measured fundamental period can differ depending on which waveform feature is being tracked, especially when the formants change rapidly. It can be seen in Figure 13.11 how the detailed variation during each waveform cycle differs on a cycle-by-cycle basis as the formants move, including the fine detail of the main positive peaks that are often used to identify each cycle. They also note that measurements based on zero crossings will produce small perturbations in the f_0 output especially when there is noise present in the input signal due, for example, to a breathy voice quality.

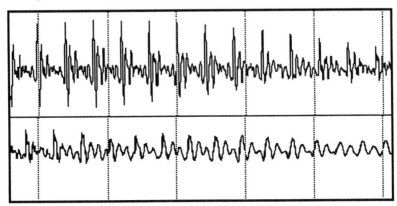

Figure 13.11 Waveform for portion of /ai/ where the formants move rapidly. The lower waveform is a continuation of the upper. (y-axis: acoustic pressure; x-axis: time calibrated as 10 ms per division.)

Frequency domain f_0 estimation techniques take advantage of the fact that a periodic signal has a series of regularly spaced peaks, or harmonics, in the frequency spectrum and a non-periodic signal has a continuous spectrum with no regularly spaced peaks. This can be observed in Figure 13.10 by comparing spectral plot B for /s/ (voiceless: non-periodic) with spectral plot D for /a:/ (voiced: periodic). The periodicity exhibited in the waveform of /a:/ is reflected in its spectrum as a number of peaks that are the individual harmonics themselves occurring at integer multiple of f_0. Frequency domain f_0 estimation tends to be based on finding and tracking either: (a) the f_0 component itself; or (b) the frequency difference between any two adjacent harmonics (= f_0); or (c) the f_0 which best 'fits' all the harmonics present. Particular problems can occur with each method as follows: with (a) when the fundamental is very weak compared to the other harmonics, particularly when the first formant frequency is high in a vowel such as /a:/ and the estimated f_0 jumps up an octave to the second harmonic (as discussed earlier, the second harmonic has a frequency that is twice that of f_0 by definition, which is equivalent to a pitch increase of one octave); with (b) when individual harmonics are weak due to the relative formant positions or variations in the cycle-by-cycle nature of vocal fold excitation; and with (c) in finding a best fit f_0, particularly if short cuts are required to save on processing time.

In general, frequency domain techniques cannot be used when an accurate cycle-by-cycle estimate of f_0 is required because of the need for a finite length of the input signal, known as a time window, which must be at least as long as one cycle from which to compute the spectrum. This results in some averaging of the f_0 value, which it is particularly important to note when f_0 is changing rapidly and high, because a high f_0 has a short fundamental period and the analysis window will therefore encompass a larger number of cycles. Frequency domain techniques tend, however, to be more resilient in the presence of noise, and one algorithm in particular, the *cepstral technique* (Noll, 1967), deserves a brief explanation. (The word 'cepstrum' arises from a simple reversal of four letters in the word 'spectrum'.) It is based on the idea that a spectrum that consists of harmonics, such as that shown in Figure 13.10d, is itself regularly repeating with a repetition interval of f_0. Therefore the 'spectrum' of such a spectrum, known as a 'cepstrum', would have a first 'harmonic', known as a 'rahmonic', at the fundamental 'frequency', known as 'quefrency', of the original repeating spectrum. In practice (Noll, 1967) the process involves taking the logarithm of the power spectrum of the input before taking a power spectrum again to separate the effects of the formants from the spectrum of the source.

Table 13.2 summarizes the features in the time and frequency domains that might be used in fundamental frequency estimation. Particular errors that can

Table 13.2 The nature of the features in the time and frequency domains that typify voiced and unvoiced speech and might be used in fundamental frequency estimation.

	Voiced	Unvoiced
Time domain *waveform*	Periodic *regular repeating pattern at fundamental period (Tx) where ($f_0 = 1/Tx$)*	Non-periodic *no regular repetitions*
Frequency domain *spectrum*	Line *harmonic components at ($n * f_0$) where n = 1, 2, 3, 4...*	Continuous *no harmonic components*

occur quite commonly in f_0 estimation by any means include the tracking of or sudden jumping to the second harmonic instead of the fundamental, known as pitch doubling or octave errors. Such an error can occur especially if the second harmonic is of a higher amplitude than the fundamental as can occur, for example, in vowels such as that in 'card', where the first formant is high in frequency.

Hybrid techniques make use of a combination of time and frequency domain features such that some merits of one domain might override some drawback of the other domain.

Direct measurement of larynx activity in the context of a practical f_0 estimation for clinical use includes the use of a throat microphone, often used to provide an f_0 signal for synchronous stroboscopic larynx imaging systems, and electrical impedance measurement systems, such as the electrolaryngograph and electroglottograph. These are widely used as reference f_0 estimation systems in the speech science laboratory and clinic (e.g. Hess and Indefrey, 1984; Howard, 1989; Howard et al., 1993), particularly due to their immunity to: (a) extraneous acoustic noise (that is any sound other than the desired signal), and (b) acoustic modifications to speech by the local environment, such as reverberation; both of which are common in clinical situations. These devices also generally give a more rigorous estimation than many microphone-based devices of the instant at which the boundaries between silence, voiced and voiceless sections of an utterance occur. The next section is devoted to a description of the operation of these devices due to their importance for practical voice measurement.

The larynx can be observed directly using indirect laryngoscopy (imaging the larynx with or without stroboscopic light) see Chapter 12. Very high-speed X-ray photography and photoglottography (using light to illuminate the opening and closing glottis) are also sometimes employed, however, these latter techniques are not practical for routine clinical use because they are: (a) invasive and the technique itself interferes with speech articulation, and (b) expensive on financial, time and staffing resources.

Sometimes it is necessary to smooth the output f_0 contour output to give a clearer indication of the contour shape or to lessen the presence of output errors resulting perhaps from considerable competing acoustic noise. One way of implementing f_0 smoothing is to restrict the rate of allowed change in f_0, but a very commonly used form of f_0 smoothing is median smoothing (the median being the middle value of an odd number of data points). Various lengths of median smoothing can be applied depending on the degree of smoothing desired. For example taking the median of the f_0 value itself and the f_0 value either side gives three-point median smoothing, taking the f_0 value itself and two f_0 values on either side gives five-point median smoothing, and taking the f_0 value itself and three f_0 values on either side gives seven-point median smoothing, and so on.

Electrolaryngography/electroglottography

The electrolaryngograph (Fourcin and Abberton, 1971) and the electroglottograph (e.g. Rothenberg, 1992) make use of two electrodes that are placed externally on either side of the neck at the level of the larynx, and a high-frequency constant voltage that is maintained between them. The output waveform from either device represents the current flowing between the electrodes. It should, however, be noted that although the operation of these devices is essentially identical, the electrolaryngograph output (Lx) is usually plotted with increased current positive-going (as used here), and the electroglottograph output (EGG) as the inverse. Comments made concerning the Lx waveform can therefore be applied equally well to the EGG waveform and vice versa, providing appropriate allowance is made for waveform polarity. This is illustrated in two idealized cycles of an Lx and EGG waveform plotted in Figure 13.12, where key waveform features are indicated with respect to the vibration cycle of the vocal folds.

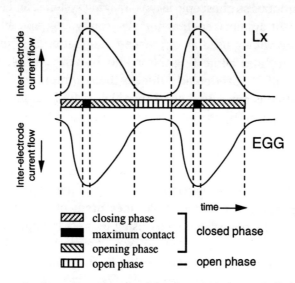

Figure 13.12 The main phases in each cycle of the electrolaryngograph (Lx) and electroglottograph (EGG) output waveforms

The current flowing between the electrodes, plotted upwards on Lx (downwards on EGG), will be higher when the vocal folds are in contact compared to that when they are apart. Variation in inter-electrode current can be interpreted in terms of changes in vocal-fold contact area. This interpretation has been confirmed by means of a number of experiments including synchronous observation of the Lx waveform alongside: high speed larynx photography (Fourcin, 1974; Baer et al., 1983; Gilbert et al., 1984); an adapted high-voltage X-flash imaging system (Noscoe et al., 1983; Fourcin, 1987); synchronstroboscopy (Leclusse et al., 1975); comparison with measured curves of glottal airflow (Rothenberg, 1981); and computer simulated Lx waveshapes based on models of vocal fold vibration during phonation (Titze, 1984; Titze et al., 1984; Childers et al., 1986).

During non-pathological modal phonation the vocal folds come together more rapidly than they part, due to the Bernoulli effect; therefore the rate of increase in vocal-fold contact area (increasing inter-electrode current flow) is greater than the rate of decrease as shown in the figure. Thus the Lx (EGG) waveforms can be marked with 'closing phase', 'maximum contact', 'opening phase' and 'open phase' as in the figure.

A number of measurements can be derived from the Lx waveform of the detailed nature of cycle-by-cycle variation in vocal fold vibration as shown in Figure 13.13 as: (i) the fundamental period (Tx); (ii) the time in each cycle for which the vocal folds are in contact, the 'closed phase' (CP); (iii) the time in each cycle for which the vocal folds are apart, the 'open phase' (OP); (iv) the rate of closing of the vocal folds (SI_c); (v) the rate of opening of the vocal folds (SI_o); and (vi) the peak to peak amplitude of each cycle (amp). SI_c and SI_o are measured as the gradient of the closing and opening slopes respectively, which are then normalized by dividing the results by that cycle's amplitude.

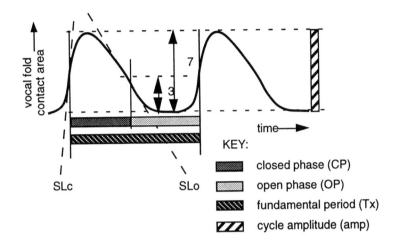

Figure 13.13 Measurements derived from the electrolaryngograph waveform

A variety of approaches are adopted by different researchers for defining the point in the cycle where the opening phase ends and the open phase starts for the measurement of OP and CP (see, for example, Howard, 1995). The key issue here is to ensure that like is compared with like, in that any comparisons made are between data derived by similar analysis techniques.

Some caveats relating to the interpretation of the Lx (or EGG) waveshape should be noted. Since the open phase is essentially indicated by the absence of (electrical) data, Baken (1987) notes that 'Lx is primarily useful for its representation of closure events and of the overall duration of the closed phase' but that 'the significance of irregularities in the open phase of Lx should be interpreted with caution'. The Lx waveform does not indicate whether the vocal folds are completely in contact or completely apart, it only indicates changes in vocal-fold contact area; therefore no conclusions can be drawn solely from the waveform as to whether or not the vocal folds contact or part completely for any particular measured voice quality. The closed and open phases and measurements derived from these should, therefore, always be interpreted with this in mind. The amplitude of the Lx (EGG) waveform is a parameter that should be treated with caution because it cannot be interpreted directly as it varies as a function of a system internal to the device itself known as automatic gain control. This is used to maintain an inter-electrode current flow that, on the one hand, is measurable and, on the other, is within an upper safety limit and its action is not instantaneous. A filter is also present to remove the effects of slowly occurring events such as vertical larynx movements, which would otherwise produce large changes in inter-electrode current flow resulting in distortion to the shape of the output waveform. This should be borne in mind when making a detailed interpretation of the output waveshape. A double-channel electroglottograph described by Rothenberg (1992) specifically enables larynx height to be tracked by means of a double set of electrodes mounted on the same neckband to provide an upper and a lower EGG system. The device makes a comparison of the two EGG output amplitudes as a basis for tracking larynx movement.

Appropriate electrode placement is crucial to assure robustness of data. These are usually placed symmetrically and externally on either side of the neck at an equal vertical height at the level of the larynx. Initially, they are adjusted by hand while the subject phonates and the output waveform is observed on an oscilloscope such that the maximum amplitude output waveform is obtained. Because the larynx moves vertically as pitch changes become more extreme, for example, if singing data are being gathered, it is important that the subject phonates across the whole f_0 range of interest while setting the electrode position. Then the neckband can be fastened tightly enough to support the electrodes firmly, but not so tight as to cause undue discomfort. If the f_0 range of interest is so wide that the Lx (EGG) waveform amplitude becomes too reduced at an extreme, then the subject could support the electrodes with the thumb and forefinger of one hand and the electrodes should be moved with the larynx.

Very occasionally it is not possible to obtain a sufficiently strong Lx (EGG) signal from speakers who have excessive adipose tissue, and the inter-electrode current path is effectively bridged by surrounding tissue such that any change in current due to vocal fold vibration becomes too small to detect. Beards very rarely present any problems for electrolaryngographic/electroglottographic analysis. The analysis of the voices of small children may require the use of special small electrodes to enable useful data to be obtained.

Some useful measures can be derived from those illustrated in Figure 13.13 as follows. The f0 of vocal fold vibration can be calculated as the number of cycles per second:

$$f_0 = 1/(Tx).\tag{13.1}$$

Larynx **closed quotient** (CQ), defined as 'the percentage of the cycle for which the vocal folds are in contact' can be derived from the CP as:

$$CQ = \left\{ \left[\frac{CP}{Tx} \right] * 100 \right\}\%\tag{13.2}$$

Similarly, larynx **open quotient** (OQ), defined as 'the percentage of the cycle for which the vocal folds are apart' can be derived from the OP as:

$$OQ = \left\{ \left[\frac{OP}{Tx} \right] * 100 \right\}\%\tag{13.3}$$

Clearly, the open phase plus the closed phase equals the period:

$$OP + CP = Tx.\tag{13.4}$$

Similarly:

$$OQ + CQ = 100\%\tag{13.5}$$

The Lx waveform itself can be observed directly, from which inferences can be made about the nature of the vibration of the vocal folds. A few cycles of Lx wave-

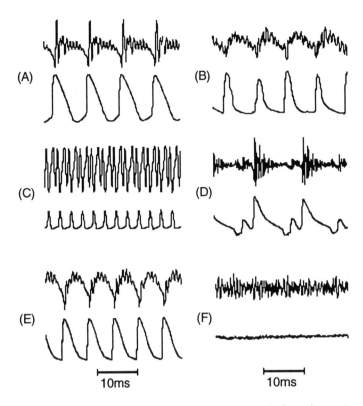

Figure 13.14 Speech pressure (upper) and electrolaryngograph (lower) waveforms for the vowel of 'spa', spoken by an adult male using: (A) modal voice; (B) breathy voice; (C) falsetto voice; (D) creaky voice; (E) harsh voice; and (F) whispered voice

form and the speech pressure waveform picked up by a microphone are illustrated in Figure 13.14 for the vowel of the word 'spa' spoken by a healthy adult male (Southern British English) using: (a) modal, (b) breathy, (c) falsetto (d) creaky, (e) harsh and (f) whispered voice qualities. It should be remembered that there is an inevitable delay (2 ms in this example for approximately 60 cm between the microphone and the lips) between the Lx and speech pressure waveforms due to the time taken for sound to travel from the glottis to the microphone. In this figure a shift of 2 ms would make appreciable difference.

Modal voice is used over most of a speaker's f_0 range. Occasionally, however, creaky voice may be used towards the lower end of the range and falsetto voice towards the upper end. In various parts of the range or for particular effect, a speaker may use breathy, creaky or harsh voice. In modal voice (Figure 13.14a), the whole body of each vocal fold vibrates giving the characteristically high Sl_c and less steep Sl_o as they snap together once per cycle. Vibration is regular. This rapid snapping together assures a rich acoustic excitation to the vocal tract, particularly in terms of the higher harmonics, which can be seen as the small rapid variations on the speech pressure waveform during each cycle.

Breathy voice arises as a result of partial abduction of the vocal folds while they are vibrating and the vocal folds do not necessarily make complete contact with each other. Breathy voice has been described as the folds 'flapping in the breeze' by Catford (1977) and as 'appearing to be simply flapping in the airstream' by Ladefoged (1975). Under these conditions no oscillation would be observed on the Lx waveform. When the folds do make contact as they vibrate, termed 'vigorous breathy voice' by Fourcin (1981), the Lx waveform reflects the oscillatory nature of the changing vocal-fold contact area (Figure 13.14b). In comparison with modal voice, Sl_c is less and OQ is longer. Due to the abduction of the folds there is a continuous flow of air through the narrowed glottis that is rapid enough for it to become turbulent, with the consequent generation of acoustic noise. This, and the increased OQ allowing air escape, produces the noise that gives the perceived breathiness to the voice. The associated speech pressure waveform shows that the formant excitation is not as marked due to the lack of variation during each cycle as compared to modal voice, and the noise element is also visible as small random variations on the speech pressure waveform.

In **falsetto voice** the vocal folds are thin and stretched to enable them to vibrate at a higher fundamental frequency. The typical Lx waveform shape (Figure 13.14c) for falsetto has a reduced amplitude due to the reduced change in contact area because it is only part or all of the upper edges of the vocal folds that come into contact. The mass of moving vocal fold tissue is reduced, and the acoustic excitation imparted to the vocal tract is not so rich in high harmonics as for modal voice. Sl_c is less steep than in modal voice. Because the fundamental frequency is high there is less time during each cycle for the formant responses to decay.

The excitation in **creaky voice** is low in pitch, and is often described as irregular, although there may be evidence of a main higher amplitude vocal fold closure-opening sequence followed by one of lower amplitude, and a less steep closing slope as in Figure 13.14d. The irregular nature of this sequence of long-short, long-short closures, gives the perceived creaky quality to the voice. This is reflected in the speech pressure waveform in which the vocal tract resonances die away considerably after each long excitation.

Harsh voice quality (Figure 13.14e) is perceived as having a hard edge to the voice with considerable breathiness. Comparing this example to the breathy voice quality uttered by the same speaker (Figure 13.14b), it can be seen that the closure for the harsh quality is more strongly defined than that for the breathy quality as Sl_c is higher and the negative-going excursions of the speech pressure waveform due to the vocal fold excitation are greater in amplitude. The speech pressure waveform shows less evidence of the decaying formants than in the modal voice example. Noise elements are visible on the speech pressure waveform in a similar manner to their appearance in breathy voice.

Whispered voice involves a narrowing of the glottis, but with no vocal fold vibration. The airflow through the glottis is turbulent, which provides the excitation in whispered speech. The example in Figure 13.14f shows that there is no vocal fold vibration since: (i) the output from the electrolaryngograph is non-oscillatory, and (ii) the speech pressure waveform is not periodic. In whispered voice, the formants are excited with acoustic noise.

Fundamental frequency data comparison

This section compares the results obtained from a number of practical f_0 measurement techniques in order to introduce: (a) the potential errors each might make, and (b) the effect of making adjustments to various user controls that are commonly provided. In each case, common input speech data is analysed. Reliable f_0 analysis depends on choosing a suitable analysis method and setting it up appropriately, a process that should be based on detailed knowledge of, and direct reference to, the intended application. It should be noted though, that it is not necessary to fully comprehend how any particular algorithm operates because, with a little practice, careful listening to the original speech and an awareness of potential errors combined with appropriate expectations for pitch variation will usually indicate which f_0 plot is most appropriate for the material in question. The output from an electrolaryngograph is used where necessary in this section to provide reference f_0 data.

The purpose of this section is not to advocate the general use of any particular device. In particular, the studies from which some of the examples are taken relate to their own particular application and they are included to provide examples. There are advantages and disadvantages of all f_0 estimation techniques in terms of:

- f_0 accuracy
- immunity to competing acoustic noise
- immunity to effects of the local acoustic environment
- accuracy in determining voicing onsets and offsets
- gain control setting
- operation with different speakers
- f_0 range
- sensitivity to microphone placement (acoustic devices only)
- sensitivity to electrode placement (electrolaryngograph/electroglottograph devices only)
- computational complexity.

Any disadvantages should be considered in terms of the effect they, and other associated issues, might have on the intended application, as some may be far more important than others. Howard et al. (1986) advocate investigating and comparing f_0 data at two levels: a macro level, where the input speech data lasts at least 2 minutes, and a micro level, where short speech inputs are used and the outputs from individual f_0 analysis systems can be inspected on a cycle-by-cycle basis. Macro and micro level discussions are presented below following a brief discussion relating to the presentation and interpretation of f_0 range data.

Fundamental frequency range data

Values are given in Table 13.1 (page 331) for f_0 ranges, and it should be noted that these are not quoted either in terms of upper and lower f_0 values, or the difference between the upper and the lower f_0 values - common practices elsewhere - because such values can be highly misleading. This is due to the way in which human hearing perceives frequency.

The human hearing system carries out a frequency analysis of incoming sound by means of the mechanical properties of the basilar membrane and the variation in maximum membrane displacement with frequency is essentially logarithmic (e.g. Pickles, 1982). **Musical intervals such as the octave (frequency ratio 2:1) or fifth (frequency ratio 3:2) are perceptually equivalent no matter where in the pitch range they occur (e.g. Howard and Angus, 1996).** A given ratio is represented as a fixed distance on a logarithmic scale, and this is the basis on which frequency relationships are perceived. Thus perceptually, f_0 ranges should be considered in terms of logarithmic frequency scales.

For convenience, the musical interval of an equal tempered semitone (1/12 of an octave) is often used, which is a number that equals 2 when multiplied by itself 12 times:

$$\text{frequency ratio for one equal tempered semitone} = \sqrt[12]{2} = 1.0595 \qquad (13.6)$$

The equal tempered semitone is usually subdivided into 100 cents for convenience, and the frequency ratio for one cent is therefore a number that equals 2 when multiplied by itself 1200 (100 * 12) times, or:

$$\text{frequency ratio for 1 cent} = \sqrt[1200]{2} = 1.000578 \qquad (13.7)$$

Figure 13.15 gives fundamental frequency values for musical notes that cover the main singing range against a four octave keyboard on which middle C is indicated by a black spot. A few points should be particularly noted:

- there are a number of notation schemes used for musical notes and the preferred one here is C4 for middle C with the numeric value changing between the notes B and C as shown in the figure;
- the frequency values given in the figure are based on the equal tempered scale referenced to the A above middle C, or A4, as 440Hz (for example, A 4 = {440 * 1.0595} Hz);
- a change of an octave up or down is equivalent to a doubling or halving in frequency respectively;
- there are 12 notes in each octave and the musical interval between each is equal to one semitone in equal tempered tuning (see, for example, Padham, 1986, or Howard and Angus, 1996, for details of unequal tempered tuning systems).

Figure 13.15 shows approximate f_0 ranges for normal conversational speech for men, women and children, and it can be seen that in each case the range is approximately 13 semitones as quoted in Table 13.1. Each is visually equivalent in length in this figure because frequency is represented logarithmically on a semitone scale. If f_0 ranges are considered in terms of the difference in frequency between the maximum and minimum f_0 values, as estimated from the figure, it becomes clear that the range for children ($\approx$ 210 Hz) is larger than that for women ($\approx$ 170 Hz), which itself is larger than that for men ($\approx$ 100 Hz), where the perceived ranges are essentially the same. **Thus the use of f0 ranges quoted in Hz can be completely misleading, a practice not uncommon in the voice literature.**

The following equations allow conversion from a frequency ratio (F1:F2) to equal tempered semitones (s-tones) and vice versa (a full derivation is given in Howard and Angus, 1996):

$$\text{s-tones} = 39.863137 * \log_{10}\left[\frac{F1}{F2}\right] \qquad (13.8)$$

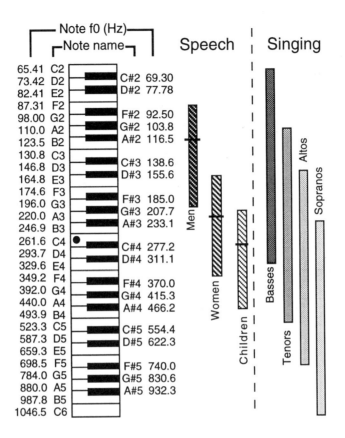

Figure 13.15 Fundamental frequency values for notes of the musical scale extending two octaves either side of middle C (marked with a black spot). Approximate fundamental frequency ranges used in singing for sopranos, altos, tenors and basses, and the speech of men, women and children, are marked

$$\left[\frac{F1}{F2}\right] = 10^{\left[\frac{s\text{-tones}}{39.863137}\right]} \qquad\qquad\qquad (13.9)$$

The following equations enable conversion from a frequency ratio (F1:F2) to equal tempered cents (c) and vice versa:

$$c = 3986.3137 * \log_{10}\left[\frac{F1}{F2}\right] \qquad\qquad\qquad (13.10)$$

$$\left[\frac{F1}{F2}\right] = 10^{\left[\frac{c}{3986.3137}\right]} \qquad\qquad\qquad (13.11)$$

Figure 3.15 also shows approximate fundamental frequency ranges expected from singers, and it can be seen that these are considerably greater than those that singers will habitually use in their speech. The range for a bass extends both above and below the average speaking f_0 range for an adult male, and that for a tenor extends a considerable way above the speaking range. A similar trend can be noted for the range of the alto and soprano compared to the average speaking f_0 range for adult females.

Macro level comparison

Statistical presentation of data at the macro level is in common use in the clinic and elsewhere by means of a histogram of f_0. Barry et al. (1990) note that an f_0 histogram stabilizes in terms of its mean being 'settled' after approximately 90 s of speech input if spoken at at least an average rate, which suggests that at least 90 s of speech should be used for any macro analysis of f_0. Associated summary statistics, such as f_0 mean, f_0 standard deviation, f_0 mode and f_0 median, can be calculated from histogram data. It is often forgotten that standard statistical approaches apply in terms of the nature or shape of the underlying distribution, which for f_0 can vary considerably with speaker and voice quality, and its potential effect on such summary statistics. An f_0 distribution is often far from being normal in the statistical sense and therefore due caution and appropriate measures should be applied when quoting summary statistics.

Three orders of f_0 histogram, or Dx plot, that are commonly used for f_0 analysis based on the output from the electrolaryngograph (Lx), known as first, second and third order, are described by Fourcin (1981) and Abberton et al. (1989) Figure 13.16. The f_0 axis of the histogram is logarithmic (for the reasons discussed above) and the probability axis is also usually logarithmic. In a first order analysis, the

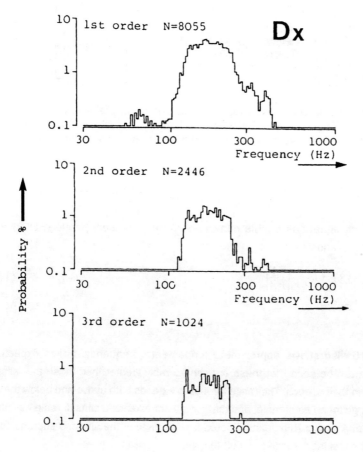

Figure 13.16 First, second and third order f_0 histogram plots from the electrolaryngograph output for a healthy adult female speaker reading a 2-minute passage. (From Howard et al., 1986)

histogram is built up from all Tx values measured (see Figure 13.13). For second and third order analysis, Tx values are taken in successive pairs for second order (triplets for third order) and an entry is only made in the histogram if both (all three for third order) values fall within the same histogram analysis bin.

The use of second and third order histograms provides a method by which f_0 irregularity can be investigated because successive Tx pairs (or triplets) will tend not to fall within the same histogram bin as irregularity increases. This effect can be seen in the Dx plots presented in Figure 13.16 (from Howard et al., 1986) for a passage read by a healthy adult female speaker, particularly in terms of the disappearance of the entries below 100 Hz in the second and third order Dx plots due to creaky voice. Summary statistics are given in Table 13.3 for these Dx plots where the ranges and standard deviation (s.d.) extremes have been converted to semitones using equation 3.8.

Table 13.3 Summary statistics for first, second and third order f_0 histogram plots shown in Figure 13.16. Ranges and standard deviation (s.d.) extremes have been converted to semitones using equation 3.8. (Data from Howard et al., 1986)

	Order		
	1	2	3
Mode (Hz)	167	167	134
Mean (Hz)	176	183	184
S.d. (log Hz)	0.158	0.112	0.108
S.d. (Hz-Hz)	122-253	141-230	143-236
S.d. (semitones)	12.63	8.47	8.67
Median (Hz)	175	180	181
80% range (Hz-Hz)	127-353	134-342	134-240
80% range (semitones)	17.70	16.22	10.09
90% range (Hz-Hz)	111-313	129-303	130-290
90% range (semitones)	17.95	14.78	13.89
Sample size	8055	2446	1824

Another macro analysis that has been found to be useful, particularly in the investigation of f_0 irregularity, is a *scattergram* or cross-plot of f_0 values, in which each f_0 value is plotted against the previous f_0 value, known as a Cx plot (Abberton et al., 1989). Both axes in such a plot are logarithmic, and example Cx plots are shown in Figure 13.17. The density of points on the scattergram indicates the probability of transition between the values plotted. When f_0 changes smoothly, the differences between successive f_0 values is quite small and the points on the Cx plot will therefore lie close to the main diagonal ($f_{01} = f_{02}$). Any successive f_0 values that differ greatly, for example when a creaky voice quality is used, will result in points plotted well away from the main diagonal. The length of the main diagonal ($f_{01} = f_{02}$) on the plot measured on either axis, therefore, gives the f_0 range and this is equivalent to the first order Dx range; and the degree of scatter away from this diagonal indicates f_0 irregularity. Creaky voice quality tends to show up on a Cx plot as points scattered away from the main ($f_{01} = f_{02}$) diagonal around and below the lower f_0 limit, which can be clearly observed in the figure.

Macro level analyses such as Cx can be used as a basis for comparison of the operation of various f_0 analysis systems against a reference system, usually the electrolaryngograph. Figure 13.17 shows Cx plots from the f_0 outputs from four analysis devices for a healthy 7-year-old girl reading a short passage from Howard (1989). Two of the acoustic devices operate in the time domain, a peak-

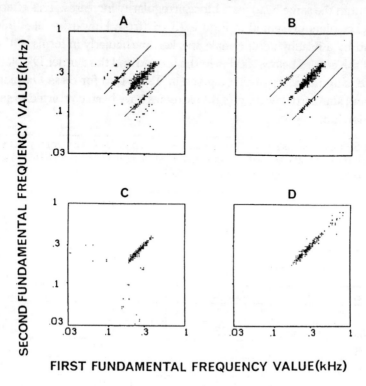

Figure 13.17 Fundamental frequency scattergrams (Cx) from four devices for a healthy 7-year-old girl reading a short passage: (A) electrolaryngograph; (B) peak-picker; (C) Gold–Rabiner algorithm; and (D) cepstrum. (From Howard, 1989)

picker (Howard and Fourcin, 1983; Howard, 1989) and the Gold–Rabiner algorithm (Gold and Rabiner, 1969), and the other is the cepstrum technique (see above), which operates in the frequency domain (Noll, 1967) and incorporates output f_0 smoothing. The additional lines drawn on the plots for the electrolaryngograph and peak-picker outputs are where there is an octave difference between consecutive f_0 values (i.e. where $f_{01} = [2 * f_{02}]$ and $f_{02} = [2 * f_{01}]$). They are provided to illustrate that this is probably a genuine feature in this recording as there are points along these lines in the output from the electrolaryngograph, which is being taken as the reference. Howard (1989) also notes that the output from the electrolaryngograph also has islands of points where f_0 changes by a factor of 3 that are not shown in the output from the peak-picker. The other two devices do not exhibit this octave scattering. The widths of the main diagonal are greater for the electrolaryngograph and peak-picker than for the other two devices. Some low frequency scatter is exhibited by the Gold–Rabiner device, and the high frequency values referred to above with respect to the output from the cepstral device are clearly shown in the Cx plot where they lie on or close to the main diagonal.

Micro level comparison

An f_0 analysis over a short stretch of speech is often desired and commonly presented, and this can usefully be termed a microanalysis. In many experiments, f_0 data relating to steady sustained vowels are presented. Much can be gained from comparing directly the periodic structure of the acoustic pressure waveform itself on a cycle-by-cycle basis with the output from an f_0 analysis system, from which it is generally clear when an analysis system is making serious errors. An f_0 cycle-by-cycle analysis is also the basis of the measurement of *jitter* or frequency perturbation which is the relationship of the period of each cycle to that which it follows. If there were no involuntary changes in f_0 then the only changes to be measured would be those related to intended intonation variation, and jitter would be zero. Hence jitter measurements are used as an index of vocal stability. The perception of 'roughness' or 'harshness' is associated with raised jitter values in relation to the mean f_0 of the sample. Considerations in regard to the practical measurement of jitter are exactly those discussed in this section in relation to micro level comparison. Baken (1987) reviews the usefulness of jitter measurement in evaluation of laryngeal and vocal pathologies.

Two examples are shown in Figures 13.18 and 13.19 for the vowel in spa, spoken by a healthy adult male with a modal voice quality and a creaky voice quality respectively. In both figures, the acoustic pressure and Lx waveforms are presented along with the fundamental period marker output from the peak-picker, the Gold–Rabiner algorithm and the cepstrum device. The actual operating prin-

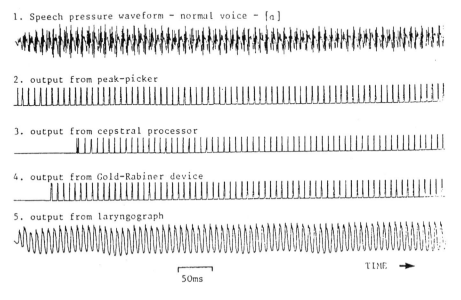

Figure 13.18 Acoustic pressure waveform, fundamental period markers from the peak-picker, cepstral device and Gold-Rabiner algorithm, and the electrolaryngograph output waveform for the vowel of spa, spoken in an anechoic room by a healthy adult male speaker in modal voice

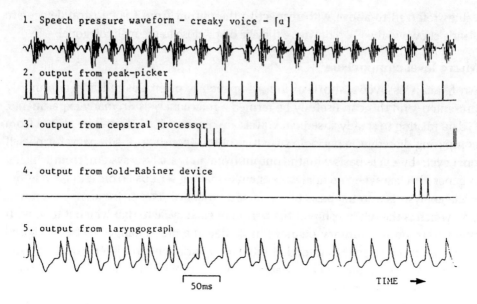

Figure 13.19 Acoustic pressure waveform, fundamental period markers from the peak-picker, cepstral device and Gold–Rabiner algorithm, and the electrolaryngograph output waveform for the vowel of spa, spoken in an anechoic room by a healthy adult male speaker in creaky voice

ciples behind the devices themselves are immaterial because the intention is to provide a basis for understanding micro level comparisons in terms of their desirability, methodology and interpretation.

In these figures, it should be noted that the outputs from the acoustically-based devices are plotted so as to include any processing delay in the system itself, and it can be seen that the processing delays in these particular implementations of the cepstral and Gold–Rabiner systems from the late 1970s are approximately 80 ms and 44 ms respectively. Of course, reduction in processing delay is only important if a real-time analysis is required, for example, in the case of a real-time visual feedback of f_0 for speech or singing training. Any delay greater than approximately 25 ms in a real-time visual display system will be noticeable.

The outputs from each of the three acoustically-based devices appear to indicate appropriate fundamental period markers for the vowel spoken in modal voice (Figure 13.19) in that they agree with the output from the electrolaryngograph. The vowel is the pure acoustic output from the speaker's lips unmodified by any acoustic environment as it was recorded with a high quality microphone in an anechoic room where there are no acoustic reflections from the walls, floor or ceiling. The creaky voice recording (Figure 13.19) was made under identical conditions. The Lx waveform has the large closure-opening sequence followed by a secondary smaller amplitude closure-opening sequence, which occur irregularly, giving the perceived creaky quality to the voice. The acoustic result of these can be observed on the acoustic pressure waveform.

The outputs from the three acoustically based f_0 estimation systems demonstrate the basic difference between systems, which make some decision about whether the input speech is voiced or voiceless based on the regularity of the input waveform or importance of harmonics in the spectrum. The fundamental period outputs from the Gold-Rabiner and cepstral techniques do not indicate a voiced output for this input creaky voice quality. This is due to their in-built post-processing rules that govern what constitutes voiced speech. The peak-picker, on the other hand, has no post-processing rules, and its output in this case is quite close to that from the electrolaryngograph. However, the lack of such post-processing rules can place the peak-picker and similar devices at some disadvantage when the input speech is produced in the presence of competing acoustic noise or in a reverberent environment.

In a real acoustic environment such as a voice clinic, conditions are never anechoic. The acoustic pressure waveform heard by a listener or picked up by a microphone is a combination of the direct sound and reflections from the room boundaries (e.g. see Howard and Angus, 1996). This has a direct effect on the nature of the acoustic pressure waveform input to the f_0 analysis system, and it can serve to obscure the periodicity of a voiced speech waveform. Figure 13.20 shows the result of f_0 analysis by the four devices for the vowel of 'spa', spoken in a reverberant office by a healthy adult male with a lip to microphone distance of 50 cm. It can be seen that the periodicity of the acoustic pressure waveform is significantly less distinct than the anechoic version. The output from the electrolaryngograph is presented in the form of pulses to make it more directly comparable with those from the acoustically-based devices. The f_0 output from the cepstral device is the only one that is smooth, clear and uninterrupted. The outputs from the other two

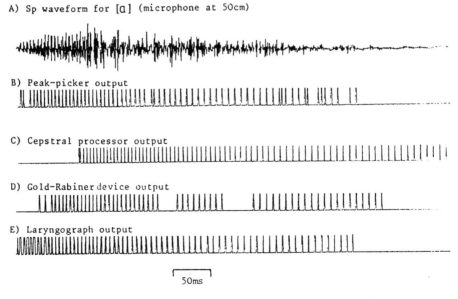

A) Sp waveform for [ɑ] (microphone at 50cm)

B) Peak-picker output

C) Cepstral processor output

D) Gold-Rabiner device output

E) Laryngograph output

50ms

Figure 13.20 Acoustic pressure waveform, fundamental period markers from the peak-picker, cepstral device and Gold–Rabiner algorithm, and the electrolaryngograph output waveform for the vowel of spa, spoken in a reverberant office by a healthy male adult speaker in modal voice with a lip microphone distance of 50 cm

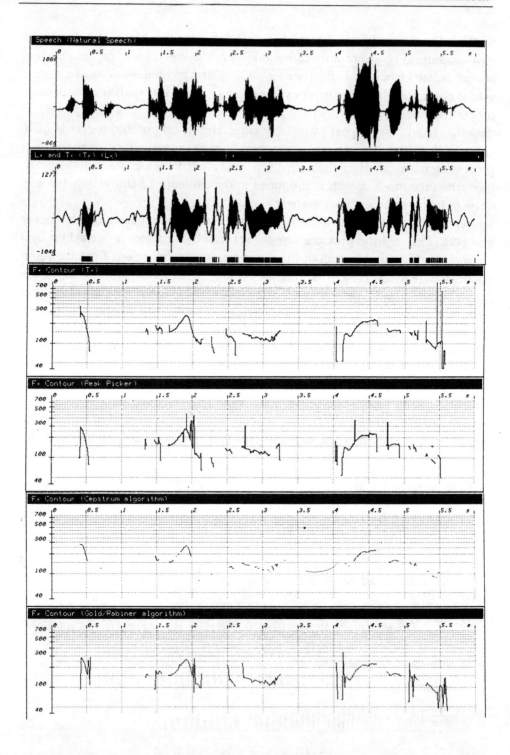

Figure 13.21 Acoustic pressure waveform, electrolaryngograph output waveform and period markers derived from it, and f_0 contours from the electrolaryngograph, peak-picker, cepstral device and Gold–Rabiner algorithm for the sentence 'Speech is so familiar a feature of daily life that we rarely pause to define it', spoken by a healthy adult female speaker

acoustically-based devices are not smooth. The output from the peak-picker misses some markers and adds in some additional markers, and that from the Gold–Rabiner device is smooth in places but with gaps, occurring presumably as a result of its post-processing rules. *Therefore of the acoustically-based devices, the cepstral algorithm provides the most appropriate fundamental period indication, which suggests that it is less affected by the waveform distortion resulting from reverberation than are the other two devices represented.*

These plots demonstrate the importance of microphone placement in terms of its distance from the speaker. To provide an f_0 analysis system with an acoustic pressure waveform that is as close to anechoic as possible, the microphone should be placed as close to the speaker's lips as is practically possible. However, it should be kept to one side of the main airstream to avoid the 'popping' sounds often associated with plosive sounds, such as the consonants in 'bee' and 'pea', when they are spoken into a microphone directly in front of the lips. Whenever possible, microphones should not be clipped to the clothing of the speaker as: (a) the speaker's voice will sound rather 'boomy' because the upper frequencies will be reduced in amplitude with respect to the lower frequencies due to the increased directionality from the lips for higher frequencies, and (b) additional 'microphonic' sounds will be picked up if the position of the microphone cable is disturbed as the speaker moves or fiddles with the cable.

Plots of fundamental period markers are extremely useful for evaluating and becoming aware of the nature of the output from f_0 estimation systems at a micro level. However, they are not particularly useful, and in many cases not available, in a practical voice measurement situation for evaluating changes in f_0 where a plot of f_0 against time is the most commonly used data presentation format. Such contours allow utterances longer than single vowels to be investigated, but f_0 contours can usually be time zoomed to reveal detail at a micro level and thus can enable many of the comparisons described with fundamental period markers to be carried out locally.

Figure 13.21 shows a plot of f_0 against time for the sentence 'Speech is so familiar a feature of daily life that we rarely pause to define it', spoken by a healthy adult female with the acoustic pressure waveform, the electrolaryngograph output waveform and period markers derived from it, and f_0 contours derived from the electrolaryngograph output, the peak-picker, the cepstrum device and the Gold–Rabiner algorithm. Considering that the electrolaryngograph output was unavailable for a moment and viewing the f_0 contours from the acoustically-based devices as a group, the output based on the cepstral technique provides overall the smoothest and cleanest f_0 contour, which might suggest that it is the most appropriate contour on which to base the analysis for this sentence. The other two devices have a number of jumps in their f_0 contours, which makes them rather visually messy and indicates of errors. In the case of the peak-picker, some of these look like octave errors, while in the case of the Gold–Rabiner algorithm it is not obviously octave errors that are being made, but there are jumps in the output f_0 contour that suggest errors are being made, even without access to a reference contour.

Considering now the reference f_0 contour derived from the output from the electrolaryngograph (the upper contour in the figure), it is convenient to number the individual fragments of the f_0 contour to aid comparison, using underlining to indicate the voiced segments, as shown in Table 13.4. Between each voiced segment during a sentence there is a voiceless segment or silence, indicated in the table as the non-underlined letters of the words appearing at the end and/or the start of each V+ segment indicated, except between segments four and five between which the speaker made use of a glottal stop.

Table 13.4 The voiced segments (underlined) that relate to each of the 13 f_0 contour fragments in the f_0 contour derived from the electrolaryngograph output shown in Figure 13.21 for the sentence 'Speech is so familiar a feature of daily life that we rarely pause to define it', spoken by a healthy adult female. The presence/absence of each reference fragment in the outputs from the acoustically-based devices is indicated with multiple snippets in a reference fragment being indicated by numbers in brackets.

f_0 fragment in reference	V+ segment (underlined)	Peak-picker	Cepstrum	Gold–Rabiner
1	Sp<u>ee</u>ch	✓	✓	✓
2	<u>is</u>	✓	✗	✓
3	s<u>o</u>	✓	✓	✓
4	f<u>amiliar</u>	✓	✓ (5)	✓
5	<u>a</u>	✓	✓	✗
6	f<u>ea</u>	✓	✓	✓
7	<u>ture of daily life</u>	✓ (2)	✓ (9)	✓
8	th<u>at</u>	✓	✗	✓
9	<u>we rarely</u>	✓	✓ (4)	✓
10	p<u>ause</u>	✓	✓	✓
11	t<u>o</u>	✓	✓	✓ (11 & 12
12	d<u>e</u>	✓	✓	combined)
13	f<u>ine</u> it.	✓ (3)	✓ (4)	✓

For f_0 fragment 1 it can be seen from the reference that the vowel of the first word 'speech' is uttered with a falling pitch over a range of about two octaves (f_0 falls from approximately 290 Hz to 70 Hz, which is equivalent to a pitch change of 24.6 semitones using equation 13.8), and that it is well separated from the next word in the sentence, 'is'. All three acoustically-based devices produce an output for this fragment, but the peak-picker is closest to the reference in terms of its duration and frequency extent. All devices except the cepstrum indicate fragment 2. Fragment 3 is output by all devices and the Gold–Rabiner provides the contour closest in shape to the reference. The fall/rise fragment 4 has its peak represented by all three acoustically-based devices, but the cepstrum produces a greatly shortened and broken-up contour in five sections, while the other two produce outputs that exhibit large pitch jumps at a similar instant. Fragment 5 is represented most appropriately by the peak-picker as it is very short in the cepstrum output and non-existent in the Gold–Rabiner output. Fragments 6 and 7 are best represented in the Gold–Rabiner output in terms of duration and frequency change; they are shorter in the other two outputs and broken up in the latter. The cepstrum misses fragment 8, and of the other two, the Gold–Rabiner output has a more appropriate frequency change in this rapid fall in pitch. The peak-picker tracks fragment 9 most appropriately, closely followed by the Gold–Rabiner device, and the cepstrum contour is broken up again. The Gold–Rabiner gives a very close version of fragment 10, closely followed by the peak-picker and again, the cepstrum output is short. The peak-picker tracks fragments 11 and 12 well, closely followed by the cepstrum output, which is again shorter than the reference, while the Gold–Rabiner device has linked them together across a clear (see the electrolaryngograph waveform) short break in voicing. Fragment 13 is broken in both the peak-picker and cepstrum outputs, and the Gold–Rabiner output exhibits large pitch jumps but is not broken up. Notice also that the reference output exhibits some very large pitch jumps in this last fragment.

This detailed examination of the outputs from three acoustically-based f_0 estimation systems is provided to indicate the differences that can occur at a micro level between successive voiced fragments during a speech utterance. In this case, bearing in mind that these devices have been selected simply to demonstrate differences and not to make any recommendations, each acoustically-based system has provided the most as well as the least appropriate f_0 output for at least one of the 13 fragments presented. This further highlights and complicates the business of making an informed choice of f_0 estimation system for a particular application, and indicates that any system is likely not to be the most appropriate even within the bounds of a single sentence.

Some general conclusions can be drawn in terms of the outputs from these devices.

The f_0 post-processing used in this implementation of the cepstrum technique tends to produce shorter durations for voiced segments and f_0 always changes smoothly, which might suggest it is the most suitable to use. However, Table 13.4 shows that for this utterance, there are four fragments out of 13 that are broken into smaller sections and two that are missing altogether. If an indication of the number of voiced (and voiceless) sections in this sentence is important, Table 13.4 shows that the cepstrum output indicates that there are a total of 29 voiced sections, the Gold–Rabiner indicates 11 and the peak-picker indicates 16 where the reference indicates 13. In terms of providing the most appropriate indication of change in f_0, this too varies between the acoustically-based devices even for successive fragments during the utterance, and a choice between a heavily smoothed f_0 output as opposed to one that produces some pitch jump errors would depend on what the f_0 output is to be used for. If a macro level statistical analysis is to be made as a summary, then pitch jumps such as those exhibited by the peak-picker and Gold–Rabiner devices in Figure 13.21 would have no effect at all on the median or mode, and providing they do not occur too often, little or no noticeable effect on the mean, standard deviation or range(s).

Caveat on the use of an electrolaryngograph reference

Throughout the preceding sections, use has been made of the output from the electrolaryngograph as a reference, a practice endorsed by Hess (1983), Hess and Indefrey (1984) and Howard (1989). There are, however, occasions when there is evidence of vocal-fold vibration provided by the electrolaryngograph output that is not reflected in the acoustic pressure waveform and vice versa. This could have a bearing on comparisons made at the micro level, particularly if the number of fundamental periods output by the reference and another system are compared directly or the exact instant to within one cycle of voicing onset and offset is required. Howard and Lindsey (1988) have noted this effect particularly at the offset of voicing, and they present examples in which: (1) a periodic electrolaryngograph output continues strongly while periodic variations in the acoustic pressure waveform greatly reduce in amplitude; (2) periodic variations in the acoustic pressure waveform continue strongly while periodic variations in the electrolaryngograph output waveform greatly reduce in amplitude or are not apparent; and (3) periodic variations in both signals terminate simultaneously.

Figure 13.22, taken from Howard and Lindsey (1988), shows a marked drop in the acoustic pressure waveform at the vowel offset while the electrolaryngograph output waveform continues more strongly for the vowel of spa, spoken by a healthy adult male speaker with a falling intonation. Howard and Lindsey suggest that this is due to a breathy offset to the vowel, which results in a longer open phase and a decrease in the sharpness of vocal-fold closure, and a significant reduction in acoustic excitation energy to the vocal tract. This effect appears to be speaker-dependent. Consider Figure 13.23, taken from the same speaker, in which the converse cessation pattern is observed. Howard and Lindsey suggest that here, the vocal folds are 'vibrating sufficiently to generate acoustic energy but with insufficient contact to register on the electrolaryngograph output waveform' or 'flapping in the breeze', to use Catford's (1977) term to describe breathy voice. The data presented in these figures were recorded in an anechoic room and the potential lengthening effects of reflected waves in an enclosed space on the acoustic pressure waveform are clearly also relevant when considering a detailed cycle-by-cycle micro level examination of f_0 data.

These examples are given to provide an indication that in practical voice measurement work, one should endeavour to keep in perspective the signal being measured, the path that signal has taken and the basis on which the measurement system operates. It is rarely necessary to have a deep knowledge of the algorithms themselves, but much can be gained from careful observation of the results obtained from analysing signals whose origins are known, and from comparing the outputs obtained with the input waveforms themselves at a micro level. The next section considers the effects of different settings of typical parameters often made available to the user. Once again it is the potential differences in f_0 output that are considered as there is no one setting on any particular system that will always provide the most appropriate f_0 contour in all situations.

Effects of user-adjustable parameters

Most f_0 estimation algorithms have an optimum range of input speech pressure waveform amplitudes at which they produce the most reliable outputs. As there is no way of predicting the amplitude level of speech, the input signal level to the system, often known as the input gain, is adjustable. In most systems that operate in real-time (i.e. the f_0 contour is plotted such that it appears to be simultaneous with the input acoustic signal) the input gain is set to an appropriate value by the user, often by means of a level meter similar to that found on a tape recorder. Alternatively, the setting can be automatic, particularly when operation is non-real-time, when it is known as an automatic gain control. Instead of input gain,

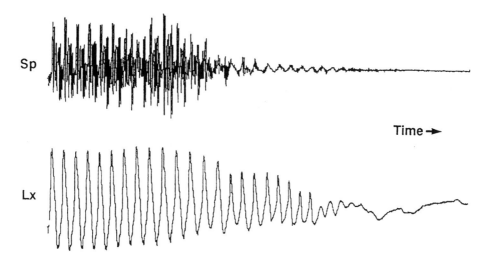

Figure 13.22 Acoustic pressure waveform and electrolaryngograph output waveform for the vowel of 'spa', spoken by a healthy adult male speaker. (From Howard and Lindsey, 1988)

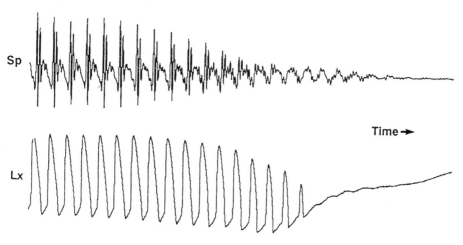

Figure 13.23 Acoustic pressure waveform and electrolaryngograph output waveform for the vowel 'spa', spoken by a healthy adult female speaker. (From Howard and Lindsey, 1988)

some systems have a threshold setting that can be varied and which adjusts the level at which f_0 processing is carried out internally to the algorithm itself; in terms of the observed f_0 output, the effect has many similarities with the effects of varying input gain.

Figure 13.24 shows the effect produced when the peak-picker is run with a number of different gain settings for the sentence 'Speech is so familiar a feature of daily life that we rarely pause to define it', spoken by a healthy adult female speaker (same recording as in Figure 13.21). The gain settings are the percentage of the maximum amplitude of the input acoustic pressure waveform: 5%, 7.5%, 10%, 15% and 20%. At lower gain settings the f_0 output misses some voiced fragments altogether, and these are the ones whose acoustic pressure waveform amplitudes are the lowest. As the gain setting is increased, f_0 outputs are produced for more of the voiced fragments and there comes a point in this example where f_0 outputs appear for non-voiced fragments such as the initial and final consonants of the first word 'speech' for gains of 15% and 20%. Selecting the appropriate gain value is a case of balancing the errors against the overall f_0 contour produced, and a gain of 10% was chosen for this sentence for the comparisons made with respect to Figure 13.21. It is interesting to note that had a gain setting of 15% been employed, fragment 13 would have been a very close representation of the reference instead of being broken into three sections, but there would have been output errors for the consonants of the first word.

Vocal tract response measurement

Background

Each speech sound has unique acoustic patterns by which it is perceived and these acoustic patterns are related to the acoustic output from both the sound source and the sound modifiers (see Figure 13.1). The acoustic properties of these vary as different sounds are articulated, and subtle acoustic differences will be apparent even in the same sound produced by a particular speaker on more than one occasion. It is often important to analyse the acoustic nature of a sound in terms of its frequency components, from which properties of the vocal tract response can be usefully inferred. However, when considering the results gained from such an analysis of the acoustic pressure waveform, it must always be remembered that they represent the combination of the acoustic spectrum of the voice source with the vocal tract response at that instant of time. There are methods that are designed to analyse either the voice source or the vocal tract response more directly, but these usually rely on an assumption that the acoustic nature of the voice source remains fairly consistent. While this may be a fair first approximation when considering the speech of a vocally healthy individual, it is an assumption that should be made with caution when analysing the speech from persons with voice disorders. This should not imply that nothing useful can be gained from an analysis of the acoustic pressure waveform when nothing is known about the acoustic consequence of the voice source itself. Indeed, much of the knowledge about acoustic cues in speech gained over many years of research is based on a frequency analysis of the speech output from the lips on the assumption that the frequency spectrum of the voice source itself remains essentially constant.

Speech spectrography

Formant frequencies change as different articulation gestures are made and tracking these changes is an important requirement of a practical vocal tract response measurement system. Idealized spectra for two vowels are shown in Figure 13.8. The spectrum is one form of output from a device known as a speech spectrograph, sound spectrograph or just spectrograph.

For spectrum analysis a vital consideration is the accuracy with which

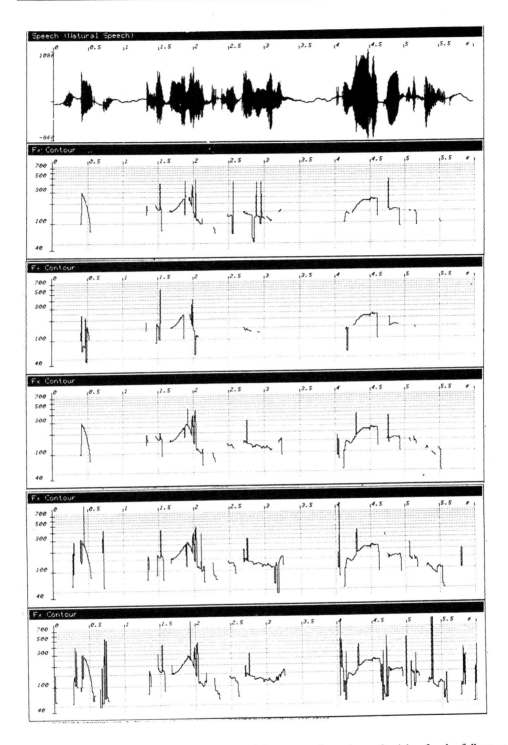

Figure 13.24 Acoustic pressure waveform and f_0 contours from the peak-picker for the following gain settings: 5%, 7.5%, 10%, 15% and 20% for the sentence 'Speech is so familiar a feature of daily life that we rarely pause to define it' spoken by a healthy adult female speaker. (The gain values themselves are arbitrary in the sense that they are multipliers internal to the algorithm itself.)

frequency can be analysed. The relevant parameter available to the user on a spectrograph is the *analysis filter bandwidth*, which is usually indicated as 'wide' or 'narrow'. These terms refer to whether the filter bandwidth is wider or narrower than the f_0 of the speech being analysed. Good frequency resolution is offered by narrow band analysis.

Figures 13.25 and 13.26 illustrate the frequency resolution effect for the idealized spectrum of the vowel of the word 'bee', taken from Figure 13.8 when analysed by a narrow and a wide band filter respectively. Frequency analysis by spectrography is represented in the figures by the centre diagram, which represents the concept of a moving analysis filter. Bearing in mind that the spacing between the harmonics of the input idealized vowel spectrum is equal to f_0, it can be seen that the bandwidths of the filters are narrow and wide with respect to f_0 in their representation in each figure.

In effect, the analysis filter is 'slid' over the input speech spectrum plotting its components as the output spectrum. One way of accomplishing this in practice is to play the input speech through the analysis filter repeatedly as the filter is moved from low to high frequencies, while plotting the amplitude of the resulting output signal from the filter to produce the output spectrum in the lower diagram of each figure. In this example, the output spectrum from the narrow band filter indicates the individual harmonics clearly, but that from the wide band filter blurs the harmonics together. They are not resolved individually after wide band analysis because the filter bandwidth is greater than the spacing between the harmonics by definition of 'wide'. Thus the narrow band analysis gives the better frequency resolution. The output spectrum produced by the narrow band filter is not an exact representation of the speech spectrum input to the analysis system because each component in its output spectrum is coloured by the shape of the analysis filter itself. This suggests that **the narrower the filter bandwidth, the better the frequency resolution**, which is true, but there is a practical limit that is explored below.

Five spectra of the vowel of 'spa', spoken by a healthy adult male, each analysed with a different filter bandwidth, are shown in Figure 13.27. The f_0 in this example is approximately 100 Hz, and therefore the spectra analysed with filter bandwidths of 20 Hz, 30 Hz and 40 Hz can be considered as being of narrow bandwidth, and those analysed with bandwidths of 125 Hz and 200 Hz as being wide. This can be inferred by comparison with Figures 13.25 and 13.26. As the analysis filter becomes wider, the frequency components in the spectrum also become wider as they are increasingly coloured by the shape and bandwidth of the analysis filter. The formant positions can be seen in all these spectra, and the wide band spectra appear to offer the clearest indication of formant frequencies visually. This is because the blurring of the harmonics by the wide band filter leads to the visual appearance of an envelope across the harmonic peaks. However, this can be misleading, particularly if accurate formant frequency measurements are required, because the output from the wide band filter is the sum of the amplitudes of the components that happen to fall within it (see Figure 13.26). Therefore the frequency positions of the peaks are rarely accurately related to the formant centre frequencies directly, because they

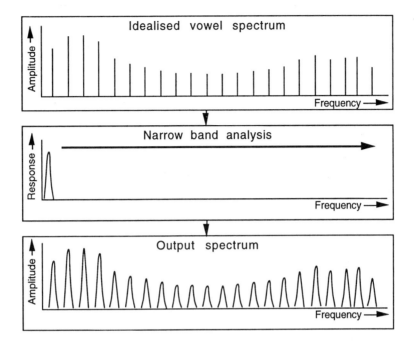

Figure 13.25 Frequency analysis of the idealized spectrum of the vowel in 'bee', using a narrow band filter

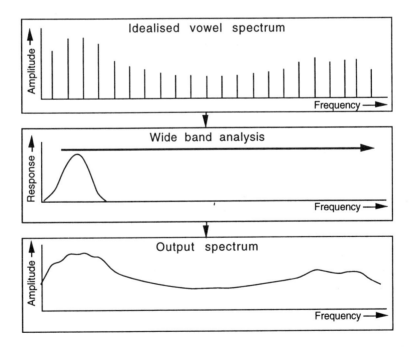

Figure 13.26 Frequency analysis of the idealized spectrum of the vowel in 'bee', using a wide band filter

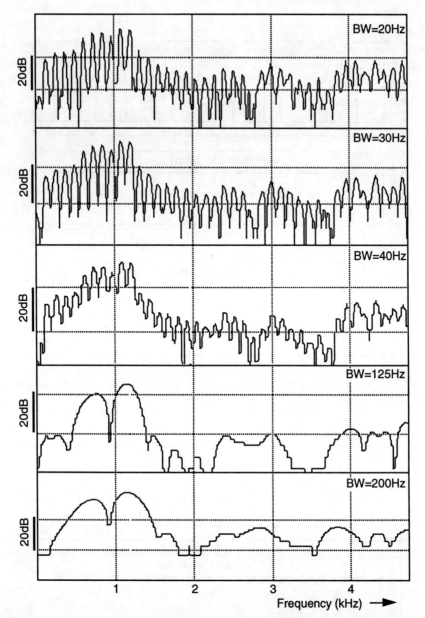

Figure 13.27 Spectra of the vowel of 'spa', spoken by a healthy adult male in modal voice analysed with filters of the following bandwidths: 20 Hz, 30 Hz, 40 Hz, 125 Hz and 200 Hz

vary as a function of the amplitudes of individual harmonics that could be quite distant (in frequency) from the actual format peak. Formant frequencies can be measured from the narrow band spectrum by estimating the position of the formant peaks visually from the harmonic peaks, in effect by tracing the vocal tract response curve out over the output spectrum (c.f. the discussion relating to Figure 13.9).

The acoustic nature of the speech signal is changing all the time (it would be little use for communication purposes if it did not!). While the spectrum provides a clear basis on which to measure the amplitudes of the frequency components, it corresponds to just a single time instant. The spectrograph also provides a spectro-gram **output that plots how the spectrum changes with time as the variation in amplitude** (blackness of marking) of the frequency (y axis) components in the speech signal against time (x axis). Modern computer-based spectrographic analysis systems allow the use of colour to represent different amplitude levels. However, the use of a grey scale is to be preferred because it provides even visual transitions as amplitude changes, whereas colour scales have visually distinct boundaries where the colours change that are misleading because the amplitude does not change in distinct steps. Further details of spectrographic analysis can be found in, for example, Fry, (1979); Baken, (1987); and Rosen and Howell (1991).

The time dimension requires similar consideration to that given to frequency in terms of its resolution, and the same principles apply in terms of the analysis by means of a moving wide or narrow band filter. To appreciate the effect of different filter bandwidths and their time resolution, consider the analysis of a single short acoustic event in time, such as a hand clap, when analysed by filters of different bandwidths. Figure 13.28 shows an idealized waveform for a short acoustic pressure pulse, the response curves of a wide and a narrow band analysis filter, and the resulting output waveforms from these filters for the input pressure pulse. The centre frequency of the filter in each case is f_c. The output from both filters consists of a sinusoidal vibration that decays in amplitude, and the frequency of the sinusoid is the centre frequency of the filter itself (f_c). In the figure it is shown as the period of the output waveforms as ($1/f_c$) (see Note 3).

Two important effects characterize the time responses of filters with wide and narrow bandwidths: (1) the narrower the bandwidth the longer the decay time of the output sinusoid waveform for an input pulse, or the longer the filter continues ringing, and (2) the narrower the bandwidth the lower the peak amplitude of the output. In effect, the energy of the input pulse is spread out in time and reduced in amplitude to a greater degree as the bandwidth of the filter is made narrower. **The wide band filter therefore has a better time resolution than the narrow band filter** because: (1) its short ringing time means that it responds to an input event rapidly and is ready more quickly to respond to the next event in the input, and (2) its response is greater in amplitude and thus pulse-like events, for example, the bursts in plosives, such as the consonants in bucket and dog, are better preserved in the output. In order to analyse time or frequency accurately by means of spectrography, a wide or narrow band spectrogram should be used respectively. **It is therefore customary to consider both wide and narrow band spectrograms of a given input with bandwidths set in appropriate relation to the f0 of the speech being analysed.**

Figure 13.29 shows the acoustic pressure waveform as well as narrow and wide band spectrograms for short snippets of the vowel in spa, spoken by a healthy adult male using modal, breathy, falsetto, creaky, harsh and whispered voice qualities. A look at the overall form of each spectrogram shows that the detailed fine structure of the narrow band spectrogram is mainly horizontal and that of the wide band spectrogram is mainly vertical. The horizontal structure of the narrow band spectrogram is providing detail that relates to the vertical axis (frequency) and blurring

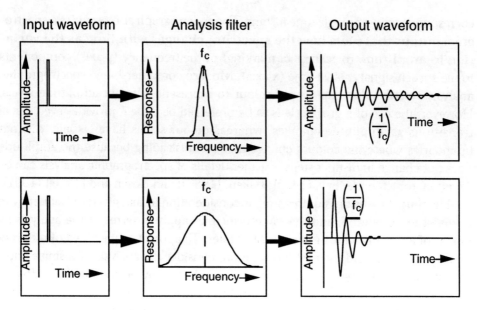

Figure 13.28 The effect on the output waveform from an analysis filter (centre frequency f_c) with two bandwidth settings for an input short pressure pulse

of detail along the horizontal axis (time), and vice versa for the wide band spectrogram. This directly reflects the better frequency and time resolution of the narrow and wide band spectrograms respectively with regard to each other. The harmonics of the modal vowel can be seen in the narrow band spectrogram, and in the wide band spectrogram the closely spaced vertical lines represent the acoustic pressure pulses resulting from each individual vocal-fold closure, termed striations. The f_0 can be measured from a spectrogram by measuring either the harmonic spacing on the narrow band spectrogram, generally by measuring the frequency of, say, the tenth harmonic and dividing by 10 for increased accuracy, or by measuring the time between striations. It should be noted that the accuracy of the latter cannot be improved by measuring over a number of striations if f_0 is varies during the time interval over which the measurement is made.

Conclusions can be drawn from the spectrograms for each voice quality about the nature of the vocal-fold excitation and the voice quality itself, as well as the positions of the formants. Regularity of vocal-fold vibration is shown on spectrograms by unbroken harmonics in the narrow band and by regular unbroken striations in the wide band. This is particularly clear during *modal* voice.

During the *falsetto* example the harmonics are clear and widely spaced on the narrow band spectrogram indicating the high f_0, which can be seen to be approximately 430 Hz by observation of the position of the tenth harmonic. Striations are not clear on the wide band spectrogram for this falsetto example because the bandwidth of the analysis filter (200 Hz) is narrow compared to f_0 and therefore the output shows some harmonic structure, but each harmonic is coloured by the width of the analysis filter.

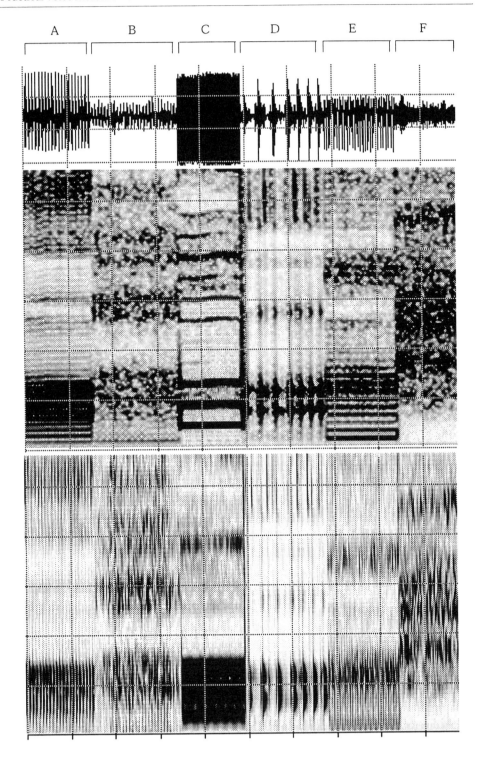

Figure 13.29 Acoustic pressure waveform, narrow band (40 Hz bandwidth) and wide band (200 Hz bandwidth) spectrograms for the vowel in 'spa', spoken by a healthy adult male voice using (A) modal; (B) breathy; (C) falsetto; (D) creaky; (E) harsh; and (F) whispered voice qualities. These examples are taken from the same tokens as those plotted in Figure 13.14

During *harsh* voice the narrow band spectrogram indicates that for this example the harmonic structure is clearly defined at frequencies up to approximately 2 kHz, while at high frequencies the harmonics appear to be broken up in an irregular manner. This is the way in which acoustic noise excitation is represented, indicating that this harsh voice incorporates noise excitation at high frequencies that is not apparent in the modal example. The same conclusion can be reached from the wide band spectrogram, where the striations are spaced regularly in the low frequency region, but successive vocal-fold closures are not as similar in amplitude (blackness of marking) as in the modal example, and are less well defined at high frequencies.

Noise excitation with no vocal-fold vibration is the acoustic source during *whispered* voice and the spectrograms show this clearly. There are no harmonics or striations apparent in either the narrow or wide band spectrograms respectively, and the underlying detail, although it is horizontal and vertical respectively, is broken up in an irregular manner.

The *breathy* voice example incorporates mainly acoustic noise excitation. Even though the folds are vibrating, there is no evidence of well defined vocal fold closures in the striations on the wide band spectrogram. Reference to the breathy voice waveforms plotted in Figure 13.14b for the same utterance shows that the vocal fold closures are less rapid as shown by the electrolaryngograph output waveform than for modal voice, and that this results in a less well defined associated excursion in the acoustic pressure waveform than in the modal example.

In the *creaky* example irregularity of vocal fold vibration is indicated very clearly by the striations (wide band), and the secondary closures can be seen clearly as the fainter striations between the dark ones. The narrow band output shows striations also because the filter is responding to each individual vocal-fold closure almost completely before the next. The filter bandwidth (40 Hz) is not narrow with respect to f_0 in this creaky example, which varies between approximately 28 Hz and 35 Hz (estimated from the fundamental period between successive major striations in the wide band spectrogram), and therefore it is acting as a wide band filter. The striations are blurred in time compared with the output from the wide band (200 Hz) analysis due to the difference in time resolution between the filters.

To locate the formants on spectrograms, particularly for single steady vowels, it is helpful to have an approximate idea where they might be expected to lie. Table 13.5 gives selected typical formant frequency values for the first three formants based on data from Peterson and Barney (1952).

From the table, typical formant frequencies for the vowel in 'bard', uttered by an adult male are: 730 Hz, 1100 Hz and 2450 Hz. These then give approximate formant positions for the vowel shown in the spectrograms shown in Figure1 3.29, and they are most clearly seen in these examples in the wide band spectrogram for creaky voice. This is because each individual acoustic excitation is clearly separated in time in creaky voice, and the ringing response of each formant to each excitation pulse can be observed immediately following the striation itself. (It should be noted

Table 13.5 Typical frequency values for the first (F1), second (F2) and third (F3) formants in speech. (Data from Peterson and Barney, 1952)

Vowel	F1 (Hz)			F2 (Hz)			F3 (Hz)		
	Men	Women	Children	Men	Women	Children	Men	Women	Children
bee	270	300	370	2300	2800	3200	3000	3300	3700
bet	530	600	700	1850	2350	2600	2500	3000	3550
bat	660	860	1000	1700	2050	2300	2400	2850	3300
bard	730	850	1030	1100	1200	1350	2450	2800	3200
bought	570	590	680	850	900	1050	2400	2700	3200
boot	300	370	430	850	950	1150	2250	2650	3250

that formant ringing is in fact illustrated in Figure 13.28, as the acoustic excitation is a pressure pulse, and a formant itself is a band-pass filter.) The lower two formants are clear, but the third formant is not particularly well defined in this creaky example. The formants can be seen in the modal example, and comparison with the spectra for an instant during this utterance in Figure 13.27 shows that the third formant is around 2400 Hz but low in amplitude, which explains why it is not clearly represented on this spectrogram. In the breathy, falsetto and harsh examples the frequency region of the first two formants can be observed, but not easily measured, and once again the third is not clear. The wide band spectrogram of the falsetto example, for which it has been pointed out that the filter bandwidth is narrower than the f_0, demonstrates how an erroneous analysis could be made. In the region of the first two formants there appear to be three horizontal black bars that have a width which is similar to the formant width exhibited in the modal example. Comparison with the narrow band spectrogram shows that these three bars are the first three harmonics and they appear so wide due to the colouration by the wide band analysis filter.

This falsetto example demonstrates how formant analysis can become increasingly difficult with high f_0 values (c.f. Figure 13.9). Analysis of the speech of women and children is more difficult than for that of men because their f_0 values are raised to a greater extent relative to their formant centre frequencies than are those of men. The resulting harmonic spacing is, therefore, relatively greater compared with the formant frequencies for women and children than for men. One analysis strategy is to use filters with a bandwidth of around 600 Hz to keep it wide with respect to f_0, but the blurring effect of the filter itself begins to obscure individual formants, particularly when they are close to each other in frequency.

The dynamic patterns of moving formants are considerably easier to track on spectrograms than static formants. Figure 13.30 shows narrow and wide band spectrograms of 'speech matters to you', spoken by a healthy adult male. Harmonics and striations are clear on the narrow and wide band spectrograms respectively. The formant transitions can be seen on both spectrograms, but notice how the harmonics have similarities to the formants, particularly when they move in the same direction as in the vowel of the word 'speech'. It would be impossible to measure the higher formant frequencies from the narrow band spectrogram during this vowel, but it would be possible on the wide band spectrogram. The dominant high frequency energy in the voiceless fricative sounds that start and end the first word 'speech', are clear in both spectrograms. Again it is possible to see that this energy is represented horizontally and vertically in the narrow and wide band spectrograms respectively as a result of the time/frequency responses of the analysis filters themselves. The release of the 't' in 'matters', almost dead centre in these spectrograms, is cleanly defined in time on the wide band spectrogram but spread out in time on the narrow band spectrogram. It is only possible from the wide band spectrogram to assess its energy distribution as having a peak around 4.3 kHz in this particular example. The formant transitions in the vowels of 'to you' are clearly defined in the wide band spectrogram again, but they are apparent on the narrow band where again, care should be taken in assessing the visual contribution of harmonic movement as f_0 changes.

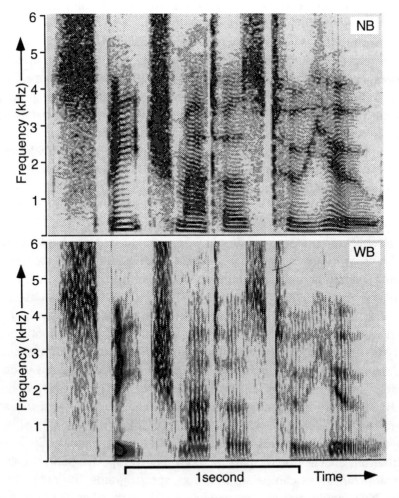

Figure 13.30 Narrow (upper) and wide (lower) band spectrograms of 'Speech matters to you', spoken by a healthy adult male

In a practical spectrograph system, a feature that is usually provided is *pre-emphasis*. This is an electronic filter that emphasises the input speech signal prior to spectrographic analysis. Its purpose is to counteract the overall -6 dB per octave average spectral shape of voiced speech (see Figure 13.7) so that the signal has an approximately flat spectrum prior to analysis. This ensures that spectral detail at higher frequencies is not lost in the spectrogram or spectrum by being at too low a level with respect to the low frequency components to appear on the spectrogram. However, there may be occasions when it is not desired, for example, if experimental interest is focused on the actual relative levels of spectral components. In such cases it should be turned off and any related discussion should clearly state that this is the case.

Linear predictive coding (LPC)

Linear predictive coding (LPC), or linear prediction, is a technique that is often available with practical voice measurement systems on modern computer based packages. It has particular application in formant estimation, and it also provides a basis for f_0 estimation. LPC analysis is a time domain technique that is applied to digitally time sampled speech. More detailed discussions of the LPC technique are given by Witten (1982) and Markel and Gray (1976).

The output speech signal can be modelled as a sound source and sound modifiers (see Figure 13.1) and assumptions can be made about the nature of the sound source itself. The linear prediction technique is based on the idea that if the sound source is modelled as remaining constant in terms of its spectral shape then the effect of the sound modifiers on the output speech waveform can be predicted. Figure 13.7 shows that the average spectral shape in speech of the voiced sound source is -12 dB per octave, of the sound modifiers is 0 dB per octave and of the lip radiation is +6 dB per octave. In linear prediction it is most convenient to assume a sound source spectrum that is flat or with a 0 dB per octave shape and a 0 dB per octave shape for the sound modifiers, the change in the sound source being compensated by a -6 dB per octave equalization in place of the lip radiation. The overall output therefore remains at -6 dB per octave (0 dB/octave + 0 dB/octave + -6 dB/octave). Such an arrangement enables linear prediction to be used for voiced as well as unvoiced speech analysis because the acoustic noise excitation associated with unvoiced speech also has an average 0 dB per octave spectral shape (see Figure 13.5).

Linear prediction assumes an ideal pulse as the acoustic excitation from each vocal fold closure with an overall 0 dB per octave spectral shape, and based on this assumption, the nature of the output ringing waveform from each formant can be predicted (see Note 3, Figure 13.28 and the discussion relating to time response of the spectrographic analysis filters). This formant ringing is predictable as a sinewave at the formant frequency whose amplitude decays exponentially dependent on the bandwidth of the formant. In effect, the caption to Figure 13.28 could equally well read: 'The effect on the output waveform from a vocal tract formant (centre frequency f_c) with two bandwidth settings for an input acoustic excitation short pressure pulse', with the centre column labelled 'formant' rather than 'analysis filter'. Each individual output sample from a formant can therefore be predicted mathematically from known previous output samples from the formant. In terms of the output voiced speech pressure waveform itself, it can be considered as the result of adding the outputs from each individual formant. This is the basis of linear prediction, which relies on five key assumptions: (i) the ringing of the formants during voiced speech production is purely due to the most recent vocal fold excitation acoustic pressure pulse; (ii) the formant frequencies remain constant during each cycle; (iii) the formant bandwidths remain constant during each cycle; (iv) the vocal tract response can be completely modelled in terms of formants for all speech sounds; and (v) the acoustic excitation to the vocal tract can be modelled as being spectrally flat (0 dB per octave).

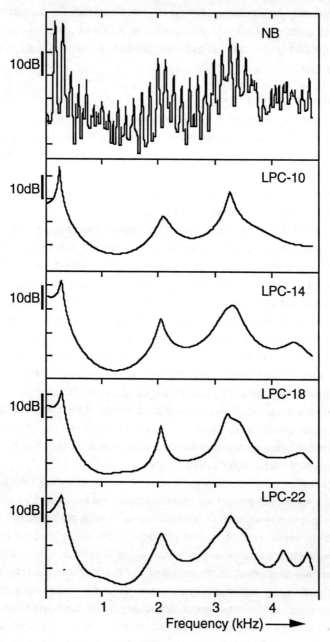

Figure 13.31 Narrow band spectrum (NB) and LPC analyses of orders 10, 14, 18 and 22 of the vowel in feed, spoken by a healthy adult male

None of these assumptions is fully upheld during all voiced speech sounds, and the potential limitations of the method based on the five assumptions above are as follows: (i) remains true while f_0 is low enough, but as f_0 increases there comes a point where the ringing due to one excitation has not fully died away before the next acoustic pressure pulse arrives; (ii) formant frequencies are constantly changing and this can be particularly rapid during formant transitions; (iii) formant bandwidths change during each vocal-fold vibrating cycle due to increased damping of acoustic energy absorbed by the subglottal spaces and the lungs during the open phase compared to the closed phase, termed subglottal damping; (iv) speech sounds such as those that make use of the nasal cavity in parallel with the oral cavity by means of a lowered velum (see Figure 13.1) cannot be modelled with only formants; and (v) the spectrum of the acoustic excitation to the vocal tract due to vocal-fold vibration varies dynamically as conditions local to the folds themselves, such as saliva and air flow, alter with successive closures. LPC analysis is, therefore, usually carried out on input frames of speech which are 10 ms to 25 ms in duration, on the basis that over such short times most of these aspects remain fairly static. In conjunction with an electrolaryngograph, LPC analysis can be carried out only during the closed phase of the vocal-fold vibration cycle, known as closed phase LPC analysis, providing a useful technique for countering problem (iii). LPC remains a widely used and extremely useful technique for formant estimation, but it is one which requires some caution in the interpretation of results.

The main parameter usually made available to the user is the order or number of poles of the LPC analysis. One order is needed for the equalization and a further two are required to model each formant. LPC is usually carried out with orders between 11 and 15, corresponding to five and seven formants respectively, chosen with respect to the number of formants expected. Too low an order may result in several formant peaks being combined into a single peak, and too high an order can result in output peaks being placed over individual harmonics. These effects are illustrated in Figure 13.31, which shows the results from a narrow band spectrum (NB) and LPC analyses of orders 10 (LPC-10), 14 (LPC-14), 18 (LPC-18) and 22 (LPC-22) for the vowel in 'feed', spoken by a healthy adult male. It can be seen that the number of peaks indicated by each LPC analysis increases as the order increases. In some cases there will be peaks lying close together resulting in a broader output peak overall, as for example around 3.2 kHz in the LPC-14 example. As the order increases, peaks appear in the frequency region above 4 kHz in this example.

Inverse filtering

If the effect of the sound modifiers could be somehow removed from the output speech pressure waveform, the result should represent the sound source itself. One method is to exactly filter out the effect of the sound modifiers, and this is the basis of an analysis method known as inverse filtering. A filter with a response curve that is exactly the inverse of that of the sound modifiers is used and this neutralizes the effects of the formants to give a waveform that represents the glottal pressure or glottal airflow waveform. In principle, this is an extremely useful technique, but it is one that is rather difficult to implement readily in practice.

A widely used device for inverse filtering is the Rothenberg flow mask

(Rothenberg, 1973), which consists of a face mask with an airflow transducer. The output from this airflow transducer for the vowel in 'spa', spoken by a healthy adult male is shown in the upper waveform in Figure 13.32. Associated with the mask is an electronic inverse filter that the user sets by hand in terms of the formant frequencies and bandwidths of F1 and F2. Formants higher than F2 are not involved in this inverse filtering system because its overall frequency response is limited to below approximately 1.5 kHz due to the effects of the mask itself. The crux of inverse filtering is the setting of the inverse filter itself, which is based on nulling out the effects of the formant ringing. The inverse filter controls are adjusted such that the resulting waveform shows little or no evidence of formant ringing. An example is shown in Figure 13.32 where the effect of inverse filtering only F2 and only F1 is plotted, as well as the resulting waveform when F1 and F2 are inverse filtered, which is assumed to represent closely the airflow waveform at the glottis. Notice that the effects of the formants are not apparent in the glottal airflow waveform, and that the effect of F1 or F2 can be seen when only F2 or F1 is inverse filtered respectively.

The underlying difficulty with inverse filtering is that it relies on having some knowledge of the likely shape of the glottal airflow output waveform itself in order to set up the inverse filter. In other words, assumptions have to be made about the result to carry out the analysis. If the assumptions are erroneous, for example, the glottal airflow may have ringing associated with it, then the output will be unreliable. Inverse filtering can be carried out automatically where, for example, the

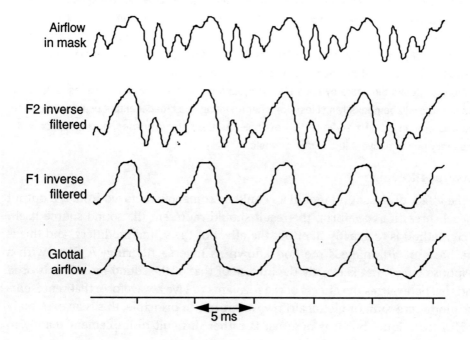

Figure 13.32 Acoustic pressure waveform and outputs when F2 only, F1 only is inverse-filtered, and the glottal airflow waveform that results when F1 and F2 are inverse-filtered, of the vowel in 'spa', spoken by a healthy adult male

inverse filter is set up after LPC analysis, or closed phase LPC analysis of the speech waveform has been first carried out to identify the positions of the formants. As LPC analysis itself makes assumptions about the nature of the voice source that may not be appropriate, and the five key assumptions listed above are not always upheld, the results of inverse filtering based on LPC analysis need to be considered with considerable care.

Hearing modelling

Knowledge of the manner in which the peripheral hearing system analyses sound has advanced alongside developments in available computational processing power to the extent that there now exist systems that can provide a spectrographic representation of speech that is based on human hearing. A review of the human hearing system can be found in Pickles (1982), Moore and Glasberg (1983) and Howard and Angus (1996).

The frequency analysis capability of each ear can be modelled as a bank of band-pass filters operating in parallel whose bandwidths vary as a function of their centre frequencies as shown in Figure 13.33. The human hearing system effectively has narrow band filters at low frequencies, which become wider as frequency increases. **Thus the human hearing system exhibits 'good' frequency resolution at low frequencies and 'good' time resolution at high frequencies.**

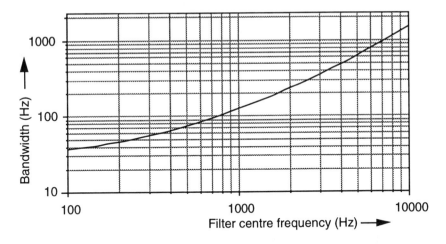

Figure 13.33 Variation in auditory filter bandwidth as a function of its centre frequency based on the equivalent rectangular bandwidth , or ERB, scale of Moore and Glasberg (1983)

Figure 13.34 shows the output in spectrographic form from the real-time hearing model (Swan et al., 1994), which consists of a bank of 64 filters whose bandwidths are determined by the curve shown in Figure 13.33 for the vowel of 'spa', spoken by a healthy adult male using (a) modal, (b) breathy, (c) falsetto, (d) creaky, (e) harsh and (f) whispered voice qualities as used in Figures 13.14 and 13.29 (upper plot), and 'Speech matters to you', spoken by a healthy adult male as used in Figure 13.30 (lower plot).

The 'good' frequency and time resolution of the GammaTone spectrogram can be seen at low and high frequencies as clear harmonics and striations respectively. This is particularly clear in the modal voice quality (a) example in the upper plot of Figure 13.34 as well as throughout the spectrogram of the sentence in the lower plot. The frequency axis is related to the filter bandwidths (see Figure 13.33), with each filter output receiving an equal distance on the y axis. This has the effect of compressing the high frequencies with respect to the low frequencies in a manner that is fairly similar to a logarithmic scale. The perceptual weight of the different frequency regions is represented in these spectrograms, which has the effect of spreading the lower formants out and compressing the high frequency information. The lower three harmonics in the falsetto example are clear and the striations in the creaky example become thinner at high frequencies, demonstrating the increased time resolution towards high frequencies. Another interesting example of this is shown at the very end of the spectrogram where the final 'click' of the editing process is smeared in time at the bottom, but not at the top, of the spectrogram. Other features can be compared with the traditional spectrograms of these voice qualities plotted in Figure 13.29.

In the sentence, the unvoiced fricatives at either end of the first word 'speech' are very clear, and the different frequency balance of each can be seen. Throughout the voiced regions, the lowest three to five harmonics can be clearly seen, with striations becoming apparent above approximately 1 kHz. The last fricative of 'matters' is devoiced, which can be seen as the harmonics at its start gradually disappear. The formant transitions are clearly illustrated, especially in the final voiced section of the words 'to you'.

By way of comparison, Figure 13.35 shows an eighteenth order LPC spectrogram of the same utterance, 'Speech matters to you', for which a spectrogram

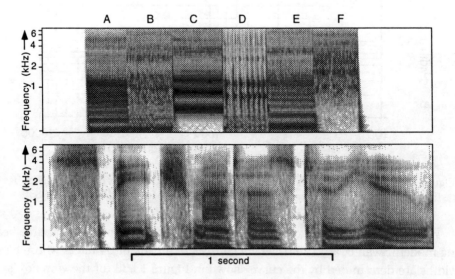

Figure 13.34 Spectrograms from the human hearing model based on ERB spaced Gamma-Tone filters for: (upper) the vowel in 'spa', spoken by a healthy adult male voice using (A) modal, (B) breathy, (C) falsetto, (D) creaky, (E) harsh and (F) whispered voice qualities, the same data as in Figures 13.14 and 13.29; and (lower) 'Speech matters to you', spoken by a healthy adult male, the same data as in Figure 13.30

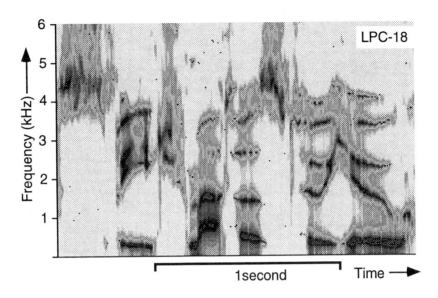

Figure 13.35 Eighteenth order LPC analysis of 'Speech matters to you', spoken by a healthy adult male. This can be compared directly with the spectrograms in Figures 13.30 and 13.34

based on a human hearing model is plotted in Figure 13.34 and traditional narrow and wide band spectrograms are plotted in Figure 13.30. The frequency scales in Figures 13.30 and 13.34 are linear. It is left to the reader to make comparisons between these various representations of the acoustic patterns of the utterance, providing an opportunity to see the potential benefit of using an analysis based on the human hearing system in terms of how it combines the features found particularly in the narrow and wide band spectrograms.

Notes

1. The ratio of two pressure values P1 and P2 is expressed in decibels (dB) as follows
$dB = 20*\log_{10}\{P1/P2\}$.
If $P2 = 4*P1$, then this is equivalent to: $20*\log_{10}\{1/4\}$ dB $= 20*(-0.6021)$ dB $= -12.042$ dB.
2. One way of thinking about this is that a non-repeating waveform has a period that is infinite because it consists of just one cycle when extended for ever. The Fourier theorem states that the spectrum will consist of harmonics that are spaced by the f_0, where $f_0 = (1/period)$. In this case, $f_0 = (1/infinity) = zero$. Therefore the spacing between its harmonics must be zero Hz, or they must be infinitesimally close together, which is the nature of a continuous spectrum.
3. This description applies equally well to the formants themselves when they are excited by the acoustic pressure pulses arising from vocal-fold closure, as a single formant has the same characteristics as the analysis filter of the spectrograph. It, too, can be described in terms of its centre frequency, or formant frequency, and a

bandwidth, and its output resulting from each vocal-fold closure is a sinewave at the formant frequency that decays in amplitude depending on the formant bandwidth, otherwise described as ringing (see Figure 13.28). Evidence of ringing during each cycle can be seen in the speech pressure waveforms plotted in Figures 13.10, 13.11 and 13.14.

Glossary relating to topics covered in chapter 13

Given the highly multi-disciplinary nature of the voice clinic, one of the main purposes of this chapter is to provide an introduction to practical voice measurement to those working on voice whose main field of study was not acoustics. There are a number of terms relating to practical voice measurement which are in common use in the literature and elsewhere, and the purpose behind providing this glossary is to list some of those that are commonly found. Such a list can never be exhaustive, but it is hoped that it can serve as a useful guide to readers who are more unfamiliar with this area of voice work.

(Items in italics have their own entry in the glossary.)

AGC	Acronym for automatic gain control.
ALC	Acronym for automatic level control, synonymous with automatic gain control.
amplify	Increase to *amplitude*
amplitude	The value quantity, for example of a *waveform* as it varies with time
attenuate	Reduce in *amplitude*
automatic gain control	An electronic circuit which holds its output *amplitude* essentially constant despite variations in its input.
band-pass filter	A *filter* which passes components with frequencies in a band between two cut-off frequencies, and stops those with frequencies outside this band.
band-stop filter	A *filter* which stops components with frequencies in a band between two cut-off frequencies, and passes those with frequencies outside this band.
bendwidth	The *frequency* band within which a device operates.
cepstrum	A word formed by letter reversal in' *spectrum*', it refers to the spectrum of the logarithm of the power *spectrum* of a signal.
CQ	Acronym for larynx closed quotient.
C_x	Fundamental frequency scattergram.
cycle	A single complete variation of a repeating quantity.
D_x	Fundamental frequency histogram.
decibel (dB)	The unit most commonly used in comparisons of acoustic power; defined as: 10 x the logarithm of the ratio between two sound pressures.
EGG	Acronym for the electroglottograph or its output waceform.
electroglottograph	A device which monitors the area of vocal fold contact electrically giving a positive voltage output for decreasing vocal fold contact area.
electrolaryngograph	A device which monitors the area of vocal fold contact

	electrically giving a positive voltage output for increasing vocal fold contact area.
equivalent rectangular bandwidth	The *bandwidth* of an auditory filter which varies as a function of its centre *frequency*.
ERB	Acronym for equivalent retangular bandwidth.
F₀	Shorthand for fundamental frequency.
F₁, F₂, F₃, etc	Shorthand for first *formant*, second *formant*, third *formant* etc
filter	A device which attenuates the *amplitudes* of components in certain *frequency* ranges (stop bands) whilst leaving the *amplitudes* unchanged of components in other *frequency* ranges (pass bands).
formant	A vocal tract acoustic resonance.
Fourier theorem	Any periodic waveform can be built up from a series of sinewaves whose frequencies are integer multiples of a *fundamental frequency*
frequency	The number of *cycles* of a periodic quantity that occur in a second.
fricative	Speech sound whose acoustic source is non-periodic noise.
fundamental frequency	The number of cycles per second of a periodic quantity which is equal to the reciprocal of its period {i.e. fundamental frequency = (1/period)}. It is also the lowest frequency component that can be present in a spectrum of a periodic quantity.
gain	The increase in *amplitude* provided by an electronic *amplifier* circuit.
glottis	The space between the open vocal folds.
harmonic	A sinewave component that is an integer (1, 2, 3, ..) multiple of a *fundamental frequency*.
Hertz	The unit of *frequency*, equivalent to the number of cycles per second.
high-pass filter	A *filter* which stops components with *frequencies* below its cut-off frequency, and passes those with *frequencies* above its cut-off frequency.
inverse filtering	The process of filtering the *speech pressure waveform* with a *filter* which has a response that is equal and opposite to that of the vocal tract in order to recover the acoustic source signal.
jitter	Cycle-by-cycle variation in the *fundamental period* during *voiced* speech.
larynx closed phase	The time in each cycle of vocal fold vibration for which the vocal folds are in contact.
larynx closed quotient	The percentage of each cycle of vocal fold vibration for which the vocal folds are in contact.
larynx open phase	The time in each cycle of vocal fold vibration for which the vocal folds are apart.
larynx open quotient	The percentage of each cycle of vocal fold vibration for which the vocal folds are apart.
low-pass filter	A *filter* which passes components with *frequencies* below its cut-off frequency, and stops those with *frequencies* above its cut-off frequency.
Lx	The output *waveform* from an electrolaryngograph.
LPC	Acronym for linear predictive coding.
linear predictive coding	A mathematical technique that enables future samples of a digital speech pressure waveform to be estimated from previous samples.

mean	The mean is the sum of a number of samples divided by their total number.
median	The median is the value middle in position in a series of values.
mode	The mode is defined as the centre frequency of the bin containing the highest number of samples.
octave	The musical interval formed between a signal and another produced by doubling (octave up) or halving (octave down) its *fundamental frequency*.
OP	Acronym for larynx open phase.
OQ	Acronym for larynx open quotient.
period	The duration of a complete *cycle* of a periodic quantity.
pitch	Human perception on a scale of 'low' to 'high' of sounds with different *fundamental frequencies*.
quefrency	A word formed by letter reversal in '*frequency*', it refers to the quantity plotted on the X-axis of a *cepstrum*.
rahmonic	A word formed by letter reversal in '*harmonic*', it refers to a component found in a *cepstrum* that has the properties of a *harmonic* in a *spectrum*.
semitone	The musical interval equal to one twelfth of an octave in equal tempered tuning.
shimmer	Short-term variation in the *amplitude* of *the speech pressure waveform*.
sinewave	A *waveform* with the shape of the sin function.
SL_c	The rate of closing of the vocal folds.
SL_o	The rate of opening of the vocal folds.
spectrogram	Output plot from a spectrograph.
spectrograph	A device which produces a time/frequency/amplitude of an acoustic signal.
spectrum	A plot of the *amplitude* of the *frequency* components of a signal.
spectral trend	A description of the variation of amplitude with frequency, usually from a spectrum.
speech pressure waveform	A plot of the acoustic pressure variation picked up by a microphone during speech.
sub-glottal damping	The increase in absorption of acoustic energy by the sub-glottal cavities during the larynx open phase as compared to the larynx closed phase in *voiced* speech as a result of the increase in acoustic damping of the *formants*.
threshold	The value of a quantity above which some activity is triggered.
T_x	Shorthand for fundamental period.
unvoiced	Adjective used to describe speech sounds produced with non-vibrating vocal folds.
voiced	Adjective used to describe speech sounds produced with vibrating vocal folds.
waveform	A plot of the variation of a quantity as it varies with time.

References

Abberton ERM, Howard DM, Fourcin AJ (1989) Laryngographic assessment of normal voice: a tutorial. Clinical Linguistics and Phonetics 3: 281-296.
ANSI (1960) American standard acoustical terminology. New York: American National Standards Institute.

Baer T. Löfquist A., McGarr NS (1983) Laryngeal vibrations: a comparison between high-speed filming and glottographic techniques. Journal of the Acoustical Society of America 73: 1304-1308.

Baken RJ (1987) Clinical measurement of speech and voice. London: Taylor and Francis.

Barry WJ, Goldsmith M, Fourcin AJ, Fuller H (1990) Larynx analyses on normative reference data. Alvey Project MMI/132: Speech technology assessment.

Catford JC (1977) Fundamental problems in phonetics. Edinburgh University Press.

Childers DG, Hicks DM, Moore GP, Alsaka YA (1986) A model for vocal fold vibratory motion, contact area, and the electrolaryngogram. Journal of the Acoustical Society of America 80: 1309-1320.

Dejonckere PH, Hirano M, Sundberg J (1995) Vibrato. San Diego: Singular Publishing Group.

Fourcin AJ (1974) Laryngographic assessment of vocal fold vibration. In Wyke B (Ed.) Ventilatory and phonatory control systems. Oxford University Press.

Fourcin AJ (1981) Laryngographic assessment of phonatory function. Proceedings of the Conference on the Assessment of Vocal Pathology, ASHA Report 11, pp. 116-127.

Fourcin AJ (1987) Electrolaryngographic assessment of phonatory function. Journal of Phonetics 14: 435-442.

Fourcin AJ, Abberton ERM (1971) First applications of a new laryngograph. Medical and Biological Illustration 21: 172-182.

Fry DB (1979) The physics of speech. Cambridge University Press.

Gilbert HR, Potter CR, Hoodin R (1984) The laryngograph as a measure of vocal fold contact area. Journal of Speech and Hearing Research 27: 178-182.

Gold B, Rabiner LR (1969) Parallel processing techniques for estimating pitch periods of speech in the time domain. Journal of the Acoustical Society of America 21: 487-495.

Hess W (1983) Pitch determination of speech signals: algorithms and devices. Berlin: Springer.

Hess W, Indefrey H (1984) Accurate pitch determination of speech signals by means of a laryngograph. Proceedings of the IEEE International Conference on Acoustics, Speech and Signal Processing, ICASSP-84, pp. 1-4.

Howard DM (1989) Peak-picking fundamental period estimation for hearing prostheses. Journal of the Acoustical Society of America 86: 902-910.

Howard DM (1995) Variation of electrolaryngographically derived closed quotient for trained and untrained adult singers. Journal of Voice 9: 163-172.

Howard DM, Angus JAS (1996) Music technology: Acoustics and psychoacoustics. Oxford: Focal Press.

Howard DM, Collingsworth J (1992) Voice source and acoustic measures in singing. Acoustics Bulletin 17: 5-12.

Howard DM, Fourcin AJ (1983) Instantaneous voice period measurement for cochlear stimulation. Electronics Letters 19: 776-779.

Howard DM, Hirson A, French JP, Szymanski JE (1993) A survey of fundamental frequency estimation techniques used in forensic phonetics. Proceedings of the Institute of Acoustics 15: 207-215.

Howard DM, Lindsey GA (1988) Conditioned variation in voicing offsets. IEEE Transactions on Acoustics, Speech and Signal Processing 36: 406-407.

Howard DM, Maidment JA, Smith DAJ, Howard IS (1986) Towards a comprehensive quantitative assessment of the operation of real-time speech fundamental frequency extractors. IEE Conference Publication 258: 172-177.

Kent RD, Read C (1992) The acoustic analysis of speech. San Diego: Singular Publishing Group.

Ladefoged P (1975) A course in phonetics. New York: Harcourt Brace Jovanovich.

Lecluse FLE, Brocaar MP, Verschurne J (1975) The electroglottography and its relation to glottal activity. Folia Phoniatrica 27, 215-224.

Markel JD, Gray AH (1976) Linear prediction of speech. Berlin: Springer-Verlag.

Moore BCJ (1982) An introduction to the psychology of hearing. London: Academic Press.

Moore BCJ, Glasberg (1983) Suggested formulae for calculating auditory-filter bandwidths and excitation patterns. Journal of the Accoustical Society of America 74: pp 750-753.

Noll AM (1967) Cepstrum pitch determination. Journal of the Acoustical Society of America 41: 293-309.

Noscoe NJ, Fourcin AJ, Brown MA, Berry RJ (1983) Examination of vocal fold movement by ultra-short pulse X radiography. British Journal of Radiology 56: 641-645.

Padham CA (1986) The well-tempered organ. Oxford: Positiv Press.

Peterson GE, Barney HE (1952) Control methods used in the study of vowels. Journal of the Acoustical Society of America 24: 175-184.

Pickett JM (1980) The sounds of speech communication. Baltimore: University Park Press.

Pickles JO (1982) An introduction to the physiology of hearing. London: Academic Press.

Rabiner LR, Cheng MJ, Rosenberg AE, McGonegal CA (1976) A comparative performance study of several pitch detectors. IEEE Transactions on Acoustics Speech and Signal Processing ASSP-24: 399-413.

Rosen S, Howell P (1991) Signals and systems for speech and hearing. London: Academic Press.

Rothenberg M (1973) A new inverse-filtering technique for deriving the glottal waveform during voicing. Journal of the Acoustical Society of America 53: 1632-1645.

Rothenberg M (1981) Some relations between glottal airflow and vocal fold contact area. In Ludlow CO, Hart MO (Eds) Proceedings of the Conference on the assessment of vocal pathology. ASHA Report 11, pp 88-96.

Rothenberg M (1992) A multichannel electroglottograph. Journal of Voice 6: 36-43.

Swan C, Tyrrell AM, Howard DM (1994) Real-time transputer simulation of the human peripheral hearing system. Microprocessors and Microsystems 18: 215-221.

Titze IR (1984) Parameterization of the glottal area, glottal flow, and vocal fold contact area. Journal of the Acoustical Society of America 75: 570-580.

Titze IR (1994) Principles of voice production. New Jersey: Prentice Hall.

Titze IR, Baer T, Cooper D, Scherer R (1984) Automatic extraction of glottographic waveform parameters and regression to acoustic and physiologic variables. In Bless DM, Abbs JH (Eds) Vocal fold physiology: contemporary research clinical issues. San Diego: College Hall, pp. 146-154.

Van den Berg J (1958) Myoelastic-aerodynamic theory of voice production. Journal of Speech and Hearing Research 1: 227-244.

Wells JC, Colson G (1971) Practical phonetics. London: Pitman.

Witten IH (1982) Principles of computer speech. London: Academic Press.

Index

abdominal breathing 159, 167, 227–9, 237
abdominal muscles 59–61, 129, 163–5, 224
Accent Method 164, 166, 167–71, 188, 189, 192, 195, 230
accessory muscles 57–8
ACE inhibitors 268
adolescent psychogenic dysphonia 200–1
adrenalin and emotional state 160
ageing
   drug treatment for 277
   effect on larynx 84, 107
airstream, egressive/ingressive 325
alcohol 276
   excessive intake, effect of 99
Alexander technique 116, 156
allergens 271
analysis filter bandwidth 362–5
anger, suppressed 160, 247
ankylosing spondilitis 100, 103
anterior strap muscles 28–30
antero-posterior supraglottic compression 85
antero-posterior supraglottic contraction 194–7
antibiotics 274–5
antihistamines 271
antitussives 268
anxiety 160, 198, 247
anxiety disorder 248
archiving 10
aryepiglottic folds 176–7
aryepiglottic narrowing 181
aryepiglottic sphincter 181
aryepliglotticus muscle 27, 74
arytenoid adduction 301
arytenoid cartilage 19, 67–8, 115
arytenoid position 153
arytenoid tips 194
aspirate onset 165

assessment 98ff
assessment protocols 9
asthma 99, 159
   drug therapy 271–3
   in singers 218, 272
autonomic/voluntary nervous system, overactivity of 248–9

belting 181, 234
Bernoulli effect 326
Bernoulli principle 327
body language 98
'Bogart-Bacall' Syndrome 194-7
breath, top-up 166
breath before tone 165, 196
breath control 166
breath/voice coordination 165–6
breathing 106, 158
   and habitual emotional state 160
   structural/pathological problems 62–3
breathing exercises 161
breathing patterns
   alterations to 159
   habitual 146
   in singers 221
breathy voice 223, 343–4, 368
bronchodilator 272

candidiasis, oesophageal 218, 272
cartilages 16–20
cathartic techniques 253
central nervous system and dysarthria 100
cepstral technique 338, 352–3
cerebrovascular accident 155
cervicodorsal shelf 84, 104, 105–6
   correction of 119
chest wall 62
children, dysphonic 154–5
chronic obstructive pulmonary disease 99, 159

medial compression 74
medializing procedures 299
nodule 41
palsy 141
paresis 179, 199
pathology 92
polyp 42
positioning 66
stretching, inappropriate 153;
  long-term 98
structure 34ff
tension 222
tightening 79
vibration 158, 304–5;
  myoelastic aerodynamic theory 327
vocal gesture 141
vocal ligament 20, 21
Vocal Profile Analysis 152
vocal quality 141
vocal range 180–1
  exercises for 235
  and passaggio 233
vocal stamina 141
vocal symptoms, patients' reported 140–1
vocal tract
  discomfort 141
  freeing 231
  response measurement 360–77
vocalis muscle 36, 76
  fatigue 190
  and visor 95

voice
  measurement 323ff
  pitch locked 84
voice clinic
  administration of 3
  appointments 8
  financing 7
  initial interview 4
  multidisciplinary nature 5
  personnel 1–3
  referrals to 2, 6–7
  role of singing teacher 208–9
  role of speech therapist 145–7
  teamwork 5
voice production patterns 145
voice quality 141
voice rest 218–19
voice types 242–4
voice/breath coordination 165
voicing patterns 83–7

waveform, non-periodic 329
webs 296
Wegener's granulomatosis 47
whispered voice 344, 368
white noise 330
widow's hump *see* cervicodorsal shelf

X-ray, high-speed 314
xeroradiography 314

yawn-sigh technique 174, 192, 193, 232